Principles of Sterile Product Preparation

E. Clyde Buchanan

Barbara T. McKinnon

Douglas J. Scheckelhoff

Philip J. Schneider

Correspondence to the authors should be sent in care of the publisher, American Society of Health-System Pharmacists, 7272 Wisconsin Avenue, Bethesda, MD 20814.

The information presented herein reflects the opinions of the authors and reviewers. It should not be interpreted as official policy of ASHP or as an endorsement of any product(s).

The authors and ASHP have made every effort to ensure the accuracy and completeness of the information presented in this book. However, the reader is advised that the publisher, authors, contributors, editors, and reviewers cannot be responsible for the continued currency of the information, for any errors or omissions, and for any consequences arising therefrom.

Produced by the American Society of Health-System Pharmacists' Product Development Office.
Cover and page design: Hector L. Coronado.

ISBN: 1-879907-57-7

Contents

Appendices 139

Glossary 181

Introduction

Principles of Sterile Product Preparation is a textbook of fundamentals. Nevertheless, the basic information supplied in this book has been lost to many in the profession of pharmacy. While our profession has gained much expertise in providing patient-oriented services during the past two decades, we have lost ground in the skill of compounding sterile products.

Highly publicized incidents involving patient injury and death caused by pharmacy-compounded sterile products have prompted professional pharmacy organizations to refocus their attention on this area. After all, pharmaceutical compounding is still the unique right and responsibility of pharmacists and pharmacy technicians among health care professionals.

OBJECTIVES OF THIS BOOK

The objectives of *Principles of Sterile Product Preparation* are to

- ❏ Enable pharmacists, pharmacy technicians, and pharmacy students to understand the new, stricter, sterile compounding guidelines adopted by the pharmacy profession.
- ❏ Supplement other educational materials on pharmacy-prepared sterile products published by the American Society of Health-System Pharmacists (ASHP).
- ❏ Provide pharmacy personnel with a reliable reference for compounding and dispensing safe and effective sterile products.

This text is suitable as both a teaching guide and a reference for pharmacists, pharmacy technicians, and students. Although it is a comprehensive review of the fundamentals of preparing sterile products, it also indicates other sources of information on stability and incompatibility. Moreover, this book applies to sterile product preparation regardless of the pharmacy setting—hospital, home care, or community.

ORGANIZATION OF THIS BOOK

Principles of Sterile Product Preparation is composed of two main sections, chapters and appendices. There is also a glossary of sterile product terms.

The chapters cover topics essential to the pharmacy professional's understanding of why and how to prepare safe and effective sterile products. Each chapter begins with an outline that facilitates locating information within it.

Chapters 1 and 2 present background on pharmacy compounding of sterile products and the extent to which pharmacists and technicians are required to learn this skill. Chapters 3–11 develop the compounding process—from formulation through facilities and equipment, garb, aseptic technique, and batch production.

Chapters 12–15 describe the dispensing process, including expiration dating, labeling, storing, and handling of products. Then Chapters 16–19 cover quality-assurance methods of process validation and end-product evaluation, as well as documentation of preparation and procedures.

The seven appendices reproduce the most recent professional standards for sterile product preparation published by the Food and Drug Administration, the National Association of Boards of Pharmacy, ASHP, and the United States Pharmacopeial Convention.

ACKNOWLEDGMENTS

On behalf of the authors, I express sincere appreciation to the Special Projects Division staff of ASHP, particularly Michael Soares, the project coordinator. This group helped us organize some good ideas into a text that should inspire the profession of pharmacy to revisit its roots in compounding. We also hope that this book will guide pharmacists and technicians in producing the quality and variety of sterile products needed by their patients.

E. Clyde Buchanan, M.S., FASHP
May 15, 1995

Authors

E. Clyde Buchanan, M.S., FASHP
Director of Pharmaceutical Services, Emory Hospitals, Emory
University System of Healthcare, Atlanta, GA
Adjunct Professor, School of Pharmacy, Mercer University,
Atlanta, GA

Barbara T. McKinnon, Pharm.D., BCNSP
Director of Development, Pharmacy Services, Nova Factor, Inc.,
Memphis, TN
Assistant Professor of Clinical Pharmacy, College of Pharmacy,
University of Tennessee, Memphis

Douglas J. Scheckelhoff, M.S.
Associate Director of Pharmacy, University of Kentucky Hospital,
Lexington
Clinical Assistant Professor, College of Pharmacy, University of
Kentucky, Lexington

Philip J. Schneider, M.S., FASHP
Associate Director of Pharmacy, The Ohio State University Medical
Center, Columbus
Clinical Associate Professor, Division of Pharmacy Practice and
Pharmaceutical Administration, College of Pharmacy, The Ohio
State University, Columbus
Clinical Associate Professor, Department of Surgery, College of
Medicine, The Ohio State University, Columbus

Contributors

The authors and ASHP gratefully acknowledge the following individuals who donated their assistance in the development of this book:

Kenneth N. Barker
Toby Clark
Deborah Mangum
Roger Rose
Howard W. Switzky

Reviewers

The authors and ASHP gratefully acknowledge the following individuals who donated their expertise in reviewing the chapters for this book:

Crady Adams

Michael J. Akers

Elizabeth L. Allan

Kenneth E. Avis

Kenneth N. Barker

Kevin Bebout

J. Joseph Belson

Curtis D. Black

Harold J. Black

Jeffrey A. Bourret

Ken Breslow

Patrick N. Catania

William W. Churchill

Bart Clark

Toby Clark

James Craddock

Mary Louise Degenhart

Kathryn Ellis

Vince Galletta

Douglas L. Gill

Harold N. Godwin

Mark Gross

Donald A. Holloway

Mick Hunt

Rolley E. Johnson

Bonnie Kirschenbaum

Jack G. Kitrenos

Jane Kwan

Dennis V. Lau

J. W. Levchuk

Edward Madden

Ed Mansfield

Philip Naut

David W. Newton

Robert E. Pearson

Larry Pelham

Pamela A. Ploetz

Robert P. Rapp

Lois Reynolds

Beverly A. Rose

Patricia Sands

Ann Seidel

Rita Shane

Larry K. Shoup

Patricia Simms

Greg Snyder

Gene L. Stauffer

J. Grady Strom

Howard W. Switzky

Lawrence A. Trissel

Salvatore J. Turco

Jeffrey W. Wadelin

Chapter 1
Concepts and Guidelines in Preparing Sterile Products

E. Clyde Buchanan

The preparation of sterile products is an integral part of any health system setting. However, preparation procedures vary widely nationwide.[1] This lack of uniformity, combined with changing technology in sterile product preparation and delivery, has led to serious medication errors and, therefore, recommendations for new practice guidelines.

UNNECESSARY EVENTS

In 1990 and 1991, some serious and highly publicized medication errors challenged the pharmacy profession to review its policies and procedures for sterile products. Four cases involved admixing the wrong ingredients. In one of these cases, three premature infants died because a pharmacy technician—whose work had been checked by a pharmacist—accidentally substituted potassium chloride injection for an IV flush solution of heparin, dextrose, and water.[2] In two of the other cases, a woman died after receiving magnesium sulfate during eye surgery[3] and a child died after receiving a TPN solution without dextrose.[4] In the fourth case, two premature infants died after receiving an antibiotic incorrectly prepared by a pharmacy technician. This technician's work also had been checked by a pharmacist.[5]

Poor aseptic technique caused three other incidents. In one, two adults died and six other patients suffered infections resulting from cardioplegia solutions contaminated during batch preparation in the pharmacy.[6] In a separate incident, four patients died due to contaminated sodium glutamate–potassium aspartate solution during open heart surgery.[3] In a less critical incident, 13 patients developed eye infections from contaminated (and subpotent) indomethacin eye drops prepared by a community pharmacy.[7]

These incidents of improper sterile product preparation are not isolated. In 1994, two patients died and two others suffered respiratory distress after receiving incorrectly mixed total nutrient admixtures. The TPNs contained amino acids, carbohydrates, and lipids as well as calcium, phosphates, and other nutrients.[8] Apparently, calcium phosphate precipitated after compounding with an automated compounder. The autopsies revealed diffuse microvascular pulmonary emboli containing calcium phosphate.[9]

MORE CHALLENGES AHEAD

The cited incidents illustrate the danger inherent in admixture procedures. While many institutions have developed practices to prevent these dangers, new technologies and procedures are challenging the pharmacist's abilities to compound, package, and label appropriately.[10,11]

New Technologies

New technologies, such as syringe pump infusion systems and patient-controlled analgesia (PCA) pumps, require pharmacists to repackage injectables into syringes, increasing the chance of errors.[12] Infusion pumps that allow a pharmacist to place multiple intermittent doses into a single IV bag also increase the risks of incorrect preparation, packaging, and labeling. Portable pumps and indwelling medication reservoirs permit longer infusion periods and higher product temperatures, possibly leading to mistakes in expiration dating.[13,14] Elastomeric infusion devices, which are simple to use but require special storage conditions, may lead to dosing errors.[15]

New Procedures

The use of high-risk routes of administration (e.g., intrathecal) also increases the danger level. Additionally, the use of more toxic sterile products—highly concentrated injections of potassium chloride, dextrose, lidocaine, and doxorubicin—has led to fatal medication errors. The preparation of sterile drugs from nonsterile ingredients also increases the level of risk. Common examples include concentrated morphine injection for epidural analgesia and reservoirs, alum for bladder irrigation,[16] and caffeine for neonatal respiratory distress.

Another technical, and possibly legal, issue for pharmacists is the use of automated compounders:

- ❏ How do such large devices affect laminar airflow in a hood?
- ❏ How does a pharmacist ensure that the right additives are hung on individual stations?[17]
- ❏ How does a pharmacist ensure that the pump is measuring ingredients accurately?[18,19]

Other complexities arise because pharmacy-prepared sterile products are now used in numerous settings, including patients' homes, physicians' offices, and long-term care facilities. In these settings, pharmacists must ensure the efficacy and safety of any product they compound or check.

FDA AUTHORITY AND ACTIONS

The technological and procedural issues described here have led to action by the Food and Drug Administration (FDA), which has the authority to regulate the quality of drug products prepared in pharmacies. Since 1990, FDA has sent warning letters to retail pharmacies that may manufacture, distribute, and promote unapproved drugs for human use outside the bounds of licensed pharmacy practice.[20] FDA's position was stated in a 1980 compliance guide (see Appendix 1).[21]

After recognizing some serious pharmacy errors in batch compounding, in 1990 FDA formally reminded pharmacists that they are responsible for adhering to good manufacturing practices and safe packaging.[22] In March 1992, then FDA Commissioner David Kessler addressed the American Pharmaceutical Association (APhA) convention and discussed the compliance guide on manufacturing by state-licensed pharmacies. The guide stated that "pharmacists may prepare very limited quantities of drugs before receiving valid prescriptions, provided they can document a history of receiving valid prescriptions that have been generated solely within an established professional practitioner–patient–pharmacist relationship and provided further that they maintain the prescription on file for all such products dispensed at the pharmacy as required by law"[20] (see Appendix 2).

Under its authority to regulate "new" drugs, FDA allows physicians to prescribe "an unusual preparation that requires compounding by a pharmacist from drugs readily available for other uses and which is not generally regarded as safe and effective for the intended use"[23] (see Appendix 3). However, processing and repackaging of approved drugs by pharmacists for resale to hospitals, other pharmacies, etc., are subject to premarket approval by FDA as new drug products.[23] FDA's regulatory authority over extemporaneous and batch compounding is interpreted by its inspectors, who generally do not examine state-licensed pharmacies.

In the fall of 1992, four professional pharmacy organizations—APhA, American Society of Health-System Pharmacists (ASHP), American Association of Colleges of Pharmacy (AACP), and American Society of Consultant Pharmacists (ASCP)—met with FDA officials to ask for clarification of its compliance guideline 7132.16.[20] These organizations gave 10 examples of pharmacy compounding that could be misconstrued by an FDA inspector as manufacturing. FDA did not accept all 10 scenarios, but the matter is not closed.[24] The guideline was challenged in court by Professionals and Patients for Customized Care (P2C2). However, a March 1994 decision by a Houston federal court upheld the FDA guideline, ruling that it is not a blanket prohibition against pharmacist compounding but is aimed at "drug manufacturing that takes place in pharmacies."[25]

In response to the 1994 calcium phosphate precipitate deaths, FDA sent a Safety Alert letter to hospital pharmacists, nutritional support teams, home health pharmacists, physicians, and other health care providers.[26] This letter recommended seven ways to prevent and detect precipitates of calcium phosphate.

Clearly, pharmacists are embarrassed by compounding errors and are concerned that FDA will increase inspections. Concurrent with the publicity and FDA actions, three pharmacy organizations have published new guidelines to help pharmacists improve sterile compounding procedures.

NABP ACTIONS AND GUIDELINES

The National Association of Boards of Pharmacy (NABP) says that prescription compounding is a pharmacist's responsibility and should be regulated by state boards.[27] To distinguish between compounding and manufacturing, NABP defined these terms in its Model State Pharmacy Practice Act:[28]

> *"Compounding—the preparation, mixing, assembling, packaging, or labeling of a drug (including radiopharmaceuticals) or device (i) as the result of a practitioner/patient/pharmacist relationship in the course of professional practice, or (ii) for the purpose of, or as an incident to, research, teaching, or chemical analysis and not for sale or dispensing. Compounding also includes the preparation of drugs or devices in anticipation of prescription drug orders based on routine, regularly observed prescribing patterns.*
>
> *Manufacturing—the production, preparation, propagation, conversion, or processing of a drug or device, either directly or indirectly, by extraction from substances of natural origin or independently by means of chemical or biological synthesis, and includes any packaging or repackaging of the substance(s) or labeling or relabeling of its container, and the promotion and marketing of such drugs or devices. Manufacturing also includes the preparation and promotion of commercially available products from bulk compounds for resale by pharmacies, practitioners or other persons."*

NABP has published two model regulations or guidelines about the preparation of sterile products. One is Good Compounding Practices Applicable to State Licensed Pharmacies[28,29] (see Appendix 4), a general compounding document for state boards of pharmacy that was prepared at the request of FDA. The other is Model Rules for Sterile Pharmaceuticals[30] (see Appendix 5). Both guidelines, to be incorporated into NABP's Model State Pharmacy Practice Act, apply to pharmacy practice regardless of the setting (e.g., home, hospital, and nursing home). However, NABP model regulations do not have the force of law. They merely serve as a basis for individual state boards to develop rules and regulations. Many state boards circulate NABP model regulations in their newsletters.

These appendices should be studied to gain a thorough understanding of these model regulations. Neither guideline distinguishes among levels of product risk to patients. (See discussion of risk levels under ASHP Actions and Guidelines.) In summary, NAPB guidelines have eight key points:

- ❏ A policy and procedure manual should be established for compounding, dispensing, and delivery of sterile pharmaceutical prescription orders.
- ❏ Pharmacists and supportive personnel should be trained and have sufficient reference materials about sterile products.
- ❏ Drugs and supplies should be stored, labeled, and disposed of properly.
- ❏ Sterile compounding should be done in an area separate from other activities. (However, a "cleanroom" environment is not specified.)
- ❏ Personnel should adhere to hygienic and aseptic techniques.
- ❏ Documentation should specify when and why manufacturer-labeled expiration dates are exceeded.
- ❏ Pharmacists should check finished products.
- ❏ Records of compounding should be carefully maintained as part of a documented, ongoing quality-assurance program.

ASHP ACTIONS AND GUIDELINES

ASHP has continually promoted appropriate pharmacy compounding in the institutional setting. In 1990, ASHP developed a multistep action plan to encourage and teach pharmacists to compound safe and effective sterile products.

Letter and Survey

The first step of this plan was to send a letter to pharmacy directors, assistant directors, and IV supervisors nationwide, urging them to review and revise their sterile product techniques.[31] In the second step, ASHP sent a survey to a representative sample of hospital pharmacy directors to assess the quality of sterile product procedures.[32] Some key findings were[1]

- ❏ Almost 96% of hospital pharmacies extemporaneously compounded sterile products; 61% also batch prepared such products.
- ❏ Almost all pharmacists (99.4%) who prepared sterile products used a laminar-airflow hood.
- ❏ About 75% of respondents used laminar-airflow hoods in limited-access areas.
- ❏ About 50% of respondents said that their hoods were certified every 6 months and that prefilters

were changed monthly.

❑ Less than 33% of respondents reported sampling the environment in and around the hood for microbial contamination.

❑ About 33% of pharmacists used final filtration to sterilize some products prepared extemporaneously, and 16% of pharmacists filtered products in batch compounding.

Nearly half of the survey respondents never tested the chemical purity, drug concentration, sterility, or pyrogenicity of sterile products. Less than a third of the pharmacies tested their pharmacists or technicians, either by written exam or process validation, on aseptic technique. In other words, the majority of hospital pharmacists did not determine whether they were compounding safe and effective sterile products. ASHP concluded that certain quality-assurance procedures for sterile products needed major improvement.

Conference

The third step in ASHP's plan was to invite key persons to participate in a conference;[33] its purpose was to list apparent problems with pharmacy-prepared sterile products and to identify possible solutions. Attendees included representatives from the FDA, United States Pharmacopeial Convention (USP), American Hospital Association (AHA), NABP, Intravenous Nurses Society, Association for Practitioners of Infection Control, American College of Apothecaries, Joint Commission on the Accreditation of Healthcare Organizations (JCAHO), AACP, Parenteral Drug Association, Pharmaceutical Manufacturers Association, American Biological Safety Association, Canadian Society of Hospital Pharmacists, American Nurses Association, and some members and staff of ASHP.

Conference participants listed 12 problems with pharmacy sterile compounding practices. These problems may be categorized into four groups:

1. A lack of appropriate policies and procedures.
2. A lack of personnel training and education materials.
3. A lack of consistent regulatory definitions, standards, and enforcement by professional and governing groups.
4. A lack of commercially available sterile products.

Twenty-six ideas were suggested for resolving the problems.

Educational Programs and Publications

ASHP began the fourth step of its plan with educational programs and publications to teach pharmacy personnel how to prepare safe and effective sterile products. One of the first programs was an open hearing at ASHP's 1991 Midyear Clinical Meeting. Related open hearings have continued at other ASHP meetings. Several articles and editorials also have been published in the *American Journal of Health-System Pharmacy* (formerly the *American Journal of Hospital Pharmacy*).[34–43]

Finally, ASHP developed a practice standard for the quality assurance of pharmacy-prepared sterile products. These guidelines were first drafted for public comment in February 1992,[44] and approximately 75 written remarks were received. ASHP worked with key practitioners to incorporate comments and revise the guidelines. At its April 1993 meeting, the ASHP Board of Directors changed the guidelines to a draft technical assistance bulletin (TAB).[45] A TAB has less power than a professional standard but offers specific, detailed advice.[46] Therefore, a governmental or judicial authority would have less success holding a pharmacist or pharmacy to the requirements in a TAB.

The final version of the TAB on sterile product preparation was published in November 1993[47] and is required reading for an understanding of the following concepts (see Appendix 6). A summary of its highlights follows. Subsequent chapters give more detail on why practices are specified in the TAB and how to implement good compounding techniques.

Risk levels

The ASHP Technical Assistance Bulletin on Quality Assurance for Pharmacy-Prepared Sterile Products designates three levels of risk to patients, increasing from the least (Risk Level 1) to the greatest (Risk Level 3) potential for harm. Risk levels are defined, and examples of sterile products in each level are given. Quality-assurance practices for patient safety and product effectiveness also are listed for each level. This categorization by risk levels allows pharmacists to match sterile compounding procedures to the products they prepare. When compounding a product under conditions that do not meet risk level requirements, pharmacists are required to use their best judgment of risk to benefit for the patient.

Cleanrooms

One controversial part of this TAB pertains to a suitable environment (or controlled area) for sterile compounding. While Risk Level 1 products require a separate, clean space of sufficient size, Risk Levels 2 and 3 require "cleanrooms." This concept, although new for many pharmacists, means a separate room that houses the laminar-airflow hood; the room receives air filtered to a standard level of cleanliness (expressed in airborne particles per cubic foot). Airborne particles are the main vectors for microbes that contaminate products during processing.

The special environment requirement is controversial because of its cost–benefit ratio. The key is to ensure that airborne microbes do not enter the laminar-airflow hood workspace. One study showed that simple changes in operating procedures can produce a cleanroom environment without costly architectural changes.[48] Finally, a laminar-airflow hood suited to the compounded products is the most important equipment, but it must be properly used and maintained to prevent contamination.

Garb

A discussion on garb (clothing, masks, gloves, and shoe covers) also is an integral part of the TAB. Operators should wear garb that sheds low levels of particulates, wash their hands frequently, and use proper hygiene.

Process validation and key points

The TAB also describes the need for process validation to determine whether an operator, working under the most challenging situation, can consistently produce a sterile product. Growth media are substituted for normal ingredients in the compounding process to validate the environment, equipment, supplies, and aseptic technique. Process validation (sometimes referred to as "media fills") is better than end-product sterility sampling, which can lead to accidental contamination, delayed results, and higher costs. The TAB stipulates process validation for individual operators in Risk Level 1, for each compounding process in Risk Level 2, and for each product in Risk Level 3.

Other key points in the TAB include

- ❏ Development and maintenance of up-to-date procedures.
- ❏ Training and competency testing of personnel.
- ❏ Storage and handling of closures, containers, and supplies.
- ❏ Product stability (compatibility and physical and chemical stability) at the time of use.
- ❏ Expiration dating of products compounded outside of the manufacturer's labeling.
- ❏ Labeling requirements.
- ❏ Final product inspection (sterility, nonpyrogenicity, accurate drug concentration, and stability).
- ❏ Documentation of all sterile compounding processes.
- ❏ Documentation of employee testing and validation, refrigerator temperatures, hood certification, batch control testing, and quarantine records.

USP ACTIONS AND GUIDELINES

Long before any highly publicized pharmacy compounding errors, USP decided that preparation of sterile IV products for home use involved special concerns (e.g., extended product storage and patient manipulations prior to use). Therefore, USP established a Home Health Care Advisory Panel in 1989 to draft a monograph or guideline on compounding sterile products for home use. The first draft of this monograph was published in March 1992.[49] Following the review of 22 written comments, the Panel published a second draft for public comment in May 1993.[50] The final draft was published in November 1993,[51] and it now appears in the 1995 *United States Pharmacopeia/National Formulary*[52] (see Appendix 7).

Again, this standard should be read for comparison and contrast to the NABP model rules and the ASHP TAB. Like ASHP, USP defined three risk levels to patients, a low-risk and two high-risk categories. However, USP risk levels do not include preservatives, storage temperatures, and time limits between preparation and completion of administration. Because risk levels are defined differently than in the ASHP TAB, some product types do not match ASHP's corresponding risk levels.

Table 1-1 offers examples of what products fit into corresponding risk levels of the ASHP and USP documents. The USP monograph places less emphasis on categorizing processes and procedures by risk level because it covers only home use sterile drugs. Unlike ASHP, USP guidelines do not use the term "batch." USP lists requirements for written, approved policies and procedures.

COMPARISON OF GUIDELINES

Ignorance and carelessness cause the most errors in compounding accuracy as well as product contamination. However, NABP, ASHP, and USP guidelines do not emphasize the teaching of aseptic technique and cleanroom procedures. While ASHP categorizes educational guidelines by risk level, USP does not. But USP explains storage and handling, especially once the sterile product arrives in a patient's home.

NABP, ASHP, and USP specify that sterile products be compounded in an area separate from other pharmacy activities. ASHP calls this place the controlled area; USP, the buffer room; and NABP, the designated area. ASHP does not mention an anteroom to the controlled area until Risk Level 2, but USP requires an anteroom at all three risk levels.

Cleanrooms are classified by the measured level of airborne particles larger than 0.5 µm/cu ft; therefore, a Class 10,000 cleanroom is 10 times as "clean" as a Class 100,000 cleanroom. ASHP specifies the need for a Class 100,000 cleanroom in Risk Level 2 and a Class 10,000 in Risk Level 3. USP requires Class 100,000 for the low-risk level and Class 10,000 for both high-risk levels. All three guidelines require laminar-airflow hoods to create a Class 100 environment for the actual performance of aseptic technique. Both ASHP and NABP specify that the hoods be recertified every 6 months, while USP requires rou-

Table 1-1. *Examples of Sterile Products by Risk Level Category*

ASHP TAB	USP Monograph
Risk Level 1 Single-patient admixtures Single-patient ophthalmics with preservatives Single-patient syringes without preservatives used in 28 hr Batch-prefilled syringes with preservatives	**Low-Risk Category** Sterile drug products transferred from vials or ampuls into sterile final containers with syringe and needle Sterile drug products transferred into sterile elastomeric infusion containers with aid of mechanical pump and appropriate sterile transfer device, with or without subsequent addition of sterile drug products with sterile syringe and needle Sterile nutritional solutions combining dextrose injection and amino acid injection via gravity transfer into sterile empty containers, with or without addition of sterile drugs to final container with sterile syringe and needle
Risk Level 2 TPNs for administration after 7 days Injections for use in portable pump or reservoir Batch-reconstituted antibiotics without preservatives Batch-prefilled syringes without preservatives	**High-Risk Category I** Sterile nutritional solutions compounded with automated compounder, involving repeated attachment of fluid containers to proximal openings of compounder tubing set and of empty final containers to distal opening Additive transfers into filled final container from individual drug product containers or from pooled additive solution Ambulatory pump reservoirs prepared by adding more than one drug product, with evacuation of air from reservoir prior to dispensing Ambulatory pump reservoirs prepared for multiday (ambient temperature) administration
Risk Level 3 Alum bladder irrigations Morphine injections made from powder or tablets TPNs made from dry amino acids Autoclaved IV solutions TPNs sterilized by final filtration	**High-Risk Category II** Injectable morphine solutions prepared from nonsterile morphine substance and suitable vehicles Sterile nutritional solutions prepared from nonsterile ingredients, with initial mixing in nonsealed or nonsterile reservoir

tine certification only every 12 months. ASHP lists environmental cleaning intervals, but USP and NABP do not.

None of the guidelines offers advice about quality assurance in the use of automated compounding machines, yet several fatal errors have occurred with these compounders. Pharmacists who use automated devices for compounding should follow manufacturers' instructions and use special controls to prevent major errors (e.g.,

refractometers and scales to verify dextrose content).

ASHP and USP have similar garb requirements. However, gloves are not required by ASHP until Risk Level 2 but are required in all three risk levels by USP. NABP has no specifications for garb. All three guidelines similarly describe aseptic technique, but each guideline has some unique features.

Both ASHP and USP require process validation for individual operators in the lowest risk level, for each type of product (e.g., home TPN and ambulatory pump reservoirs) in the second risk level, and for each product in the highest risk level. While ASHP designates little about methods of process validation, USP discusses types of media, incubation times, and sample sizes of media fills. ASHP states that personnel are to be revalidated annually; however, USP specifies quarterly revalidation. NABP does not mention process validation.

According to the USP guidelines, expiration dates, unless otherwise stated in product labeling, should not exceed 30 days. Labeling is not stressed by USP, but patient/caregiver training and monitoring are emphasized.

All three guidelines require pharmacists to test extensively when sterile products are compounded from nonsterile ingredients and containers. These products must be quarantined until tests prove them to be quantitatively accurate, sterile, and nonpyrogenic. USP elaborates on product quality assurance during transit to and time in a patient's home. USP also says more on the appropriate use of compounding equipment. Once a sterile product leaves the pharmacy, both USP and NABP place responsibility on the pharmacist to ensure quality control. ASHP's TAB applies *only* to sterile product preparation in the pharmacy.

For the most part, all three organizations have similar requirements for documentation. Only USP does not require personnel education and competency evaluation to be documented. However, USP requires a second person to initial all component measurements during compounding, and ASHP and NABP do not. NABP is alone in requiring lot numbers of all components to be recorded, presumably even for simple admixtures.

Both USP and NABP specify that pharmacists are responsible for training patients and caregivers on the handling and use of sterile products at home. ASHP guidelines are limited to training pharmacy personnel. USP offers the only guidance on monitoring and tracking patient experience with sterile products. All three guidelines require a formal quality-assurance program for the entire sterile compounding operation.

SUMMARY

Pharmacists who are responsible for compounding sterile products face a host of issues unknown 10–15 years ago. With current publicity, governmental scrutiny, and technological changes, pharmacists have a difficult challenge to meet this responsibility.

To compound sterile products appropriately, pharmacists must understand the guidelines of NABP, ASHP, and USP. Each guideline has a unique perspective and offers some information not covered in the other two. However, professional judgment is required in applying these guidelines to individual practice settings.

REFERENCES

1. Crawford SY, Narducci WA, Augustine SC. National survey of quality assurance activities for pharmacy-prepared sterile products in hospitals. *Am J Hosp Pharm.* 1991; 48:2398–413.
2. Pharmacist blamed for fatal medication error. *Am Druggist.* 1990; 202 (Aug):21.
3. ASHP gears up multistep action plan regarding sterile drug products. *Am J Hosp Pharm.* 1991; 48:386–9.
4. Gebhart F. Test hyperal solutions? Fla. mom says yes. *Hosp Pharm Rep.* 1992; 6 (2):35.
5. Two infants die in Dallas hospital accident. *Atlanta Journal-Constitution.* 1991; Feb 24:A4.
6. Two deaths in Nebraska. *Am Druggist.* 1990; 202 (Aug):21.
7. Eye drop injuries prompt an F.D.A. warning. *NY Times.* 1990; 140 (Dec 9): Sec 1, 39.
8. Gannon K. FDA issues TPN safety alert after two die in Hawaii. *Hosp Pharm Rep.* 1994; 8 (5):1, 8.
9. Food and Drug Administration. Safety alert: hazards of precipitation associated with parenteral nutrition. *Am J Hosp Pharm.* 1994; 51:1427–8.
10. Kwan JW. High-technology i.v. infusion devices. *Am J Hosp Pharm.* 1991; 48 (Suppl 1):S36–51.
11. Kwan JW, Anderson RW. Pharmacists' knowledge of infusion devices. *Am J Hosp Pharm.* 1991; 48 (Suppl 1):S52–3.
12. Mulye NV, Turco SJ, Speaker TJ. Stability of ganciclovir sodium in an infusion-pump syringe. *Am J Hosp Pharm.* 1994; 51:1348–9.
13. Stiles ML, Tu Y-H, Allen LV Jr. Stability of morphine sulfate in portable pump reservoirs during storage and simulated administration. *Am J Hosp Pharm.* 1989; 46:1404–7.
14. Duafala ME, Kleinberg ML, Nacov C, et al. Stability of morphine sulfate in infusion devices and containers for intravenous administration. *Am J Hosp Pharm.* 1990; 47:143–6.
15. Kaye T. Prolonged infusion times with disposable elastomeric infusion devices. *Am J Hosp Pharm.* 1994; 51:533–4.
16. Levchuk JW. Rapid preparation of alum bladder irrigation. *Hosp Pharm.* 1991; 26:577. Letter.
17. Davis NM. Unprecedented procedural safeguards needed with the use of automated i.v. compounders. *Hosp Pharm.* 1992; 27:488. Editorial.
18. Brushwood DB. Hospital liable for defect in cardioplegia solution. *Am J Hosp Pharm.* 1992; 49:1174–6.
19. Murphy C. Ensuring accuracy in the use of automatic compounders. *Am J Hosp Pharm.* 1993; 50:60. Letter.
20. Office of Enforcement, Division of Compliance

Policy. Manufacture, distribution, and promotion of adulterated, misbranded, or unapproved new drugs for human use by state-licensed pharmacies. FDA Guide 7132.16. Washington, DC: Food and Drug Administration; Mar 16, 1992:Chap 32.

21. Division of Field Regulatory Guidance. Hospital pharmacies—status as drug manufacturer. FDA Guide 7132.06. Washington, DC: Food and Drug Administration; Oct 1, 1980:Chap 32.

22. Bloom MZ. Compounding in today's practice. *Am Pharm.* 1991; NS31 (Oct):31–7.

23. Office of Enforcement, Division of Compliance Policy. Regulatory action regarding approved new drugs and antibiotic drug products subjected to additional processing or other manipulations. FDA Guide 7132c.06. Washington, DC: Food and Drug Administration; Jan 18, 1991:Chap 32c.

24. Myers CE, Director, Professional Practice Division, American Society of Hospital Pharmacists, Bethesda, MD. Apr 21, 1994. Personal communication.

25. FDA compounding compliance policy guide upheld by Houston federal court. *FDC Rep "The Pink Sheet."* 1994; 56 (May 23):T&G-19.

26. Lumpkin MM, Burlington DB. FDA safety alert: hazards of precipitation with parenteral nutrition. Washington, DC: Food and Drug Administration; Apr 18, 1994. Letter.

27. Delegates approve 20 resolutions at annual meeting, resolution No. 89-1-93. *NABP Newsl.* 1993; 22:57.

28. Good compounding practices applicable to state licensed pharmacies. Part I. *Natl Pharm. Compliance News.* 1993; May:2–3.

29. Good compounding practices applicable to state licensed pharmacies. Part II. *Natl Pharm. Compliance News.* 1993; Oct:2–3.

30. Model rules for sterile pharmaceuticals. Chicago, IL: National Association of Boards of Pharmacy; 1993:12.1–3.

31. ASHP urges review of sterile drug product procedures. *ASHP Newsl.* 1991; 24 (Jan):1.

32. Next step in sterile product action plan: a survey of hospital pharmacists. *ASHP Newsl.* 1991; 24 (Feb):1.

33. ASHP invitational conference on quality assurance for pharmacy-prepared sterile products. *Am J Hosp Pharm.* 1991; 48:2391–7.

34. Zellmer WA. Upgrading quality assurance for pharmacy-prepared sterile products. *Am J Hosp Pharm.* 1991; 48:2387–8. Editorial.

35. Tormo VJ. Perspective on sterile compounding practices and the draft guidelines. *Am J Hosp Pharm.* 1992; 49:946–7.

36. Reynolds LA. Guidelines for the preparation of sterile ophthalmic products. *Am J Hosp Pharm.* 1991; 48:2438–9.

37. American Society of Hospital Pharmacists. ASHP technical assistance bulletin on pharmacy-prepared ophthalmic products. *Am J Hosp Pharm.* 1993; 50:1462–3.

38. McKinnon BT, Avis KE. Membrane filtration of pharmaceutical solutions. *Am J Hosp Pharm.* 1993; 50:1921–36.

39. Chandler SW, Trissel LA, Wamsley LM, et al. Evaluation of air quality in a sterile-drug preparation area with an electronic particle counter. *Am J Hosp Pharm.* 1993; 50:2330–4.

40. Favier M, Hansel S, Bressolle F. Preparing cytotoxic agents in an isolator. *Am J Hosp Pharm.* 1993; 50:2335–9.

41. Trissel LA. Compounding our problems. *Am J Hosp Pharm.* 1994; 51:1534. Editorial.

42. Hasegawa GR. Caring about stability and compatibility. *Am J Hosp Pharm.* 1994; 51:1533–4. Editorial.

43. Mirtallo JM. The complexity of mixing calcium and phosphate. *Am J Hosp Pharm.* 1994; 51:1535–6. Editorial.

44. American Society of Hospital Pharmacists. Draft guidelines on quality assurance for pharmacy-prepared sterile products. *Am J Hosp Pharm.* 1992; 49:407–17.

45. American Society of Hospital Pharmacists. Draft technical assistance bulletin on quality assurance for pharmacy-prepared sterile products. *Am J Hosp Pharm.* 1993; 50:1440–52.

46. Hicks WE. Development of ASHP practice standards. *Am J Hosp Pharm.* 1993; 50:878, 880.

47. American Society of Hospital Pharmacists. ASHP technical assistance bulletin on quality assurance for pharmacy-prepared sterile products. *Am J Hosp Pharm.* 1993; 50:2386–98.

48. Lau D, Shane R, Yen J. Quality assurance for sterile products: simple changes can help. *Am J Hosp Pharm.* 1994; 51:1353. Letter.

49. Dispensing practices for sterile drug products intended for home use. *Pharmacopeial Forum.* 1992; 18:3052–75.

50. Sterile drug products for home use. *Pharmacopeial Forum.* 1993; 19:5380–409.

51. Sterile drug products for home use. *Pharmacopeial Forum.* 1993; 19:6554–84.

52. Sterile drug products for home use. In: United States pharmacopeia, 23rd rev./national formulary, 18th ed. Rockville, MD: United States Pharmacopeial Convention; 1994:1963–75.

Chapter 2
Personnel Education, Training, and Evaluation

Philip J. Schneider
E. Clyde Buchanan

Attention to the quality of pharmacy-prepared sterile products prompts an assessment of how well pharmacists are educated to perform this function. With the current emphasis on clinical practice, traditional subject matter is being deemphasized. Therefore, pharmacy schools, professional organizations, and employers must verify that adequate training on sterile product preparation is offered to their students, pharmacists, and technicians.

This chapter first examines the current status of pharmacy school training on sterile product preparation. The technician's role in this area and the current level of technician training are then presented. The need for employers to train and evaluate all employees in sterile product preparation is then discussed, followed by a brief description of the importance of such training to pharmacy licensure.

PHARMACY SCHOOL TRAINING

Professional Perceptions

In 1991, the American Society of Hospital Pharmacists (ASHP, now the American Society of Health-System Pharmacists) held a conference on quality assurance for pharmacy-prepared sterile products.[1] Attendees included representatives from the Food and Drug Administration (FDA), National Association of Boards of Pharmacy (NAPB), and the United States Pharmacopeial Convention (USP) as well as practitioner-based organizations. Conference proceedings noted several apparent problems related to pharmacist training on this subject:[1]

❑ Many pharmacists and pharmacy technicians lack education and training on the preparation of sterile products.

❑ Many pharmacists receive little or no formal education and training in pharmacy schools on the preparation of sterile products.

❑ Many pharmacists and pharmacy technicians do not understand applicable quality-assurance principles.

❏ Mere experience in the preparation of sterile products does not impart the knowledge and understanding necessary to ensure their accurate and safe preparation.

❏ Few pharmacy school faculty members have the knowledge and skill to teach others about this subject area.

❏ Instructional materials are not readily available.

Several ideas for resolving these problems were identified at the conference:

1. The American Association of Colleges of Pharmacy and the American Council on Pharmaceutical Education (ACPE) should reassess the present curricula of colleges of pharmacy. Sterile product preparation should be a required component.

2. The knowledge and skill of college faculty in sterile product preparation should be upgraded, perhaps through videotapes at the teaching site.

Student Perceptions

A recent study evaluated graduating pharmacy students' knowledge of aseptic technique and attempted to determine if specific factors influenced this knowledge base.[2] Results indicated that

❏ Student performance on a test of this knowledge varied widely.

❏ Students reported limited exposure to sterile product preparation as part of their academic programs.

❏ Only about 19% of the experiential training was in this area.

❏ Two percent of the students said that they had no exposure to sterile products in classes.

❏ Twenty-seven percent of the students said that they had no exposure in their internships.

❏ Thirteen percent of the students said that they had no exposure during their externships.

❏ Eighty-one percent of the students did not take any elective courses in sterile product preparation.

Practitioner Perceptions

Another study on this issue surveyed hospital externship preceptors and a selected group of home care pharmacists.[3] Its purpose was to address concern regarding inadequate parenteral product and IV therapy instruction in the core curriculum in spite of the in-

creased use of these products in both the hospital and ambulatory settings.

According to this study's findings, subjects related to sterile products are neglected at many colleges of pharmacy. The topic is often covered in a fragmented fashion, and proper equipment (e.g., cleanrooms and laminar-airflow hoods) is not available. The current emphasis on therapeutics and clinical practice has occurred at the expense of science and technology, so new pharmacy graduates are inadequately prepared to make sterile products.

Changing the Curriculum

The inadequate exposure to sterile product preparation in colleges of pharmacy will not be an easy problem to solve. These institutions make changes slowly and face many curricular issues. Nevertheless, given the attention being devoted to pharmacy-prepared sterile products by the FDA and the public, it seems prudent for colleges to revisit their commitment to this area of practice.

If a three- or four-credit course with laboratory experience is offered, this problem may be resolved. Some educators also recommend creating residencies in sterile products in strategically located schools with the necessary faculty, facilities, and equipment.[3] The curriculum could emphasize both manufacturing and admixture technologies. Such course work is becoming even more relevant with the increased involvement of community practitioners and the growth of the home infusion industry. At a minimum, the subjects covered in this book should be in the core curriculum for any course on sterile product preparation.

PHARMACY TECHNICIAN TRAINING

Technician Involvement in Sterile Product Preparation

Pharmacy technicians are actively involved in all aspects of pharmaceutical care. The Scope of Pharmacy Practice Project[4] found that 26% of technicians' time is spent in

Table 2-1. *Percentage of Pharmacy Technicians Who Participate in Sterile Compounding by Product Type*[5]

Sterile Product	Pharmacy Technician Participation in Extemporaneous Compounding, %
Unit dose injections	60
Large volume parenteral admixtures	81
TPNs	57
IV piggybacks	85
Chemotherapy agents	31
Narcotic infusions	38

collecting, organizing, and evaluating information. The second most time-consuming functions (total of 21%) involve preparing, dispensing, distributing, and administering medications.

A smaller survey identified what percentage of hospital pharmacy technicians prepare certain sterile products (see Table 2-1) and where these technicians are trained. According to this survey, 75% are trained on the job, 9% are trained in formal hospital-based programs, 2% are trained in formal academic centers (e.g., community colleges), 7% are trained in military courses, and 7% are trained in a combination of settings.[5]

The results of both studies indicate the need for formal training of technicians in sterile product preparation.

Training Competencies

To help fulfill the identified need for technician training in sterile product preparation, ASHP published outcome competencies and training guidelines for institutional technician programs.[6] According to this 1982 bulletin, technicians should be able to

1. List five possibilities for contamination of an injectable solution during its preparation as well as a precaution that would prevent each possibility.
2. Demonstrate proper technique for using a syringe and needle for aseptic withdrawal of the contents of a rubber-capped vial and a glass ampul.
3. Demonstrate proper technique for aseptic reconstitution of an antibiotic injection.
4. Describe when hand washing is required and demonstrate proper technique.
5. Demonstrate correct techniques and procedures for preparing at least three parenteral admixtures, including the label and control records.
6. Identify major components of a laminar-airflow hood and state their functions.
7. Define and describe (1) microbial growth and transmission; (2) origin, pharmacologic effect, and prevention of pyrogens; (3) sterility; (4) heat sterilization; and (5) cold sterilization.
8. Designate, from a list of 10 sterile preparations, those that may be safely heat treated.
9. Demonstrate proper technique for visual inspection of parenteral solutions.

Additional competencies should now be added to this list. Examples include

❒ Compounding of chemotherapy and other cytotoxic products.
❒ Operation of automated compounders.

❒ Filling of pump reservoirs.
❒ Work in cleanroom environments.

Accreditation

To help ensure these competencies in sterile product preparation, ASHP encourages the formal training of pharmacy technicians, either in hospitals or academic settings, by means of ASHP-accredited programs. Accreditation is the process of granting recognition or vouching for conformance with a standard and usually is conferred on a specific institution.

To be accredited, pharmacy technician training programs must be surveyed according to ASHP regulations[7] and meet the accreditation standard.[8] This standard states that technicians should have a working knowledge of aseptic compounding and parenteral admixture operations. By mid-1995, ASHP's Commission on Credentialing had accredited 46 pharmacy technician training programs. Although this number is small, ASHP accreditation is the only established mechanism for ensuring a minimum quality for these programs.

Certification

Another mechanism to ensure the quality of pharmacy technician education is certification. By the certification process, a nongovernmental agency or professional association recognizes an individual who has met certain predetermined, specified qualifications.

To be a certified pharmacy technician, a candidate must pass an examination. Two of the three currently validated technician certification examinations are administered by the Michigan Pharmacists Association (MPA) and the Illinois Council of Hospital Pharmacists (ICHP). Both examinations are voluntary, and 15–20% of their questions concern sterile product compounding.

In December 1993, ASHP, the American Pharmaceutical Association, MPA, and ICHP announced that they were jointly preparing a national voluntary certification program for pharmacy technicians.[9] As a result of this effort, the Pharmacy Technician Certification Board (PTCB) was established in January 1995. PTCB's validated examination is also voluntary and focuses on three broad functions:[10]

❒ Assisting the pharmacist in serving patients.
❒ Medication distribution and inventory control systems.
❒ Operations.

Half of this examination concerns traditional dispensing, distribution, and information management, including

❒ Calibrating equipment needed to compound medications.

❐ Compounding.
❐ Preparing IV admixtures.
❐ Documentation.

The topics covered in this national technician certification examination further indicate the need for a formalized approach to training in sterile product preparation.

EMPLOYEE TRAINING AND EVALUATION

Orientation

Because pharmacy students and technicians often are not well trained in sterile product preparation, a new employee must receive proper orientation before being given this responsibility. An orientation consists of two components: (1) providing the employee with information, and (2) measuring baseline performance.

Providing information

Regardless of a staff member's education and training before employment, some information is unique to each institution. Before preparing sterile products, a new employee should receive orientation on

❐ Dress code and garb requirements.
❐ Hand-washing techniques, including where and when to wash hands, and personal hygiene.
❐ Procedures for entering and leaving critical and controlled areas.
❐ Locations of medications and supplies.
❐ How orders are recorded and labels are generated.
❐ Documentation of work, including who made a dose and what was used.
❐ Types and locations of drug information resources.
❐ Methods for transmitting medication orders.
❐ Policies for storing prepared sterile products.
❐ Methods for sending doses to patients.
❐ Policies for reusing returned doses.
❐ Special procedures for chemotherapy agents and TPN.
❐ Quality management procedures, including process validation and environmental monitoring.
❐ Problem resolution, including spill management.
❐ Staffing and scheduling, including "safe staffing."

A checklist is recommended for documenting the satisfactory recall of this information. This checklist, with space for the employee's signature and validation by the responsible supervisor, should be placed in the employee's personnel record.

Measuring performance

Quality management requires the ongoing monitoring of an employee's technique (see Chapter 16). Therefore, a baseline evaluation of a new employee's aseptic technique, using process validation, is an important part of the orientation. While sources differ concerning how many process validation samples are needed for a baseline, USP recommendations can be considered a standard of practice.[11]

Throughout the process of education, training, and evaluation, it is important to document the attainment of competence for employees who prepare sterile products.

Continuing Education

To maintain proper quality assurance, pharmacy personnel should regularly receive didactic and experiential training and competency evaluation.[12] Tables 2-2 and 2-3 list recommended continuing education topics on sterile product preparation for pharmacists and technicians, respectively.

Although pharmacy managers generally recognize that their staffs need training, they often do not understand how adults learn.[13] Six cognitive skill levels are recognized for adult learners and should be incorporated into all education programs on sterile product preparation.

Level 1—knowledge

Knowledge includes the recall of ideas or material about sterile compounding. Although knowledge does not necessarily connote understanding, even recall is impossible without adequate training. A training course should introduce pharmacy personnel to basic and important information. Many topics for such a training course are listed in Tables 2-2 and 2-3.

The reading of this manual constitutes the transmission of knowledge of sterile compounding facts. Other texts also are available as training resources[14,15] and, of course, a pharmacy's policies and procedures for sterile compounding should be included. ASHP's *Manual for Pharmacy Technicians* has chapters on calculations and IV admixture programs.[16]

Level 2—comprehension

Comprehension of a subject—the mental grasping of ideas, facts, and concepts—is manifested by a person's ability to communicate via translation, interpretation, and extrapolation. Comprehension can be enhanced by examples, multimedia (e.g., videos), and quizzes to illustrate key points.

Table 2-2. **Pharmacist Continuing Education Topics for Sterile Product Preparation**

Aseptic technique
Critical area contamination factors
Environmental monitoring
Facilities
Equipment and supplies
Sterile product calculations and terminology
Sterile compounding documentation
Quality-assurance procedures
Proper gowning and gloving techniques
General conduct in controlled area
Good manufacturing practices
Environmental quality control
Component and end-product testing
Sterilization techniques

Table 2-3. **Technician Continuing Education Topics for Sterile Product Preparation**

Parenteral routes of administration (rationale, precautions, and problems; routes; and methods)
Equipment and systems used in parenteral administration (needles and syringes, administration sets, fluid containers, pumps, etc.)
Equipment used to prepare parenteral admixtures (laminar-airflow hoods, filters, pumps, etc.)
Aseptic compounding techniques specific to fluid system used (prefilling syringes, preparing syringes, preparing ophthalmic solutions, etc.)
Labeling and recordkeeping (bottle labels, fluid orders and profiles, compounding records, etc.)
Incompatibilities (visual and chemical incompatibilities, pH and concentration effects, reference sources, etc.)
Quality control (particulate matter inspection and monitoring of contamination)

[ASHP's recently updated video on aseptic technique includes continuing education credit testing.[17] Furthermore, ACPE maintains a continually updated data base, the "Pharmacists' Learning Assistance Network (PLAN)," of all continuing education programs offered by ACPE-approved providers. The PLAN can be contacted by telephone weekdays, 9:00 a.m. to 4:00 p.m. (central time), by calling 1-800-533-3606.[18]]

Level 3—application

Application is the ability to use and comprehend knowledge in specific and concrete ways. For example, the application of aseptic technique requires that an individual choose, organize, restructure, develop, and generalize facts and concepts.

Since adult learners must apply what they learn to retain the information, experiential training is recommended. At first, such practice should be observed by a pharmacist or technician validated in the processes being taught.

Level 4—analysis

The ability to break down systems into parts so that the organization of ideas becomes clear is termed analysis. For instance, a well-trained person can use analysis to identify ways to eliminate sources of contamination or to create more efficient processes. For quality and performance improvement, advanced learners must contribute ideas or analyses from their experience and understanding of sterile compounding.

Level 5—synthesis

Synthesis is the creation of a new system or procedure. For example, designing a new sterile compounding area based on previous analysis would show synthesis. Therefore, an expert is required to create effective training aids for teaching new learners.

Level 6—evaluation

Evaluation consists of judging (1) the value of materials and methods for achieving a goal or (2) the appropriateness of others' work. Experts evaluate performance against internal standards (e.g., environmental contamination) or external evidence (e.g., nosocomial infection rates). Evaluation of another person's technique requires an expert in the subject matter.

Adult learners are oriented to goals that will help them perform; they are primarily self-directed in learning new skills. Trainers should consider using ASHP's goals and objectives that pertain to sterile compounding for residencies in pharmacy practice and home care pharmacy practice.[19,20] Here is an example of a learning goal and the associated objectives.[20]

Goal: Prepare and dispense medications using appropriate techniques and following the home care pharmacy's policies and procedures.

Objective 1: (Application) Follow the home care pharmacy's policies and procedures to maintain the accuracy of the patient profile.

Objective 2: (Mechanism) Prepare IV admixtures using aseptic technique.

Objective 3: (Mechanism) Prepare chemotherapeutic agents observing rules for safe handling of cytotoxic or hazardous agents.

Objective 4: (Evaluation) Appraise admixture solutions for appropriate concentrations, rates, compatibilities, stability, storage, and freedom from defects (e.g., leaking and particulates).

Objective 5: (Evaluation) Determine situations when it is appropriate to compound products extemporaneously.

Objective 6: (Synthesis) Formulate a strategy for extemporaneously compounding drugs to produce the desired end product.

Objective 7: (Application) Label drug products in accordance with the home care pharmacy's policies and procedures.

Objective 8: (Comprehension) Discuss standards of practice for the preparation of drug products (ASHP and USP guidelines for preparation of sterile products).

Objective 9: (Application) Follow the home care pharmacy's quality-control standards in the preparation of drug products.

An organized sterile product training program uses learning objectives such as these for evaluating the competence of pharmacy personnel.

The trainer also should provide new learning opportunities through increasingly complex levels of cognitive skills. Furthermore, training must be combined with implementation of improved methods and reinforcement of positive results (e.g., posting team scores on process validation).[13] Enhancements to methods should be recognized and rewarded.

STATE BOARD EXAMINATION FOR PHARMACISTS

Twice a year, NABP administers a nationwide examination (NABPLEX) to pharmacists seeking licensure in 49 states plus Puerto Rico. (California has its own examination.) NABPLEX covers five areas of competency, including "Compounding and Calculation Involved in Dispensing of Prescriptions and Medication Orders." This area has a subcompetency on aseptic technique.[21]

As part of their practical examinations, some state boards require the compounding of sterile products. Compounding technique and accuracy may be evaluated via direct observation by an examiner and quantitative product analysis, respectively. Candidates should review sterile compounding prior to taking their pharmacy board examinations.

While 46 states permit pharmacy technicians to assist pharmacists, only 12 states require the licensing or registration of pharmacy technicians with the state board. Few states examine technicians or require their continuing education, but 14 states require pharmacists to train their technicians.[22]

Although 48 state boards require continuing education for pharmacist relicensure, none specifies that sterile compounding must be part of that education.[22]

SUMMARY

Pharmacists and technicians do not always receive the education and training required to prepare sterile products. Colleges of pharmacy and technician training programs should recognize the regulatory and public scrutiny being placed on the profession and its responsibility to prepare sterile products competently. Regardless of the setting, pharmacy programs should orient and train staff who are responsible for preparing sterile products and verify their skill levels initially and regularly.

REFERENCES

1. ASHP invitational conference on quality assurance for pharmacy prepared sterile products. *Am J Hosp Pharm.* 1991; 48:2391–7.

2. Brown RE, Birdwell SW, Schneider PJ, et al. Assessing factors affecting graduating pharmacy students' scores on a standardized aseptic technique test. Columbus, OH: Ohio State University, College of Pharmacy; 1993. Unpublished master's degree thesis.

3. Allen LV, Bloss CS, Brazeau GA, et al. Educational issues related to the science and technology of sterile products: academic and industrial perspectives. *Am J Pharm Educ.* 1993; 57:257–65.

4. Summary of the final report of the Scope of Pharmacy Practice Project. *Am J Hosp Pharm.* 1994; 51:2179–82.

5. Anderson RJ. Pharmacy technician survey in the state of Georgia. *Ga J Hosp Pharm.* 1993; 7 (Summer):17–9.

6. American Society of Hospital Pharmacists. ASHP technical assistance bulletin on outcome competencies and training guidelines for institutional pharmacy technician training programs. *Am J Hosp Pharm.* 1982; 39:317–20.

7. American Society of Hospital Pharmacists. ASHP regulations on accreditation of hospital pharmacy technician training programs. *Am J Hosp Pharm.* 1987; 44:2741–3.

8. American Society of Hospital Pharmacists. ASHP

accreditation standard for pharmacy technician training programs. *Am J Hosp Pharm*. 1993; 50:124–6.

9. National voluntary certification program for pharmacy technicians to be explored by four organizations. ASHP news release, Dec 6, 1993, at 28th ASHP Midyear Clinical Meeting, Atlanta, Ga.

10. National pharmacy technician certification examination: 1995 candidate handbook. Washington, DC: Pharmacy Technician Certification Board; 1995:15–7.

11. Sterile drug products for home use. In: United States pharmacopeia, 23rd rev./national formulary, 18th ed. Rockville, MD: United States Pharmacopeial Convention; 1994:1963–75.

12. American Society of Hospital Pharmacists. ASHP technical assistance bulletin on quality assurance for pharmacy-prepared sterile products. *Am J Hosp Pharm*. 1993; 50:2386–98.

13. Fitch HD. Workplace training must recognize how people learn. *CleanRooms*. 1994; 8:60–2.

14. Hunt ML. Training manual for intravenous admixture personnel, 4th ed. Chicago, IL: Pluribus Press; 1989.

15. Turco SJ, ed. Sterile dosage forms, their preparation and clinical application, 4th ed. Philadelphia, PA: Lea & Febiger; 1994.

16. Manual for pharmacy technicians. Bethesda, MD: American Society of Hospital Pharmacists; 1993.

17. Quality assurance of pharmacy-prepared sterile products. Bethesda, MD: American Society of Hospital Pharmacists; 1994. Videotape and workbook.

18. American Council on Pharmaceutical Education. Home study programs: 1994 continuing pharmaceutical education directory. Chicago, IL: American Council on Pharmaceutical Education; 1994.

19. Letendre DE, Brooks PJ. Draft ASHP pharmacy practice residency model goals and objectives. Bethesda, MD: American Society of Hospital Pharmacists; June 2, 1994. Unpublished memorandum.

20. Letendre DE, Brooks PJ. Draft ASHP home care pharmacy practice residency goals and objectives. Bethesda, MD: American Society of Hospital Pharmacists; Sept 23, 1993. Unpublished memorandum.

21. NABPLEX areas of competency. Chicago, IL: National Association of Boards of Pharmacy; June 22, 1994. General communication.

22. NABP 1993 survey of pharmacy law including all 50 states, D.C. and Puerto Rico. Park Ridge, IL: National Association of Boards of Pharmacy; 1993.

Chapter 3
Sterile Product Formulation and Compounding

E. Clyde Buchanan

The objective of formulating and compounding sterile products is to provide a dosage form of a labeled drug, in the stated potency, that is safe to use if administered properly.[1] This chapter explains the federal regulations and written procedures that should be followed during formulation and compounding. The components, containers, and closures also are described, as well as the physiologic and physical norms of preparing formulations for parenteral and ophthalmic use. However, this chapter does not cover stability and incompatibility of drugs, sterilization methods, labeling, and documentation. These topics are covered in other sections of this book.

FEDERAL REGULATIONS

When formulating and compounding sterile products, pharmacists must follow both state laws and Food and Drug Administration (FDA) regulations. State pharmacy practice acts and board of pharmacy regulations cover these activities. The FDA also regulates formulation and compounding under adulteration, misbranding, and new drug provisions of the Federal Food, Drug and Cosmetic Act (see Appendix 2).[2]

Adulteration and Misbranding

Section 501(a)(2)(B) of the Act states that a drug is adulterated if "the methods used in, or the facilities or controls used for its manufacture, processing, packing, or holding do not conform to current good manufacturing practice"[3] (see Appendix 1).

Pharmacists who prepare sterile pharmaceuticals must meet purported norms (i.e., what is implied on the label is actually true). Purported norms include identity and strength of ingredients, quality, and purity (i.e., absence of pyrogens, particulates, microbes, and other contaminants). Failure to ensure purported norms renders the product adulterated and misbranded.

New Drug Regulations

FDA Guide 7132.06 states that "a physician may prescribe an unusual preparation that requires compounding by a pharmacist from drugs readily available for other uses and which is not generally regarded as safe and effective for the intended use." If the pharmacy merely fills each prescription as received, clearance under the "new drug" provisions is not required.[3]

Preparation of investigational drugs for an investigator's use also does not require new drug registration but falls under current good manufacturing practice. If the preparation has been or will be shipped in interstate commerce for clinical trials, however, the investigator must file a new drug application. Moreover, if a pharmacist compounds finished drugs from bulk active ingredients that are not obtained from an FDA-approved facility or are not compliant with compendial standards, these finished products must be covered by a new drug application.[3]

If a pharmacist changes the strength, dosage form, or components of a commercially available product in a compounded prescription, good compounding procedures should be used.[4]

WRITTEN PROCEDURES

Any facility that formulates and compounds sterile preparations should comply with the following written procedures (see Chapter 19):

- ❒ Pharmacies must have an orderly and sanitary area for sterile compounding equipment and components that is separate from other activities.[4]
- ❒ Personnel (pharmacists and technicians) must ensure product stability by[5]
  - Using the oldest stock first and observing expiration dates.
  - Storing ingredients and finished products according to conditions stated in individual drug monographs and/or package labeling.
  - Observing products for evidence of instability.
  - Properly treating and labeling products that are repackaged, diluted, or mixed with other products.
  - Informing and educating patients about proper storage and use, including disposal of outdated prescriptions.
- ❒ Sterile compounding equipment must be appropriate in design, size, and composition so that surfaces contacting components are not reactive, additive, or absorptive. These surfaces should not alter the required safety, identity, strength, quality, and purity of the components.[4] Moreover, prescription balances and

volume-measurement devices should meet United States Pharmacopeial Convention (USP) specifications.[6]
- ❒ Dispensing pharmacists must inspect and approve or reject all formulas, calculations, substances, containers, closures, and inprocess materials.
- ❒ Pharmacists who prepare batches of parenteral products must follow a master formula sheet to reproduce products that meet all purported norms.

STERILE PRODUCT COMPONENTS

Components are any ingredients used in compounding, whether or not they appear in the final product (i.e., intermediate ingredients). Whenever possible, commercially available sterile components should be used. Commercial substances should be made in an FDA-approved facility and meet official compendial requirements. If these requirements cannot be met, pharmacists must determine if alternative substances should be procured.[4]

Vehicles

Vehicles for most liquid sterile products have no therapeutic activity or toxicity. However, they serve as solvents or mediums for the administration of therapeutically active ingredients. For parenteral products, the most common vehicle is water. Vehicles must meet USP requirements for the pyrogen or bacterial endotoxin test.[7,8] Several vehicles that are official in the compendia are discussed here.[1]

Water for injection

Water for injection (WFI) is purified by distillation or reverse osmosis and is free of pyrogens. Sterile water for injection USP (SWFI) is sterilized and packaged in single-dose containers not exceeding 1000 ml. Bacteriostatic water for injection (BWFI) is sterilized and contains one or more bacteriostatic agents in a container no larger than 30 ml.

Sterile water for inhalation is sterilized and packaged in single-dose containers that are labeled with the full name. As implied, this product cannot be used to prepare parenterals. Sterile water for irrigation is sterilized and packaged in single-dose containers with no added substances. Although this product may be packaged in containers larger than 1000 ml, it is not intended for parenteral use.

Aqueous isotonic vehicles

Aqueous isotonic vehicles are often used in sterile products. A common vehicle is sodium chloride injection, a 0.9% solution that is sterilized and packaged in single-dose containers no larger than 1000 ml. Bacteriostatic sodium chloride injection is sodium chloride injection that contains one or more bacteriostatic agents in a container no larger than 30 ml. Sodium chloride irrigation also is a 0.9% solution. However, it has no preservatives and may be packaged in a container larger than 1000 ml.

Other isotonic vehicles include Ringer's injection, dextrose injection 5%, and lactated Ringer's injection. None of these products is available in containers larger than 1000 ml.

Water-miscible solvents

Several water-miscible solvents are used as a portion of the vehicle in sterile products. These solvents (e.g., ethyl alcohol, liquid polyethylene glycol, and propylene glycol) dissolve drugs with low water solubility. Such preparations usually are administered intramuscularly.[9] Examples of drugs in cosolvent formulations include some barbiturates, antihistamines, and cardiac glycosides. When the solvent has toxic properties or produces toxic decomposition products (e.g., polyethylene glycol 300), the formulation requires extra caution (e.g., limiting cosolvent concentrations).[1]

Nonaqueous vehicles

Nonaqueous vehicles, such as fixed oils, can be used to formulate parenteral products. USP specifies that fixed oils must be vegetable (metabolizable) in origin and odorless (or nearly so) and also have no rancid odor or taste.[10] Examples include soybean, peanut, cottonseed, corn, olive, sesame, and persic oils. Some vitamins and hormones can only be solubilized in these oils. Moreover, oil-based parenterals can only be given intramuscularly. However, two emulsified oils (i.e., soybean and safflower) are marketed for their caloric contribution in IV nutrition support.

Solutes

Solutes—chemicals dissolved in vehicles—should be USP grade or better since their contaminants (especially metals) can

- ❐ Alter solubility and compatibility of other solutes.
- ❐ Cause catalytic chemical reactions.
- ❐ Cause toxicity to patients.

Many chemicals used in sterile product formulations are available in a pharmaceutical grade that meets compendial standards. The safest solutes already exist in a finished pharmaceutical product, free from microbial and pyrogenic contaminants (e.g., commercially available electrolyte additive). Solutes may be active ingredients—drugs that exert a therapeutic effect—or added substances.

Added substances can increase stability or usefulness if they are harmless in their administered amounts and do not interfere with therapeutic efficacy or responses to assays and tests.[10] Examples include antimicrobial preservatives, pH buffers, antioxidants, chelating agents, tonicity agents, and solubilizers. Although added substances may prevent a reaction or result, they can induce others. Therefore, a pharmacist must consider the total formulation of active ingredients and added substances. Moreover, no agent should be added to a sterile product solely to color it.

Antimicrobial preservatives

Antimicrobial preservatives may be added up to a concentration that is considered bacteriostatic or fungistatic. Some preservatives, however, have innate toxicity within these concentrations (e.g., phenylmercuric nitrate 0.01% and benzalkonium chloride 0.01%). Because of their toxicity, these preservatives are used mostly in ophthalmics and seldom in injectables.

Benzyl alcohol (usually 0.9%) and the parabens (methyl 0.18% combined with propyl 0.02%) are commonly used in injectables. In oleaginous products, no antimicrobial is highly effective. However, hexylresorcinol 0.5% and phenylmercuric benzoate 0.1% are reported to be moderately bacteriocidal.[9]

An antimicrobial agent may be effective in one formula of ingredients but not in another. For example, large molecule components such as polysorbate 80, polyvinylpyrrolidone, and polyethylene glycol form complexes that inactivate the parabens.[11] To select a preservative, an appropriate reference[12] should be consulted and its effectiveness should be verified. USP provides a test for the efficacy of antimicrobial preservatives.[13]

pH buffers

Buffering agents stabilize an aqueous solution of a chemical against degradation. Buffer systems are formulated at the lowest concentration needed for stability so that the body's physiologic pH is not disturbed. Acid salts such as citrates, acetates, and phosphates are commonly used as buffers.[9] For an indepth review of parenteral buffering systems, pharmacists should consult Reference 14.

Antioxidants

Antioxidants help to prevent oxidation of the component drug. The most common antioxidants are the sodium and potassium salts of metasulfite and sulfite ions.[15] However, the choice of salt depends on the pH of the system to be stabilized. Metabisulfite is used for low pH values, bisulfite for intermediate pH values, and sulfite for high pH ranges. The administration of large amounts (500 mg/L) of sodium bisulfite in peritoneal dialysis fluids causes toxicity with large volumes (10–40 L/day).[1]

Other antioxidants include acetone metabisulfite, ascorbic acid, thioglycerol, and cysteine hydrochloride.

Chelating agents

Chelating agents enhance the effectiveness of antioxidants. They form complexes with trace amounts of heavy metals, thereby eliminating the catalytic activity of metals during oxidation. The most commonly used chelating agent is edetate disodium.

Tonicity agents

Some injectable product monographs require that the osmolar concentration appear on the product's label.[16] Ideally, parenteral products are formulated to be isotonic by use of an isotonic vehicle (e.g., normal saline). When the desired concentration of the active ingredient is hypertonic, the drug must be administered by slowing the rate of injection or by infusion into a large vein (e.g., administration of TPN into subclavian vein).[1]

Solubilizers

Pharmacists must know the solubility characteristics of new drug substances (especially in aqueous systems), since they must possess some aqueous solubility to elicit a therapeutic response. To maintain some drugs in solution, pharmacists may have to include either a miscible cosolvent or a chemical solubilizer. Polyethylene glycols 300 and 400, propylene glycol, glycerin, and ethyl alcohol frequently are used. However, toxic levels of these solvents must be avoided as well as amounts that make the product too viscous for parenteral use.[1]

CONTAINERS

Containers are defined as "that which holds the article and is or may be in direct contact with the article. The closure is part of the container."[17] All containers for sterile products must be sterile, free of both particulate matter and pyrogens. These containers should not interact physically or chemically with formulations to alter their required strength, quality, or purity. Containers also must permit inspection of their contents.[10]

Container volumes are set by USP. Each container of an injection is filled with liquid, slightly in excess of the labeled size or volume that is to be withdrawn. USP provides a table showing recommended excess volumes for both mobile and viscous liquids.[10]

Single or Multiple Dose

Sterile, single-dose containers are intended for parenteral, inhalation, irrigation, otic, and ophthalmic administration. Examples are prefilled syringes, cartridges, ampuls, and vials (when labeled).

Multiple-dose containers permit withdrawal of successive portions of their contents without changing the strength, quality, or purity of the remaining portion. Sterile, multiple-dose containers may be used for preserved parenterals, ophthalmics, and otics.[18]

Glass

Glass is the most popular material for sterile product containers. USP classifies glass as[19]

- ☐ Type I (borosilicate glass).
- ☐ Type II (soda-lime-treated glass).
- ☐ Type III (soda-lime glass).
- ☐ NP (soda-lime glass unsuitable for parenteral containers).

Different glass types vary in their resistance to attack by water and chemicals. For pharmaceutical containers, glass must meet the USP test for chemical resistance.[17] Because most pharmacists do not have the time or facilities to perform glass–chemical interaction studies, they should use only Type I glass to minimize sterile product incompatibilities.[20]

Plastic

Plastic polymers can be used as sterile product containers but present three problems:

1. Permeation of vapors and other molecules in either direction through the container.
2. Leaching of constituents from the plastic into the product.
3. Sorption of drug molecules onto the plastic.

Plastics must meet USP specifications for biological reactivity and physicochemicals.[17, 21] Most plastic containers do not permit ready inspection of their contents because they are unclear. Most plastics also melt under heat sterilization.[9]

CLOSURES

Rubber closures must be rendered sterile, free from pyrogens and surface particles. To meet these specifications, multiple washings and autoclavings are required.

Closures are made of natural, neoprene, or butyl rubber. In addition, rubber contains[22]

- ☐ Sulfur as a vulcanizing agent.
- ☐ Guanidines or sulfide compounds as accelerators.
- ☐ Zinc oxide or stearic acid as an activator.
- ☐ Carbon, kaolin, or barium sulfate as a filter.

❏ Dibutyl phthalate or stearic acid as a plasticizer.
❏ Aromatic amines as antioxidants.

Thus, the rubber sealing of a vial or the plug in a syringe is a complex material that can interact with the ingredients of a formula. Rubber closures also are subject to coring. Therefore, pharmacists should consult compendial or literature standards when selecting a rubber closure for sterile product preparation.

PARENTERAL FORMULATIONS

Parenteral products are classified into five categories:[9]

1. Solutions ready for injection.
2. Dry, soluble products ready to be combined with a solvent before use.
3. Suspensions ready for injection.
4. Dry, insoluble products ready to be combined with a vehicle before use.
5. Emulsions.

Most compounded sterile parenteral products are aqueous solutions (first category). Other categories usually require the equipment and expertise of a licensed pharmaceutical manufacturer. In addition to using the appropriate vehicle, solvent, and container, the pharmacist must ensure that the final aqueous solution maintains the appropriate physiologic and physical norms.

Physiologic Norms

When injectable solutions are formulated, every effort should be made to mimic the body's normal serum values for pH and tonicity and to create a pyrogen-free product.

pH

Normal human serum pH, a measure of the hydronian ion concentration in solution, is 7.4. Drugs that are acids or bases or their salts sometimes must be buffered to a pH near normal (e.g., 3–8) to prevent pain or tissue damage. As mentioned previously, acid salts are commonly used as buffers.

Tonicity

Any chemical dissolved in water exerts a certain osmotic pressure (i.e., a solute concentration related to the number of dissolved particles—un-ionized molecules, ions, macromolecules, and aggregates—per unit volume).[23] Blood has an osmotic pressure corresponding to sodium chloride 0.9%; therefore, its common name is normal saline. Normal saline is said to be "isosmotic" with blood and other physiologic fluids.

In the medical setting, the term "isotonic" is used synonymously with isosmotic. A solution is isotonic with

a living cell if no net gain or loss of water is experienced by the cell and no other change is present when the cell contacts that solution. Very hypotonic IV products can cause hemolysis of red blood cells. Very hypertonic injections can damage tissue and cause pain on injection or crenation of red blood cells. Parenteral solutions usually exert an osmotic pressure of 150–900 mOsm/kg compared to a physiologic norm of 282–288 mOsm/kg for blood. The greater the volume of solution to be injected, the closer the parenteral product should be to isotonicity.

Pyrogenicity

Pyrogens are contaminants that are unacceptable in final compounded sterile products. Pyrogens are fever-producing endotoxins from bacterial metabolism. As large proteins, pyrogens are not removed by normal sterilization procedures and can exist for years in aqueous solution or dried form.

The sources of pyrogens in sterile products are

❏ Aqueous vehicles.
❏ Equipment.
❏ Containers and closures.
❏ Chemicals used as solutes.
❏ Touch.

If sterile water for injection is the vehicle, the risk of pyrogens in water is eliminated. Equipment, containers, and closures can be decontaminated by dry heat or by washing or soaking with acids or bases. Bulk supplies of chemicals may be specified as pyrogen free, although they usually are not. Therefore, sterile products made from bulk chemicals must undergo a USP test.[7] Touch contamination is most easily prevented with proper aseptic technique.

Physical Norms

Particulates

Parenteral solutions must be free of particulate matter—mobile, undissolved solids not intended for sterile products. Examples include lint, cellulose and cotton fibers, glass, rubber, metals, plastics, undissolved chemicals, rust, diatoms, and dandruff.[10] To determine levels of particulates, USP sets limits and provides tests.[24]

Sources of particulate matter are

❏ Vehicles and solutes.
❏ Environment.
❏ Equipment.
❏ Containers and closures.
❏ Personnel.

However, a careful choice of components, containers, and closures can minimize particulate contamination. Moreover, filtration can remove particles and bacteria from sterile products.[25] Lipid emulsions and irrigating solutions are exempt from USP's particulate matter limits.

Stability

Stability of parenteral products must be assured so that patients receive the intended dose. Hydrolytic and oxidative drug degradation are the most common forms of instability but rarely show as cloudiness, precipitates, or color changes. The rate of hydrolysis may be affected by storage temperature or pH of the solution. Oxidation is affected by temperature, pH, exposure to light, oxygen concentration of the solution, impurities (e.g., heavy metals), and concentration of the oxidizable drug.[11] Other types of degradation (e.g., racemization, polymerization, isomerization, and deamination) also can occur in solution.

Because numerous factors affect the stability of drug molecules, pharmacists who compound parenterals from bulk chemicals should use a short expiration date or know from the literature that longer stability exists. Antioxidant and/or chelation additive systems should be reserved for formulas that are verified in the literature as stable for a given period. The choice of packaging also is important for parenteral drug stability.

OPHTHALMIC FORMULATIONS

Ophthalmic products share many of the same properties as parenteral products but present additional concerns. For example, ophthalmic formulations may use different added substances (e.g., buffers, antimicrobial preservatives, tonicity-adjusting chemicals, and thickening agents). Furthermore, ophthalmic preparations include solutions (eye drops or washes), suspensions, and ointments. Since pharmacists rarely compound sterile suspensions or ointments, this discussion is limited to solutions.

Physiologic Norms

Buffers and pH

Lacrimal fluid has a pH of approximately 7.4 and limited buffering capacity. Ophthalmic solutions of weak bases (e.g., alkaloids), for which therapeutic efficacy depends on the bioavailability of the alkaloidal base, are buffered to acidity but as near pH 7.4 as possible while keeping the alkaloid in solution after instillation.[26] The buffer system (e.g., phosphate or acetate) should maintain pH within the drug's stability range for the duration of expiration dating. A moderately acidic solution does not cause discomfort on instillation unless the buffer system overcomes the buffer capacity of lacrimal fluid.

Tonicity

Lacrimal fluid has an osmotic pressure or tonicity similar to aqueous sodium chloride 0.9% solution. Eye tissue can tolerate tonicities of 0.5–1.8% without much discomfort.[26] However, the tonicity of eyewashes is more important than drops because a larger volume of solution contacts the eye. The tonicity of intraocular solutions also should be as close as possible to physiologic.

When formulating ophthalmic solutions, pharmacists should adjust the tonicity to approximate lacrimal fluid by adding a substance such as sodium chloride. Several methods can be used to calculate the amount of sodium chloride needed. The following example uses the colligative property, freezing-point depression. Lacrimal fluid lowers the freezing point of water by 0.52° C. To make a boric acid 1% solution isotonic, sodium chloride crystals are added. This acid lowers the freezing point by 0.29° C; therefore, sodium chloride must be added to lower the freezing point further by 0.23° C. To use a proportion:

$$\frac{0.52° \text{ C}}{0.9\%} = \frac{0.23° \text{ C}}{X}$$

Therefore, $X = 0.4\%$. Thus, sodium chloride crystals are added to a boric acid 1% solution to make it a sodium chloride 0.4% solution.[27]

Another easy method of calculation is to add the sodium chloride equivalent. Appendix A of Remington's Chapter 79 gives the sodium chloride equivalents, freezing-point depressions, and hemolytic effects of 274 medicinal chemicals.[23] Appendix B lists volumes of water to add to 0.3 g of 77 drugs to make an isotonic solution.

Viscosity

Viscosity is important in ophthalmic preparations. The viscosity sometimes is increased to extend contact between the solution and eye. Moreover, water-dispersible polymers (e.g., methylcellulose, hydroxyethylcellulose, hydroxypropylcellulose, and polyvinyl alcohol) are used as thickening agents. Although USP discusses use of cellulose derivatives, precautions are necessary.[28] Cellulose derivative solutions cannot be filtered. When autoclaved, the derivative precipitates from solution because of decreased water solubility at high temperatures but redissolves at room temperature.[27]

When a heat-labile drug is formulated with a cellulose derivative, all components must be sterilized separately and then recombined aseptically. The drug in solution is sterilized by filtration, and the cellulose derivative is sterilized by autoclaving.[27] Viscosity of 25–50 centipoises improves contact time with the eye, whereas higher viscosity offers no contact advantage but usually leaves a residue on eyelid margins.[26]

Sterility

To ensure sterility of ophthalmic solutions, pharmacists must prepare them in single-dose containers or use antimicrobial preservatives in multiple-dose containers. The microbe that causes great concern is *Pseudomonas aeruginosa*; however, no preservative is 100% effective against all strains of it.

The most common preservative is benzalkonium chloride (0.004–0.02%), but high concentrations of it irritate the eye. This preservative is incompatible with large anions (e.g., soaps) as well as with nitrates and salicylates. Other preservatives include phenylmercuric acetate and nitrate (0.001–0.01%), phenylethanol (0.5%), parabens (0.1%), and chlorobutanol (0.5%). Since chlorobutanol is stable only near pH 5–6, it is used only with solutions in this range.

Remington's Chapter 86 discusses different ophthalmic preservatives.[26] Some ophthalmologists prefer nonpreserved solutions because of allergic reactions to common preservatives.

Physical Norms

Required physical characteristics of ophthalmics include clarity, stability, and compatibility. Ophthalmics are made clear or particle free by filtration; nonshedding filters, containers, and closures must be used.

Stability depends on the chemical nature of the drug, product pH, preparation method (especially temperature), solution additives, and packaging. If oxidation is a problem, sodium bisulfite (up to 0.3%), ascorbic acid, or acetylcysteine can be added. Surfactants are used in low concentrations to achieve solution or suspension of active ingredients.

SUMMARY

In many cases, no commercial product is available for a final sterile preparation. Legally, pharmacists may compound these products under the regulations of the Food, Drug and Cosmetic Act. However, various sterile components (e.g., vehicles, buffers, and solubilizers) are required. It is the pharmacist's responsibility to ensure that they meet the appropriate compendial requirements.

When formulating either parenteral or ophthalmic preparations, a pharmacist should use additive components so that the final sterile product achieves both physiologic and physical norms.

❧

REFERENCES

1. Turco SJ. Composition. In: Turco SJ, ed. Sterile dosage forms, their preparation and clinical application, 4th ed. Philadelphia, PA: Lea & Febiger; 1994:11–27.

2. Office of Enforcement, Division of Compliance Policy. Manufacture, distribution, and promotion of adulterated, misbranded, or unapproved new drugs for human use by state-licensed pharmacies. FDA Guide 7132.16. Washington, DC: Food and Drug Administration; Mar 16, 1992:Chap 32.

3. Division of Field Regulatory Guidance. Hospital pharmacies—status as drug manufacturer. FDA Guide 7132.06. Washington, DC: Food and Drug Administration; Oct 1, 1980:Chap 32.

4. Good compounding practices applicable to state licensed pharmacies. Parts I and II. *Natl Pharm. Compliance News.* 1993; May:2–3 and Oct:2–3.

5. Stability considerations in dispensing practice. In: United States pharmacopeia, 23rd rev./national formulary, 18th ed. Rockville, MD: United States Pharmacopeial Convention; 1994:1957–9.

6. Prescription balances and volumetric apparatus. In: United States pharmacopeia, 23rd rev./national formulary, 18th ed. Rockville, MD: United States Pharmacopeial Convention; 1994:1952–4.

7. Pyrogen test. In: United States pharmacopeia, 23rd rev./national formulary, 18th ed. Rockville, MD: United States Pharmacopeial Convention; 1994:1718–9.

8. Bacterial endotoxins test. In: United States pharmacopeia, 23rd rev./national formulary, 18th ed. Rockville, MD: United States Pharmacopeial Convention; 1994:1696–7.

9. Avis KE. Parenteral preparations. In: Gennaro AR, ed. Remington's pharmaceutical sciences, 18th ed. Easton, PA: Mack Publishing Co.; 1990:1545–69.

10. Injections. In: United States pharmacopeia, 23rd rev./national formulary, 18th ed. Rockville, MD: United States Pharmacopeial Convention; 1994:1650–2.

11. Ravin LJ, Radebaugh GW. Preformulation. In: Gennaro AR, ed. Remington's pharmaceutical sciences, 18th ed. Easton, PA: Mack Publishing Co.; 1990:1435–50.

12. Akers MJ. Considerations in selecting antimicrobial preservative agents for parenteral product development. *Pharm Technol.* 1984; 8:36.

13. Antimicrobial preservatives—effectiveness. In: United States pharmacopeia, 23rd rev./national formulary, 18th ed. Rockville, MD: United States Pharmacopeial Convention; 1994:1681.

14. Wang YJ, Kowal RR. Review of excipients and pHs for parenteral products used in the United States. *J Parenter Drug Assoc.* 1980; 34:452–62.

15. Akers MJ. Preformulation screening of antioxidant efficacy in parenteral products. *J Parenter Drug Assoc.* 1979; 33:346–56.

16. Osmolarity. In: United States pharmacopeia, 23rd rev./national formulary, 18th ed. Rockville, MD: United States Pharmacopeial Convention; 1994:1813.

17. General notices and requirements. In: United States pharmacopeia, 23rd rev./national formulary, 18th ed. Rockville, MD: United States Pharmacopeial Convention; 1994:1–14.

18. Turco SJ. Characteristics. In: Turco SJ, ed. Sterile dosage forms, their preparation and clinical application, 4th ed. Philadelphia, PA: Lea & Febiger; 1994:28–38.

19. Containers. In: United States pharmacopeia, 23rd rev./national formulary, 18th ed. Rockville, MD: United States Pharmacopeial Convention; 1994:1781–7.

20. Turco SJ. Extemporaneous preparation. In: Turco SJ, ed. Sterile dosage forms, their preparation and clinical application, 4th ed. Philadelphia, PA: Lea & Febiger; 1994:57–78.

21. Biological reactivity tests, in-vitro. In: United States pharmacopeia, 23rd rev./national formulary, 18th ed. Rockville, MD: United States Pharmacopeial Convention; 1994:1697–9.

22. Turco SJ. Large-scale preparation. In: Turco SJ, ed. Sterile dosage forms, their preparation and clinical application, 4th ed. Philadelphia, PA: Lea & Febiger; 1994:39–56.

23. Siegel FP. Tonicity, osmoticity, osmolality and osmolarity. In: Genarro AR, ed. Remington's pharmaceutical sciences, 18th ed. Easton, PA: Mack Publishing Co.; 1990:1481–98.

24. Particulate matter in injections. In: United States pharmacopeia, 23rd rev./national formulary, 18th ed. Rockville, MD: United States Pharmacopeial Convention: 1994:1813–20.

25. McKinnon BT, Avis KE. Membrane filtration of pharmaceutical solutions. *Am J Hosp Pharm.* 1993; 50:1921–36.

26. Mullins JD, Hecht G. Ophthalmic preparations. In: Gennaro AR, ed. Remington's pharmaceutical sciences, 18th ed. Easton, PA: Mack Publishing Co.; 1990:1581–95.

27. Turco SJ. Ophthalmic preparations. In: Turco SJ, ed. Sterile dosage forms, their preparation and clinical application, 4th ed. Philadelphia, PA: Lea & Febiger; 1994:344–54.

28. Pharmaceutical dosage forms. In: United States pharmacopeia, 23rd rev./national formulary, 18th ed. Rockville, MD: United States Pharmacopeial Convention; 1994:1946.

Chapter 4
Sterile Compounding Facilities

E. Clyde Buchanan

Recently published professional guidelines (see Chapter 1 and Appendices 4–7) should persuade pharmacists to evaluate their existing sterile compounding facilities.[1-4] These guidelines specify that sterile products be compounded in an area separate from other pharmacy activities. The American Society of Health-System Pharmacists [formerly the American Society of Hospital Pharmacists (ASHP)] calls this space the "controlled area," the United States Pharmacopeial Convention (USP) calls it the "buffer room," and the National Association of Boards of Pharmacy (NABP) calls it the "designated area."

While NABP does not discuss an anteroom or cleanroom environment, both ASHP and USP do. ASHP does not mention an anteroom until Risk Level 2, but USP requires it for all three risk levels. Although ASHP does not require a cleanroom for Risk Level 1, it specifies a Class 100,000 environment for Risk Level 2 and a Class 10,000 for Risk Level 3. USP requires a Class 100,000 for its low-risk level and a Class 10,000 for both high-risk levels.

CLEANROOM SPECIFICATIONS

Air Cleanliness

To interpret the ASHP and USP guidelines, pharmacists must understand cleanroom classifications. For 30 years, Federal Standard 209 (FS 209) has defined air cleanliness in contamination control,[5] but it was not applied to pharmacy facilities (except for laminar-airflow hoods) until the ASHP and USP guidelines were published. The latest version, FS 209E, includes specifications for particulate matter for cleanrooms or clean zones (see Table 4-1).[6]

Microbial Contamination

Although FS 209E does not specify microbial limits, USP proposed a microbial classification system for cleanrooms.[7] For USP, a cleanroom is a defined space where the concentrations of (1) airborne microorganisms, (2) surface microorganisms (on equipment, walls, floors, etc.), and (3) microorganisms on personal gear (mask, gown, boots, gloves, etc.) are within specific levels for a designated class.[7]

USP classifies cleanrooms as MCB-1, MCB-2, and MCB-3; Table 4-2 summarizes these three classes as to air and surface cleanliness.

Table 4-1. Class Limits*ᵃ* in Particles per Cubic Foot (Size Equal to or Greater than Particle Sizes Shown)*ᵇ*

Class	Measured Particle Size, μm				
	0.1	0.2	0.3	0.5	5
1	35	7.5	3	1	NAᶜ
10	350	75	30	10	NA
100	NA	750	300	100	NA
1,000	NA	NA	NA	1,000	7
10,000	NA	NA	NA	10,000	70
100,000	NA	NA	NA	100,000	700

ᵃThese class limit particle concentrations are for definition only and do not necessarily represent the size distribution found in any particular situation.
ᵇReproduced, with permission, from Federal Standard 209E. Washington, DC: U.S. General Services Administration; Sept 11, 1992.
ᶜNA = not applicable.

Class MCB-1

Class MCB-1 is the critical processing area for aseptic compounding without terminal sterilization. This class includes all locations where products or containers are exposed to potential microbial contamination (e.g., transfer areas where partially stoppered or open, empty, or filled containers are exposed to the environment).

Class MCB-2

Class MCB-2 can include

- ☐ Staging area for components, containers, and bulk products, all in protected containers, used in aseptic processing.
- ☐ Room containing the critical processing area.
- ☐ Staging area for transfer of components into newer isolation-barrier systems.
- ☐ Halls and anterooms around an MCB-1 cleanroom.
- ☐ Gowning area where garments are stored and put on by operators.

Class MCB-3

Class MCB-3 includes the areas where

- ☐ Hands are washed before gowns are donned.

- ☐ Bulk solutions are prepared prior to final filtration.
- ☐ Components are assembled before steam sterilization or depyrogenation.

Regulatory Requirements

In addition to the ASHP and USP recommendations for air cleanliness and microbial contamination, two regulatory organizations have requirements for sterile product facilities. The Food and Drug Administration (FDA) requires pharmacists to use good manufacturing practices,[8] including a facility of suitable size, construction, and location to facilitate cleaning, maintenance, and proper operations. Furthermore, the Joint Commission on Accreditation of Healthcare Organizations (JCAHO) standards for hospitals state that "the preparation and dispensing of medications is in adherence to applicable law, regulation, licensure, and professional standards of practice."[9]

Although JCAHO has not adopted any professional sterile compounding standards, it expects health care organizations to identify their own and to abide by them.[10] JCAHO standards for home care state[11]

"Areas for the preparation of sterile products are functionally separate from areas for the preparation of nonsterile products and are constructed to minimize

Table 4-2. Microbial Levels for USP Cleanroom Classifications[7]

Class	Description	Airborne Microorganisms, cfu/cu ft (cfu/cu m)ᵃ	Surface Microorganisms, cfu/2 sq in (12.9 sq cm)
MCB-1	Critical processing area	0.03 (1)	3
MCB-2	Area surrounding cleanroom and anteroom	0.15 (5)	5 10 (floor)
MCB-3	Area leading to anteroom	2.5 (87)	20 30 (floor)

ᵃColony-forming units (cfu) were determined with slit-to-agar sampler. When other samplers are used, an appropriate correlation factor may be required.

opportunities for particulate and microbial contamination. A Class 100 environment is used in the preparation of sterile drugs."

The usual interpretation is that a certified laminar-airflow hood satisfies the requirement for a Class 100 environment.

MEETING CURRENT FACILITY STANDARDS

A 1991 ASHP survey indicated how hospital pharmacy departments conformed to current facility guidelines from ASHP, USP, NABP, FDA, and JCAHO (see Chapter 1).[12] Of 327 respondents, 4.9% prepared sterile products on a clean surface with no laminar-airflow hood; 28.7% used a hood in a general dispensing area; 78.6% used a hood in a limited-access room dedicated to sterile drug preparation; and 2.8% had a specifically constructed cleanroom where access, temperature, humidity, and airborne particulate contamination were strictly controlled. (The total percentages exceed 100% because some respondents prepared sterile products in more than one location.)

In short, a third (4.9% plus 28.7%) of these hospital pharmacies prepared some sterile products in facilities that did not conform with any current standard. Worse yet, a 1992 ASHP survey showed that only 67% of hospitals had a complete, comprehensive, IV admixture program.[13] As these percentages illustrate, pharmacy departments need to update their current sterile product preparation facilities.

One logical facilities planning process includes seven main steps:[14]

1. Developing a master facilities plan for the pharmacy.
2. Analyzing existing facilities.
3. Identifying functional needs.
4. Preparing architectural plans.
5. Bidding construction.
6. Building the installation.
7. Evaluating the installation.

Developing a Master Facilities Plan

The first step, development of a master facilities plan, essentially involves identifying and justifying the need for a new cleanroom.

Identifying need

Before updated facilities can be justified, the pharmacy department must determine its specific need based on patient population. Essentially, three questions can be asked to determine this need.

Table 4-3. *Common Nonsterile Ingredients Prepared as Sterile Products*[12]

Albumin alum irrigation	Glutamine injection
Apomorphine injection	Histidine injection
Brilliant green injection	Methylcellulose ophthalmic
Caffeine citrate injection	Phenol injection
Citric acid irrigation	Phosphate buffer
Cocaine ophthalmic	Renacidin irrigation
Cromolyn sodium ophthalmic	Rose bengal solution
EDTA irrigation	Talc powder suspension
Formaldehyde irrigation	Tetracaine–Adrenalin–cocaine (TAC) solution
Galactose injection	

What guidelines apply to the patient population? For hospital inpatients, ASHP guidelines should be followed. For retail pharmacy patients (where products contain suitable preservatives), NABP guidelines are appropriate. For home health care patients, USP guidelines require cleanrooms at all levels.

Will sterile products be used at room temperature or body temperature longer than 28 hr after compounding? If yes, the hospital inpatient compounding facility should be a Class 100,000 cleanroom with an anteroom and the home care compounding facility should be a Class 10,000 cleanroom with an anteroom.

Are sterile products routinely made from nonsterile ingredients, containers, or closures? If yes, the hospital inpatient or home care compounding facility should be a Class 10,000 cleanroom with an anteroom. Most pharmacies prepare some sterile products from nonsterile ingredients (see Table 4-3).[12]

Justifying need

Pharmacy directors frequently confront resistance when justifying the need to improve their facilities. Some commonly asked questions—and their corresponding answers—follow.

If admixtures are made within a laminar-airflow hood, why does its location matter? Laminar-airflow hoods do not eliminate 100% of airborne particles. These hoods remove only 99.97% of particles over 0.3 μm when operating properly.[15] Furthermore, a significant increase in airborne contamination outside the hood significantly increases contamination under the hood. Hoods also cannot prevent microbial contamination introduced by poor aseptic technique downstream from the high-efficiency particulate air (HEPA) filter (e.g., from air currents pushing room air

Table 4-4. *Effect of Airborne Microorganisms on Vial Contamination*[a]

Bacteria per Cubic Foot of Air	Number of Vials Contaminated[b]
0.01	4
2.43	22
5.31	99

[a]Adapted, with permission, from Wythe W, Bailey PV, Tinkler J. An evaluation of the routes of bacterial contamination occurring during aseptic pharmaceutical manufacturing. J Parenter Sci Technol. 1982; 36:102–7.
[b]Approximately 9000 vials filled per condition.

into the hood). Table 4-4 shows the effect of increased airborne bacteria on aseptic processing contamination.

If the hood is already in a separate room, do you really need a cleanroom? A separate room minimizes unnecessary traffic near the hood but not the contamination already in a room. For example:[15]

❏ A person sitting motionless generates about 100,000 particles/cu ft/min.
❏ A person sitting down or standing up generates about 2,500,000 particles/cu ft/min.
❏ A person walking generates about 10,000,000 particles/cu ft/min.
❏ An open, nonairlocked door can add billions of particles per cubic foot per minute.

The primary functions of a well-designed cleanroom are to remove internally generated contamination and to prevent it from adversely affecting a critical area (i.e., inside hood environment).[15] Therefore, cleanrooms are recommended when product sterility is especially critical (e.g., home infusion compounding).

If pharmacy-prepared admixtures have never been implicated in nosocomial infections, why should facilities be upgraded? Pharmacy-prepared sterile products are not commonly implicated because few institutions thoroughly investigate the causes of nosocomial infections. In fact, admixtures in plastic bags prepared under pharmacy laminar-airflow hoods have shown contamination rates of 0.7–17.7%.[16–18] Even though 32.8% of hospital pharmacists perform microbial testing on samples of final products,[12] such testing cannot assure sterility of aseptically filled products.[19] In other words, pharmacists currently have no way of knowing whether their products are sterile or whether they are causing infections.

Isn't good aseptic technique more important than a cleanroom in preventing microbial contamination? In situations where sterile products are contaminated, touch contamination (as evidenced by skin bacteria) is frequently encountered.[20] However, airborne fungi and gram-negative bacteria tend

to survive and grow in IV solutions[21] and to be more pathological and difficult to cure. Cleanrooms provide an optimal environment for laminar-airflow hoods and encourage the practice of aseptic technique.

Since building a cleanroom will be so expensive, why not return the responsibility for admixture preparation to nurses? True, in admixtures prepared just prior to administration, accidentally introduced microbes have less time to grow. But one study showed that 21% of the admixtures were made incorrectly (as to ingredients, dosage, unordered admixture, or incompatibility) on nursing units.[22] Another study showed that 10.9% of the nurse-prepared admixtures in plastic bags were contaminated versus 5.6% for pharmacy-prepared admixtures in plastic bags.[17] Moreover, nurses are less well trained to make admixtures today than when these studies were published. Furthermore, since many sterile products are used for 24 hr or more (e.g., TPNs and patient-controlled analgesia syringes), microbes can easily grow to pathological levels at room or body temperature.[21] There are too many complicated sterile products as well as situations where nurses are not involved (ambulatory settings) to remove this activity from the pharmacy.

Finally, is there scientific proof that cleanrooms prevent infections? While definitive studies have not been done, the indirect evidence is so strong as to be sufficient warning to the wise. Creating a cleanroom environment need not be expensive, leaving no excuse for pharmacists not to upgrade their sterile compounding facilities. Physicians, especially surgeons, expect sterile products to be compounded in areas at least as clean as operating rooms.

Analyzing Existing Facilities

Once the need has been justified, the next important step is to determine whether a current cleanroom can be updated, a new room is needed, or a new type of facility (e.g., isolator) should be employed. Room size and environment (e.g., temperature and lighting) as well as cleanliness are important considerations.

Size and environment

Table 4-5 can be used to estimate facility size requirements.[23]

For hand washing, a sink with hot and cold running water should be in close proximity. Ventilation and room temperature control capabilities should be in accordance with manufacturer and USP product labeling requirements. In any enclosed space with heat-producing equipment, the air conditioning must keep personnel comfortable while in clean garb. Floors and active work sur-

Table 4-5. *Estimated Size Requirements for IV Admixture Center*[23]

Workload, orders/day	Floorspace, sq ft[a]
100	540
200	637
300	723
400	959
500	1118

[a] *Floorspace covers equipment, inventory, fixtures, and circulation space.*

faces (i.e., counters and shelves) should be nonporous and washable to enable regular disinfection.[1] Lighting should ensure that personnel can read packages easily (e.g., syringe gauges and drug labels) and visualize contaminants (e.g., glass fragments in ampuls and rubber cores in vials).[24]

Room cleanliness

Most hospital pharmacies compound ASHP Risk Level 2 and 3 products: long expiration-dated products, batch-prefilled syringes without preservatives, batch-reconstituted antibiotics, and a few products from nonsterile components.[12] Therefore, they need a cleanroom with an anteroom.

To handle all eventualities, a Class 10,000 environment is recommended. This environment requires a positive-pressure differential, relative to adjacent less clean areas, of at least 0.05 in of water. The anteroom to a Class 10,000 environment should meet Class 100,000 specifications. Class 10,000 or 100,000 conditions simply mean that the areas are routinely monitored to ascertain that there are no more than 10,000 or 100,000 airborne particles greater than 0.5 μm/cu ft of air, respectively.[6]

Identifying Functional Needs

The key point in functional programming is to identify every specific function—along with the required methods and systems—to be performed in the facility. After existing facilities have been analyzed, one primary decision—more than any other—has to be made. Should a custom-built cleanroom be planned or should a modular hard- or soft-wall cleanroom be purchased? Or can an existing room be remodeled or procedures be implemented to create a facility that meets cleanroom air quality standards?

Cleanrooms and anterooms

The cleanliness of surrounding air, in conjunction with an operator's aseptic expertise, is critical to maintaining Class 100 conditions in a laminar-airflow hood.[2] A high-cleanliness anteroom reduces the number of particles in the cleanroom. Appropriate activities for the anteroom include—but are not limited to—hand washing, gowning and gloving, removal of packaging, and sanitizing of hard-surface containers and supplies before they are placed in the cleanroom.[1]

USP provides further guidance for cleanroom planning.[2] Figure 4-1, modified from a USP plan, shows the important parts and spacial relationship of a cleanroom (buffer room) and anteroom (with demarcation line). Cleanroom ceilings, walls, floors, fixtures, shelves, counters, and cabinets should be resistant to sanitizing agents. Furthermore, junctures of ceilings to walls should be covered or caulked to avoid cracks and crevices where dirt can accumulate. If ceilings consist of inlaid panels, they should be impregnated with a polymer to render them impervious and hydrophobic; they also should be caulked with an elastic sealant around the perimeter and clamped to the support frame.[25]

The HEPA filter in the ceiling air supply should be placed to avoid creating air currents inside the laminar-airflow hood. Prefilters on the heating, ventilation, and air conditioning (HVAC) air blower should be changeable from outside the cleanroom.[25]

Walls may be of hard panels locked together and sealed or of epoxy-coated gypsum board or soft-wall plastic. Flooring should be a continuous, noncracking material that is mechanically and chemically robust.[26] Preferably, floors should be overlaid with wide sheet vinyl flooring with heat-welded seams and coving to the sidewall. Dust-collecting overhangs (e.g., ceiling pipes) and ledges

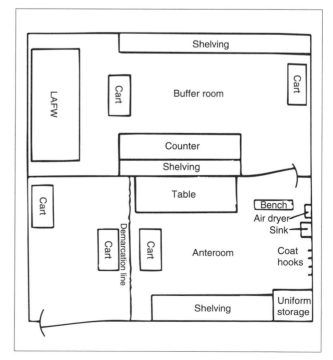

figure 4-1. *A simplified cleanroom and anteroom floorplan. (Adapted, with permission, from Reference 2.)*

(e.g., windowsills) should be avoided. The exterior lens surface of ceiling lighting should be smooth, mounted flush, and sealed. Any other penetrations through the ceiling or walls also should be sealed. The cleanroom should contain no sinks or floor drains.[2]

Access to the cleanroom should be via the anteroom door for personnel and an airlock pass through for most supplies. As supplies are moved from the anteroom into the cleanroom and then into the laminar-airflow hood, a series of cleaning steps should be followed.

1. Supply items are removed from shipping cartons prior to the demarcation line in the anteroom. Floor demarcation identifies the maximum distance into the anteroom that storeroom carts should penetrate.
2. Bottles, packages, etc., are wiped with sanitizing agent to clean the outside prior to placement in the cleanroom.
3. All items are sanitized on the outside or their wrappings (e.g., sterile syringe wrap) are removed as they are placed in the laminar-airflow hood.

A sink with air hand dryer or disposable nonshedding towels should be near the cleanroom entrance. Faucet handles should be designed so that they can be shut off with the elbows or feet. Near the cleanroom doorway, a movable bench can provide a barrier and place for personnel to don shoe covers just before entering. In the

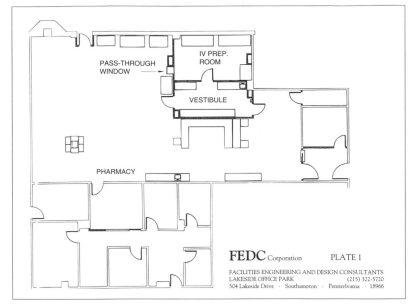

Figure 4-3. **Plans for renovated pharmacy, with cleanroom and anteroom, at Lehigh Valley Hospital, an 800-bed nonprofit community teaching hospital in Allentown, PA. (Reproduced, with permission, from Reference 28.)**

anteroom, a storage area for clean gowning supplies should be conveniently located. The cleanroom door should remain automatically, positively closed; personnel should be able to open it with elbow hooks or other means without using their clean hands.[2]

Modular cleanrooms

Many cleanroom companies install modular hard-wall cleanrooms, but costs run as high as $300/sq ft. For low-volume operations, soft-wall cleanrooms are available at a much lower cost. The pharmacy at Memorial Hospital in Carthage, IL, had a soft-wall cleanroom (see Figure 4-2) installed for under $20,000 that satisfied a JCAHO home care survey. Some facts about this cleanroom include[27]

❑ Setup of tubular frame and vinyl plastic panels took 10–12 hr for two company personnel.
❑ Dimensions are 8 ft by 16 ft, with an 8-ft ceiling height.
❑ Three "movable" walls are connected to one rigid wall. The rigid wall contains electrical and plumbing fixtures. It is made of aluminum stud supporting fire-rated dry wall and is painted with epoxy paint to provide durability and prevent particle shedding.
❑ Soft walls are made of 16-mil, replaceable, clear vinyl panels attached to a strong tubular frame.
❑ The cleanroom door is the same vinyl-on-tubular frame construction.
❑ The pass-through chamber is 16 in by 16 in.
❑ Two 2-ft by 4-ft HEPA filters are suspended in

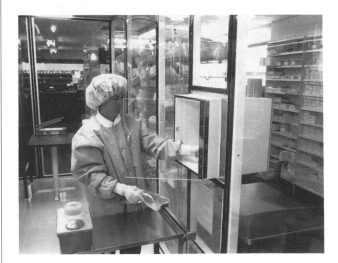

Figure 4-2. **Pharmacist in a soft-wall cleanroom at Memorial Hospital, a 67-bed hospital in Carthage, IL.**

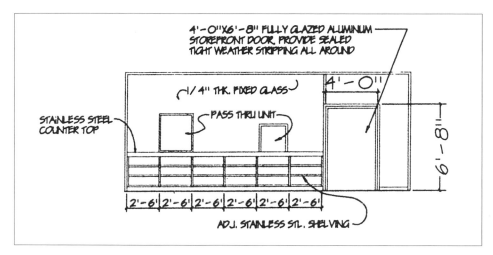

4'-0"X6'-8" FULLY GLAZED ALUMINUM STOREFRONT DOOR. PROVIDE SEALED TIGHT WEATHER STRIPPING ALL AROUND

1/4" THK. FIXED GLASS

4'-0"

PASS THRU UNIT

6'-8"

STAINLESS STEEL COUNTER TOP

2'-6' 2'-6' 2'-6' 2'-6' 2'-6' 2'-6'

ADJ. STAINLESS STL. SHELVING

Figure 4-4. *Elevation drawing of wall separating cleanroom and anteroom at University of Illinois Hospital, a 424-bed teaching hospital in Chicago, IL. (Reproduced, with permission, from Reference 29.)*

the cleanroom ceiling. Air from the pharmacy proper is blown through two standard fiberglass filters before passing through the HEPA filters into the cleanroom.

❒ Louvered dampers in the door and below the pass-through chamber permit airflow out of the positive-pressure room. They can be closed if power is lost to the blower.

❒ Ceiling tiles are vinyl-coated gypsum panels.

❒ Vinyl panels are easy to clean with detergent and water and can be replaced inexpensively if torn.

❒ A "hands free" faucet and hand dryer are just outside the cleanroom.

❒ The airborne particle count in the cleanroom is about 65 of 0.5 μm or larger, easily qualifying the environment as Class 10,000 or even Class 100. Particle counts inside the laminar-airflow hood average 5–10 of 0.5 μm or larger.

Remodeling of existing space

Kuster and Snyder described their reasons for renovating their pharmacy to create a Class 10,000 cleanroom.[28] They prepared various sterile products, including Risk Level 3 products such as glycerin and phenol injection and sterile talc injection. To lessen the chance of error due to interruptions, they placed no phone in their cleanroom and included only a foot-activated intercom for outside communications. Figure 4-3 shows a general floorplan of their pharmacy and cleanroom.

Samuelson and Clark described the planning for a Class 10,000 cleanroom with a Class 100,000 anteroom at the University of Illinois Hospital.[29] They decided to convert an existing 32-ft by 22-ft sterile products room—40% into a cleanroom and 60% into an anteroom—by constructing a wall across it. A detail of the elevation of

the cleanroom side of the wall is shown in Figure 4-4.

At the University of Illinois Hospital, the large anteroom is needed for stock storage and reference materials. The larger pass-through window is used for supplies going into the cleanroom, and the smaller window is for completed products going back to the anteroom where they are checked by a pharmacist. The glass panel around the windows preserves a sense of openness and allows the pharmacist to monitor activities in the cleanroom. Since the existing walls and floor were seamless, they could be sealed with a polymer coating. However, ventilation had to be changed to incorporate HEPA filtration of the air supply in conjunction with a new 2-in ceiling grid system. The cost of the University of Illinois renovation was about $60,000–$70,000.[30]

Another approach to remodeling was taken at University Hospital in Augusta, GA. Rather than create an enclosed cleanroom and anteroom, the pharmacy used an open architecture plan to create workspaces with the appropriate air quality. HEPA-filtered air is directed first into the space around the hoods, then through the "anteroom" area, and finally out into the pharmacy proper. During work hours, air particle counts average 946 (range of 316–1599) of 0.5 μm or larger per cubic foot in the

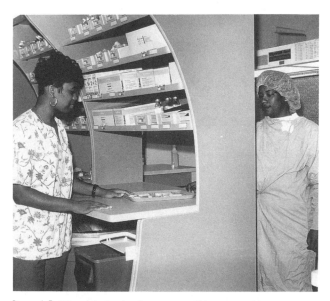

Figure 4-5. *Pharmacist in the open architecture cleanroom at University Hospital, a 700-bed teaching hospital in Augusta, GA.*

anteroom area. This airflow pattern makes the environment more efficient for traffic flow of pharmacy sterile compounding personnel (Figure 4-5). The cost of the equipment and fixtures was about $70,000–$75,000.[31]

Use of isolators

An isolator can be used to prepare cytotoxic sterile products if a cleanroom is not available.[32] This arrangement creates a Class 100 environment in a limited space and may be appropriate for small but frequent batches of Risk Level 3 products. Isolators generally cost about $8000–$20,000.

Minimal facility change

New procedures also can minimize airborne particulate matter. Lau et al.[33] described procedural changes in their large (six hood) centralized admixture room that produced a Class 10,000 environment from what was Class 100,000. Some of their changes were limiting personnel traffic, having personnel wear sterile garb, and removing cardboard containers outside the room.

Moreover, Chandler et al.[34] found that their large (four hood) sterile preparation room met Class 100,000 standards without modifications to either the room or procedures. Therefore, pharmacists should test the air quality in their sterile compounding room before embarking on expensive facility changes.

Preparing Architectural Plans

After testing their sterile compounding environment, many pharmacists will decide to improve the air quality. These pharmacists then should prepare plans with a hospital designer or architect. The pharmacist has the following roles in functional planning:[14]

- ❐ Identify functions to be performed in the cleanroom and anteroom.
- ❐ Determine workflow in the cleanroom and anteroom.
- ❐ Identify work areas to be remodeled.
- ❐ Decide how to handle workload during the renovation process.
- ❐ Specify requirements for the cleanroom and anteroom:
  - Workload.
  - Equipment and fixture types and numbers.
  - Storage.
  - Personnel types and numbers.
  - Materials handling.
  - Communications.
  - Services from other departments.
  - Security.
  - Utilities.
  - Environmental quality control (i.e., FS 209E Class 10,000) for airborne particles,

temperature, and air pressure.
- Routine cleaning of surfaces.

Details for developing these requirements are found in Reference 14. Together, the pharmacist and architect should design the optimal arrangement for work areas, find the best location, and draft schematic plans. Then the architect must develop the architectural design for floorplans, elevations, electrical fixtures, heating, venting, air conditioning, etc. Based on these functional plans, the architect can make an efficient design that is satisfying to personnel and aesthetic in appearance. The pharmacist also should have the architect make the facility flexible to accommodate future changes. And, finally, the pharmacist should review the architect's drawings and estimated costs before seeking project approval.

Bidding Construction

To renovate or construct a cleanroom or to purchase a modular cleanroom, the pharmacist and architect will have to answer numerous questions:

1. What is the maximum process exhaust air volume (e.g., from biological safety cabinet) for the cleanroom and anteroom?
2. What is the maximum process heat or power consumption of equipment in the cleanroom and anteroom, including computers, people, refrigerators, hoods, etc.?
3. What is the maximum number of individuals in the cleanroom at one time? In the anteroom at one time?
4. How many air changes are required per hour in the cleanroom (e.g., 60 in Class 10,000) and anteroom (e.g., 20 in Class 100,000)?[35]
5. What is the source of the makeup air, inside or outside?
6. What cleaning agents will be used on ceilings, walls, and floors in the cleanroom and anteroom?
7. What lighting levels are needed (in footcandles) at 30 in from the floor in the cleanroom (e.g., 100) and anteroom (e.g., 80)?
8. What flooring material (e.g., seamless vinyl or epoxy paint) is desired in the cleanroom and anteroom?
9. What wall material (e.g., modular steel, plastic vinyl, or glass) is required in the cleanroom and anteroom? (This answer may depend on how much and what kind of equipment and fixtures are to be mounted on the walls.)
10. What ceiling type (e.g., solid, panel, or walkable) is required in the cleanroom and anteroom?
11. What is the height from existing floor to ceil-

ing? What is the required ceiling height in the cleanroom and anteroom?

12. Can the ceiling and equipment (e.g., blowers, condensers, and HEPA filters) be supported by the existing room structure in the cleanroom and anteroom?

13. Are windows or viewing panels required? If so, where should they be in the cleanroom and anteroom?

14. Are pass-through chambers required? If so, where and what size should they be in the cleanroom and anteroom?

15. Where are doors to be located in the cleanroom and anteroom? What type of door (e.g., swing or sliding) should be installed?

16. Where are telephone conduits needed in the cleanroom and anteroom?

17. Where are intercom stations needed in the cleanroom and anteroom?

18. Where are duplex outlets or power strips needed in the cleanroom and anteroom?

19. Do perimeter walls require fire rating? If so, identify rating in hours for the cleanroom and anteroom.

20. Is automatic sprinkling required for fire control in the cleanroom and anteroom? If so, sprinkler heads must finish flush with the ceiling.

21. Will plenum or area above the cleanroom and anteroom need sprinkling?

22. Will smoke or fire alarms be needed in the cleanroom and anteroom?

23. Are temperature recording and monitoring required for the cleanroom and anteroom?

24. Are hot and cold water available for the anteroom? Can a sink drain be installed without threat to cleanliness?

25. Will sticky mats be used at the cleanroom entrance?

26. Must construction and service personnel be union members?

27. Is payment or performance bonding required?

28. Are permits or fees required for the construction?

29. Which of the following standard operational performance tests are required for the cleanroom and anteroom: particle count, HEPA filter integrity, temperature, humidity, light level, sound level, airborne microbial counts, and surface microbial counts?

30. Who will clean the facilities? What provision is needed for their supplies?

31. Who will remove waste material? How will hazardous and nonhazardous waste be handled?

After all drawings and specifications are prepared, construction contract documents must be drawn up. A prebid meeting should be held with potential vendors to answer questions. Bids should be sent to one or more vendors or building contractors to obtain a final cost for approval by administration. The pharmacist and architect should employ companies or contractors who are familiar with fabricating cleanroom facilities. Before construction begins, equipment should be ordered, personnel should be trained, and procedures should be written.

Building the Installation

Everyone involved in constructing a cleanroom should understand that it is no ordinary building project.[26] The microcontamination of all activities should be reviewed before they are begun.

Materials for walls, floors, and ceilings should never be stored outdoors. Packaging materials (usually doubled) cannot be torn or removed until the cleanroom contractor is ready for installation. A general wipe down of building materials with clean wipes is recommended both before and after installation.[26] After any cutting or drilling operation, the resealing should be done as soon as possible to prevent oxidation or deep contamination of building materials.

Once the floor is laid, construction workers should wear gowns and shoe covers to reduce contamination and prevent damage to the floor. No eating, smoking, chewing, etc., should be allowed in the area. All spills, filings, etc., should be cleaned up immediately. After walls and ceilings are in place (even before the air supply is turned on), the area should be restricted to authorized personnel. Finally, once the air supply is on, construction workers should be gowned like the operators will be.[26]

Evaluating the Installation

Final steps are inspecting and approving the new facility, installing and evaluating equipment, moving supplies, assessing workflow, and following up on needed changes (which are inevitable).

It is important to verify that all specifications initially outlined in the architectural plan have been achieved. The pharmacist in charge of the project also must ensure that air quality, surface conditions, environmental requirements, and working conditions (e.g., space and lighting) are as specified in the original bidding process. These requirements must be satisfied before any equipment or supplies are moved into the anteroom or cleanroom.

Furthermore, the institution's facilities management personnel must check that all policies regarding electrical fixtures, heating, ventilation, etc., have been met. Otherwise, an agreement must be reached with the contractor to rectify deficiencies before the contract can be considered satisfied.

FACILITY MAINTENANCE

Clearly, planning, building, and implementing a cleanroom facility is a detailed process. All that preparation, however, must be preserved with proper maintenance. Preventive maintenance of cleanroom and anteroom prefilters, HEPA filters, and ducts should be arranged with appropriate maintenance personnel or a service contractor. Similarly, lighting should be checked periodically and/or bulbs should be changed prior to cleaning of light fixtures.

Cleanroom

Each day, work surfaces near the hood (e.g., counter tops and carts) should be wiped clean with a freshly prepared mild detergent solution followed by a sanitizing agent approved by the pharmacist in charge. Sufficient time must be allowed for the agent to exert its antimicrobial effect. Furthermore, storage shelving should be emptied of all supplies, cleaned, and sanitized at least weekly. The sanitizing agent should be rotated with one having a different action at least quarterly. Recleaning should be performed if spillage or other events indicate the need.[2]

When no aseptic operations are in progress, floors should be mopped once daily by trained and supervised custodial personnel. Floors should not be waxed, however, since dried, worn wax adds to airborne particulates.[25] All cleaning and sanitizing agents should be approved, with careful consideration of compatibilities, effectiveness, and inappropriate or toxic residues. In addition, all cleaning tools (e.g., wipers, sponges, and mops) should be nonshedding and used only in the cleanroom (first) and anteroom.

Most wipers should be discarded after one use. If cleaning tools are reused, their cleanliness should be maintained by thorough rinsing and sanitizing and by storage in a clean environment.[2] Ceilings and walls should be cleaned monthly with a mild detergent solution followed by an approved sanitizing agent.

Trash should be collected in suitable plastic bags and removed with minimal agitation. Routine monitoring is used to control the quality of the air and surfaces in the cleanroom (see Chapter 6).

Anteroom

In the anteroom, supplies and equipment removed from shipping cartons should be wiped with a sanitizing agent, such as 70% isopropyl alcohol; this agent should be checked periodically for contamination. (Since 70% isopropyl alcohol may harbor resistant microbial spores, it should be filtered through a 0.2-μm hydrophobic filter before being used in aseptic areas.) Alternatively, if supplies are in sealed pouches (e.g., syringes), the pouches can be removed when the supplies are introduced into the cleanroom, obviating the need to sanitize individual items. No shipping or other cartons should be taken into the cleanroom.[2]

The anteroom should be cleaned and sanitized at least weekly by trained and supervised custodial personnel. However, floors must be cleaned and sanitized daily, always proceeding from the cleanroom to the anteroom. Storage shelving in the anteroom (including refrigerator interior) should be emptied of all supplies, cleaned, and sanitized at planned intervals, preferably monthly.[2] Walls and ceilings should be cleaned and sanitized at least quarterly.

SUMMARY

Facilities used for sterile product preparation play as integral a role in guaranteeing sterility as does proper aseptic technique. Therefore, pharmacy departments should assess their current facilities and, if needed, upgrade or replace them.

The essential steps in bringing facilities up to current recommended standards are

1. Developing a master facilities plan.
2. Analyzing existing facilities.
3. Identifying functional needs.
4. Preparing architectural plans.
5. Bidding construction.
6. Building the installation.
7. Evaluating the installation.

Once facilities have been brought up to current standards, a proper maintenance program for both the cleanroom and anteroom must be followed.

REFERENCES

1. American Society of Hospital Pharmacists. ASHP technical assistance bulletin on quality assurance for pharmacy-prepared sterile products. *Am J Hosp Pharm.* 1993; 50:2386–98.

2. Sterile drug products for home use. In: United States pharmacopeia, 23rd rev./national formulary, 18th ed. Rockville, MD: United States Pharmacopeial Convention; 1994:1963–75.

3. Good compounding practices applicable to state licensed pharmacies. Parts I and II. *Natl Pharm Compliance News.* 1993; May:2–3 and Oct:2–3.

4. Model rules for sterile pharmaceuticals. Chicago, IL: National Association of Boards of Pharmacy; 1993:12.1–3.

5. Fitch HD. Federal standard 209E: its evolution and

role. *CleanRooms*. 1992; 6 (9):12.

6. Federal standard airborne particulate cleanliness classes in cleanrooms and clean zones. Washington, DC: U.S. General Services Administration; 1992 (Sept):1–48.

7. Microbial evaluation and classification of clean rooms and clean zones. *Pharmacopeial Forum*. 1991; 17:2399–404.

8. Federal Food, Drug and Cosmetic Act. Section 501(a)(2)(B) of Act [21 U.S.C. 351(a)(2)(B)]. *Fed Regist*. 1978; 43:45076–7.

9. Care of patients. In: 1995 comprehensive accreditation manual for hospitals. Oakbrook Terrace, IL: Joint Commission on Accreditation of Healthcare Organizations; 1994:141–2.

10. Reid S, Home Care Surveyor, Joint Commission on Accreditation of Healthcare Organizations, Oakbrook Terrace, IL. May 5, 1994. Personal communication.

11. Pharmaceutical services. In: 1993 accreditation manual for home care, vol 1, standards. Oakbrook Terrace, IL: Joint Commission on Accreditation of Healthcare Organizations; 1992:35–43.

12. Crawford SY, Narducci WA, Augustine SC. National survey of quality assurance activities for pharmacy-prepared sterile products in hospitals. *Am J Hosp Pharm*. 1991; 48:2398–413.

13. Crawford SY, Myers CE. ASHP national survey of hospital-based pharmaceutical services—1992. *Am J Hosp Pharm*. 1993; 50:1371–404.

14. Barker KN, Allan EL, Lin AC, et al. Facility planning and design. In: Brown TR, ed. Handbook of institutional pharmacy practice, 3rd ed. Bethesda, MD: American Society of Hospital Pharmacists; 1992:149–63.

15. Greiner J. What the HEPA can and cannot do. *CleanRooms*. 1994; 7 (4):29.

16. Miller WA, Smith GL, Latiolais CJ. A comparative evaluation of compounding costs and contamination rates of intravenous admixture systems. *Drug Intell Clin Pharm*. 1971; 5:51–60.

17. Poretz DM, Guynn JB Jr, Duma RJ, et al. Microbial contamination of glass bottle (open-vented) and plastic bag (closed-nonvented) intravenous fluid delivery systems. *Am J Hosp Pharm*. 1974; 31:726–32.

18. McAllister JC, Buchanan EC, Skolaut MW. A comparison of the safety and efficiency of three intermittent intravenous therapy systems—the minibottle, the minibag and the inline burette. *Am J Hosp Pharm*. 1974; 31:961–7.

19. Frieben WR. Control of aseptic processing environment. *Am J Hosp Pharm*. 1983; 40:1928–35.

20. Ravin R, Bahr J, Luscomb F, et al. Program for bacterial surveillance of intravenous admixtures. *Am J Hosp Pharm*. 1974; 31:340–7.

21. Guynn JB Jr, Poretz DM, Duma RJ. Growth of various bacteria in a variety of intravenous fluids. *Am J Hosp Pharm*. 1973; 30:321–5.

22. Thur MP, Miller WA, Latiolais CJ. Medication errors in a nurse-controlled parenteral admixture program. *Am J Hosp Pharm*. 1972; 29:298–304.

23. Lin AC. Study of variables affecting floor space requirements for intravenous admixture compounding areas in hospitals: a computer simulation approach. Auburn University, AL: Auburn University; 1992:281–342, 359–90. Doctoral dissertation. (Available from University Microfilms, Ann Arbor, MI, Publication DA9237193.)

24. Buchanan TL, Barker KN, Gibson JT, et al. Illumination and errors in dispensing. *Am J Hosp Pharm*. 1991; 48:2137–45.

25. Kraft R. Cleanroom-construction concerns. *Am J Hosp Pharm*. 1994; 51:935. Letter.

26. Kozicki M, Hoenig S, Robinson P. Cleanrooms—facilities and practices. New York: Van Nostrand Reinhold; 1991:49–79.

27. Rose R, Director of Pharmacy, Memorial Hospital, Carthage, IL. Aug 11, 1994. Personal communication.

28. Kuster LM, Snyder GA. The future of hospital-based IV compounding. *Hosp Pharm Times*. 1993; 59 (Dec):3–8HPT.

29. Samuelson DE, Clark T. Pharmacy preparation meets the contamination control challenge. *Clean Rooms*. 1993; 7 (8):12–6.

30. Clark T, Director of Pharmacy, University of Illinois Hospital, Chicago, IL. Aug 1994. Personal communication.

31. Mangum D, Assistant Director of Pharmacy, and Severson J, Director of Pharmacy, University Hospital, Augusta, GA. Sept 1994. Personal communication.

32. Favier M, Hansel S, Bressolle F. Preparing cytotoxic agents in an isolator. *Am J Hosp Pharm*. 1993; 50:2335–9.

33. Lau D, Shane R, Yen J. Quality assurance for sterile products: simple changes can help. *Am J Hosp Pharm*. 1994; 51:1353. Letter.

34. Chandler SW, Trissel LA, Wamsley LM, et al. Evaluation of air quality in a sterile-drug preparation area with an electronic particle counter. *Am J Hosp Pharm*. 1993; 50:2330–4.

35. Center for Drugs and Biologics. Guideline on sterile drug products produced by aseptic processing. Rockville, MD: Food and Drug Administration; June 10, 1987.

Chapter 5

Equipment for Sterile Product Preparation

Philip J. Schneider

Although most sterile products are prepared using aseptic processing, some are made under nonsterile conditions and then are terminally sterilized. Both methods require the critical area to be as sterile as possible. Supplies also should be stored in a clean environment (the controlled area). Both the critical and controlled areas must be maintained appropriately (see Chapter 6), and a major determinant in their maintenance is the equipment used in them.

The most common piece of equipment used in sterile preparation areas is a laminar-airflow hood. However, automated compounding devices, refrigerators, freezers, computer terminals, shelving, chairs and tables, carts, lockers, and miscellaneous items also influence the cleanliness of critical and controlled areas.

To ensure environmental standards, as much of this equipment as possible should be separated from the critical area. Other than the laminar-airflow hood, most equipment should be stored in the controlled area or the pharmacy itself.

CLEAN AIR ENVIRONMENTS

In the critical area, air should meet Class 100 conditions. Class 100 cleanrooms can be constructed to meet this requirement (see Chapter 4). Offsite modular cleanrooms also can be purchased, but their cost may limit usage to settings where large quantities of sterile products (e.g., home care companies) or high-risk products are prepared. Two other options for maintaining a Class 100 environment are laminar-airflow hoods and gloves boxes.

Laminar-Airflow Hoods

A laminar-airflow hood—with either horizontal or vertical airflow—is a cost-effective, efficient way to provide the Class 100 environment required for pharmacy use (see Chapter 7). This hood includes a high-efficiency particulate air (HEPA) filter to retain airborne particles and microorganisms, and its use decreases the chance of product contamination.[1] According to a recent survey, nearly all (99.4%) of the pharmacies preparing sterile products had access to a laminar-airflow hood.[2]

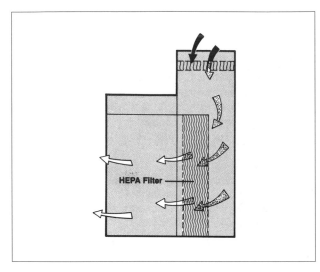

figure 5-1. *Horizontal laminar-airflow hood. (Reproduced, with permission, from Labconco Corporation, Kansas City, MO.)*

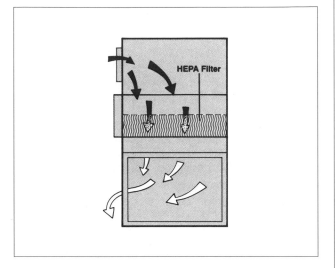

figure 5-2. *Vertical laminar-airflow hood. (Reproduced, with permission, from Labconco Corporation, Kansas City, MO.)*

Horizontal laminar-airflow hoods

Horizontal airflow hoods are used for most sterile product preparation applications because they do not require expensive venting to outside air and can be easily moved to different locations. These hoods produce air, of a specified quality, that flows horizontally over work areas (see Figure 5-1).

Horizontal hoods are available in various widths (26 in–8 ft) and with different electrical requirements (120 or 220 volts). Work surfaces are of either high-density laminated composition board or stainless steel. Although some models are for use on counter tops, others are stand-alone floor units.

Vertical laminar-airflow hoods

Since horizontal laminar-airflow hoods blow air toward the operator, vertical laminar-airflow hoods are preferred for hazardous substances (see Figure 5-2). Vertical flow hoods are part of a family of equipment called biohazard cabinets or biological safety cabinets. Three types of biohazard cabinets are available:

1. Class I cabinets have a HEPA filter on their exhaust outlet but not for inward airflow. They protect personnel and the environment but do not prevent product contamination. This class of hoods has no application in sterile product preparation.
2. Class II cabinets have HEPA-filtered inward air for product protection and HEPA-filtered exhaust air for personnel and environmental protection. They are suitable for sterile product preparation.
3. Class III cabinets are totally enclosed, vented, and gastight units. Operations are conducted

through attached rubber gloves, and the cabinet is maintained under negative pressure. These cabinets have limited applications in the preparation of sterile products.

Types of Class II cabinets. Class II cabinets are classified according to how their exhaust air is vented.

A Class II, Type A cabinet

❑ Maintains a minimum calculated average inflow air velocity of 75 ft/min through the work area access opening.
❑ Has HEPA-filtered air from a common plenum (some air is exhausted from the cabinet and some is supplied to the work area).
❑ May have air exhausted back into the controlled area.
❑ May have positive-pressure-contaminated ducts and plenums.

A Class II, Type B cabinet exhausts some or all air outside the controlled area. These cabinets are further classified as II B1, II B2, or II B3 (or A/B3) cabinets.

A II B1 cabinet

❑ Maintains an average air velocity of 100 ft/min.
❑ Has HEPA-filtered downflow air composed largely of uncontaminated, recirculated inflow air.
❑ Exhausts *most* contaminated air to the atmosphere through a dedicated duct and HEPA filter.
❑ Has all contaminated ducts and plenums under negative pressure.

A II B2 cabinet, sometimes called a total exhaust

cabinet, differs from a II B1 cabinet in that it

- ❑ Has *all* downflow air drawn through a HEPA filter from the controlled area or outside, not recirculated from the cabinet.
- ❑ Exhausts *all* air to the atmosphere after HEPA filtration, not to recirculation in the cabinet or controlled area.

A II B3 cabinet, sometimes referred to as a convertible cabinet

- ❑ Has HEPA-filtered air that is a portion of the mixed downflow and inflow air from a common exhaust plenum.
- ❑ Exhausts all air to the atmosphere after HEPA filtration.
- ❑ Can be converted from a Type B to a Type A cabinet if desired.

The airflow characteristics of different types of biohazard cabinets are shown in Figure 5-3.

Cabinet safety. The safest biohazard cabinet for sterile product preparation (e.g., chemotherapy) is a II B2 unit. It is recommended for programs where a limited number of staff handle or prepare extensive amounts of hazardous materials. However, these cabinets require expensive venting and cannot be easily located. A less expensive alternative, the Class II, Type A cabinet, does not need to be vented to the outside atmosphere if the controlled area is large and the quantity of products prepared is low.

Hood selection

Vertical laminar-airflow hoods are the preferred choice. These cabinets prevent cumulative exposure to potentially toxic medications, especially if the staff routinely prepare hazardous products for a long time.

When sterile products are prepared, aerosols can form and be blown toward the operator using a horizontal hood. Long-term exposure to cytotoxic agents as well as other drugs, especially antibiotics, is a great concern. Vertical airflow hoods, however, minimize such exposure.

The disadvantage of vertical airflow versus horizontal airflow hoods are expense and ease of use. Class II, Type B hoods are more expensive than horizontal hoods and can be very costly to install due to venting requirements. Hoods that vent air to the room (Class II, Type A) are less expensive but are still more costly than horizontal airflow hoods. Furthermore, vertical airflow hoods generally are more restrictive and may slow workflow.

When selecting a laminar-airflow hood, several

Air Flow	Recirculation to Room		Thimble Duct		Hard Duct	Hard Duct
Side View Schematic Contaminated: ➡ Room: ⇨ HEPA-Filtered: ⇨						
Class	II	II	II	II	II	II
Type	A	A/B3	A	A/B3	B3	B2
Sash Opening (inches)	10	8	10	8	8	8
Inflow (fpm)*	80	105	80	105	105	105
Downflow (fpm)*	80	80	80	80	80	60–65
% Recirculation	70	70	70	70	70	0
Exhausts To	room	room	outside	outside	outside	outside
Exhaust Duct Connection**	none	none	canopy	canopy	hard duct	hard duct

*Inflow and downflow velocities are shown at nominal fpm. **Varies according to local codes.

Figure 5-3. *Airflow characteristics of Class II vertical laminar-airflow hoods. (Reproduced, with permission, from Labconco Corporation, Kansas City, MO.)*

questions should be addressed.

Is a horizontal or vertical airflow hood (biohazard cabinet) needed? If hazardous materials are being prepared routinely, a vertical airflow hood should be utilized.

If a biohazard cabinet is required, does it need to be ventilated to the atmosphere? If large quantities of hazardous materials are being prepared regularly and the controlled area is small, operators may be exposed to high amounts of aerosols. In this case, the vertical cabinet should be vented to the outside atmosphere.

What are the counter length, depth, and height limitations in cabinet selection? These dimensions depend on the size and layout of the controlled area, workload, and number of staff working in the controlled area. Hood manufacturers readily supply cabinet dimensions on request.

What are the electrical requirements? Manufacturers offer various hoods requiring either 120 or 220 volts. Institutional policies or procedures relating to equipment voltage and the facility's capacity must be determined.

Should a counter top or stand-alone unit be purchased? This decision should be based on the space available and the work area required. Generally, smaller hoods can be placed on counter tops, but they require enough ceiling clearance to provide intake air. Door openings also must be considered when a hood is to be put in an existing cleanroom.

Glove Boxes

Glove boxes—sealed enclosures—are not extensively used for sterile product preparation in this country. All handling of items inside these boxes is carried out through long, relatively impermeable gloves secured to ports in the enclosure walls. The operator places his or her hands and forearms in the gloves from outside the box and manipulates items inside with relative freedom while viewing the operation through a window.

Glove boxes have their origins in laboratories and industries where handling in special environments is required. However, several manufacturers are now developing glove boxes that provide Class 100 conditions for aseptic transfer of sterile ingredients.

Glove boxes have the potential advantages of requiring less space and less rigorous environmental control around the box as compared to laminar-airflow hoods. For areas where a small number of doses are prepared at a time (e.g., satellite pharmacies), glove boxes may be useful. However, since glove boxes are not much less expensive than laminar-airflow hoods and curtail access to the internal environment, they may have limited applications in pharmacy-related sterile product preparation.

COMPOUNDING DEVICES

Many tools have been developed to assist personnel in preparing sterile products. Compounding devices—syringe systems, automatic systems based on peristaltic pump principles, and robotics—are frequently used for batch preparations, nutrition solutions, and cardioplegia preparations. Before these devices are employed, however, three questions should be answered:

1. Do standardized formulations lend themselves to an automated system?
2. Does the workload justify the use of the device to improve efficiency?
3. Are appropriate quality-assurance controls in place to monitor the products prepared with these devices?

Syringe-Based Devices

The Cornwall syringe, an example of a manual device, uses a two-way valve. This valve is attached to a diluting fluid and to the syringe, and spring mechanism refills the barrel after each use. This device is used for mass reconstitution of powdered drugs in vials or to add a set quantity of one ingredient to other products (e.g., electrolyte addition to nutrition formulas).

Electronically powered versions of this device also have been introduced (e.g., FasPak).

Peristaltic Pump Devices

The automated compounding device, based on peristaltic pump principles similar to infusion pumps, is a recent technological development for preparing sterile products. It is useful for complex multicomponent sterile products (e.g., nutrition formulations and cardioplegia solutions).

Automated compounding devices are available for both large volume (e.g., sterile water, dextrose, and amino acids) and small volume (e.g., electrolytes and micronutrients) components. Some devices have computer operating systems that perform calculations, record doses, maintain manufacturing records, and run the device itself.

For pharmacies preparing large quantities of complicated solutions, these devices can improve both efficiency and accuracy. Since they involve a high capital cost (over $10,000), monthly lease payments, or the purchase of expensive infusion sets, their application to small operations is limited. An organization that purchases numerous products from a company that sells an automated compounding device may be able to obtain one on a contractual basis based on product usage.

The accuracy of the final products prepared with these devices has been questioned. Patients have received formulations containing inaccurate quantities of ordered ingredients.[3–5] In most reported cases, pediatric patients received nutrition formulas containing the wrong concentration of dextrose. The accuracy of these formulations can be verified using weight or refractometry measurements,[6,7] as discussed in Chapter 17.

Robotic Devices

The next generation of automation will be robotic devices that actually prepare the final sterile product. While these devices are not yet available to pharmacists (one such device is being developed in Canada), they potentially can automate the entire process, minimizing human error and breaks in technique. These devices probably will be expensive (hundreds of thousands of dollars), however, limiting application to the largest programs or regional pharmacies.

OTHER EQUIPMENT

In addition to the cleanroom itself, many important equipment decisions have to be made concerning sterile product preparation. The relationship of equipment—from refrigerators to computers—and special precautions for their operation must be considered.

Refrigerators

Many drugs and compounded sterile products require refrigeration to maintain stability. The *United States Pharmacopeia/National Formulary (USP/NF)* defines a refrigerator as "a cold place in which the temperature is maintained thermostatically between 2 and 8 degrees centigrade (36 to 46 degrees Fahrenheit)." The *USP/NF* also defines storage conditions:

- ❏ Cold—temperatures not exceeding 8° C (46° F).
- ❏ Cool—temperatures between 8 and 15° C (46 and 59° F).

The *USP/NF* also states that articles requiring storage in a cool place (e.g., insulin) can be refrigerated unless otherwise indicated.[8]

Ordinary consumer refrigerators are often used for sterile product preparation programs. Although these refrigerators are adequate, a quality-assurance program must ensure that appropriate temperatures are maintained. At the very least, a thermometer in the refrigerator should be checked (and documented) daily.

Commercial refrigerators often are more durable and have valuable features for pharmacy applications. One desirable feature is an alarm that sounds if the temperature varies from control limits (due to power failure or equipment malfunction). Since this alarm should be monitored 24 hr/day, it should be wired to a security office.

Staff responsible for monitoring temperatures or temperature alarms should be familiar with the effects of temperature changes on stored products.

Refrigerator location

Refrigerator placement can cause pharmacy design problems. The refrigerator ventilation motor can create air movement in a controlled or critical area. If a refrigerator must be in the controlled area, it should be as far as possible from the laminar-airflow hood.

Storage refrigerators should not be in any Class 100 cleanroom. To supply refrigeration to a Class 100 cleanroom, refrigerators with two-sided, pass-through doors should be used. These refrigerators, with doors on both sides, permit access to sterile products by both operators in the controlled area and personnel outside it. If the facility is properly designed, this arrangement eliminates unnecessary entry of personnel to the controlled area to retrieve sterile products.

Refrigerator size

Since refrigerators come in many sizes, proper selection depends on the volume of drugs and final products to be stored. Having several small units instead of one large unit may be desirable because they

- ❏ Provide both a safeguard and a backup if one unit fails.
- ❏ Permit segregation of drugs and products for safety purposes (e.g., some pharmacists prefer to store chemotherapy or investigational products separately).

The simplest method to determine the refrigerator size needed is to add (1) the space required for the maximum inventory of drug supplies and final products on the busiest day of the week and (2) additional capacity for future growth. Then possible storage areas must be identified so the decision can be made between one large and several small refrigerators. Furthermore, if the facility is already built, the maximum size refrigerator that can be moved through the door and ceiling limitations must be considered. Power requirements also should be checked against institutional policies before any unit is purchased.

Freezers

Some sterile products must be kept frozen to extend their stability and shelf life. According to the *USP/NF*, a freezer is "a cold place in which the temperature is maintained thermostatically between −20 and −10 degrees centigrade (−4 and 14 degrees Fahrenheit)."[8] The same quality-control issues (e.g., monitoring temperatures) that apply to refrigerators also apply to freezers, as do concerns for location, size, and selection.

Computer Terminals and Software

To maintain records and generate labels, most sterile product preparation programs now use computers. In large institutions, these programs are part of the pharmacy computer system. Small pharmacies, however, may use commercially available software written specifically for sterile product preparation.

Computer equipment have fans to cool units and paper to print reports and labels. Both features are undesirable in the cleanroom—fans disrupt airflow and printers generate particulates. Therefore, computer equipment must be located as far as possible from the critical area and never in it. (Automated compounding devices are not considered to be computer equipment.) Space, noise, cable installation, hardware needs, and workflow should all be considered when locating computer equipment.

Shelving

Storage of supplies should be minimized in the controlled area, and no cardboard should be kept on any shelving. Shelving for plastic bags and glass containers in the controlled area should be easy to clean and provide minimal horizontal surface for particulates to settle. Stainless steel wire shelving units are ideal.

Chairs and Tables

Stainless steel furniture should be standard for the cleanroom because it can be easily cleaned and does not generate particles. For comfort, chairs may be covered with a cleanable vinyl but not porous fabric. Chairs and tables should have wheels so that they can be easily moved to clean and disinfect the flooring.

Carts

Components and final products should be moved in and out of critical and controlled areas on large, heavy duty, stainless steel carts. These carts should have 6-in swivel wheels and brakes. Their shelving should be made of heavy wire (mesh) to prevent the collection of dust and dirt on horizontal surfaces. Cardboard boxes should not be used.

Drugs and supplies should be unpacked from cardboard shipping containers outside the controlled area and then placed on these carts. Once in the controlled area, supplies and drugs can be further opened for patient-specific or batch production. These materials can be taken into the critical area on smaller stainless steel carts with smooth surfaces. As an alternative, supplies can be placed on trays or bins and then into the laminar-airflow hood.

Carts for delivery out of the controlled area (to patient areas) should be selected on the basis of size and quantity of the products involved. Large quantities of large size products should be transported on heavy duty, stainless steel wire carts, similar to those used for supplies in the controlled area.

Locker Facilities

Since personnel preparing sterile products should wear special garb (gowns, gloves, masks, etc.), they need a place to change their clothing before entering the cleanroom. This area, with individual lockable storage containers and necessary garb, should be as close to the controlled area as possible. A sink (with floor controls) and soap dispensers for hand washing also should be in this locker area.

Miscellaneous Equipment

Other items that may be useful for sterile product preparation are

- ❑ A digital readout microwave oven.
- ❑ A warming cabinet to store drugs prone to crystallization (e.g., mannitol).
- ❑ A balance (i.e., scale) for measuring compounding powders.

SPECIAL EQUIPMENT FOR CYTOTOXIC AND HAZARDOUS DRUGS

Special equipment is required when cytotoxic and hazardous drugs are prepared.[9] Shelves, carts, counters, and trays must be designed to prevent breakage. Bin shelves must have barriers at the front or other features that keep drug containers from falling to the floor. Appropriate protective apparel (e.g., disposable gloves and long sleeve gowns) must be readily available.

Other supplies such as disposable plastic-backed absorbent liners, gauze pads, cytotoxic waste disposal bags and warning labels, and plastic containers for used needles, ampuls, etc., should be conveniently located. Syringes and IV sets should have Luer-lok fittings.

Spill kits for cleaning up cytotoxic drugs also should be readily accessible. Each kit should include sealable plastic waste disposal bags (appropriately labeled), disposable dust and mist respirators, splash goggles, absorbent sheets or powders, two or more pairs of disposable gloves, and a small scoop for collecting glass fragments.

Cytotoxic drugs should be prepared in a Class II containment cabinet. Whether or not this hood must be vented to the outside atmosphere, however, is still being debated. If a Class II cabinet is unavailable, the drugs should be prepared in a quiet workspace, away from heating and cooling vents and other personnel.

SUMMARY

The maintenance of sterility depends more on technique than any other single factor. Therefore, having the appropriate equipment should not give personnel a false sense of security—there is no substitute for good aseptic technique. Nevertheless, appropriate equipment can further minimize product contamination by providing a contaminant-free environment.

The laminar-airflow hood is the most important piece of equipment used in sterile product preparation; it establishes the critical area for compounding ingredients. Other items (e.g., refrigerators, freezers, and shelving) also must ensure the proper environment for the storage of ingredients and final products.

All equipment should be selected on the basis of preventing inadvertent introduction of microbes and particulates into controlled and critical areas.

REFERENCES

1. Brier KL, Latiolais CJ, Schneider PJ, et al. Effect of laminar air flow and clean room dress on contamination rates of intravenous admixtures. *Am J Hosp Pharm*. 1981; 38:1144–7.

2. Crawford SY, Narducci WA, Augustine SC. National survey of quality assurance activities for pharmacy-prepared sterile products in hospitals. *Am J Hosp Pharm*. 1991; 48:2398–413.

3. Brushwood DB. Hospital liable for defect in cardioplegia solution. *Am J Hosp Pharm*. 1992; 49:1174–6.

4. Silverberg JM. Automix error—neonatal TPN. *Formul Inf Exch Bull Board*. 1991; Mar 20.

5. Faulty cardioplegia solution leads to $492,000 verdict. *Hosp Pharm Rep*. 1990; 4 (Aug):1.

6. Murphy C. Ensuring accuracy in the use of automated compounders. *Am J Hosp Pharm*. 1993; 50:60. Letter.

7. Silverberg JB, Webb B, Pawlak R. Specific gravity-based determination of dextrose content of total parenteral nutrient solutions for neonates. *Am J Hosp Pharm*. 1993; 50:2090–1.

8. General notices and requirements. In: United States pharmacopeia, 23rd rev./national formulary, 18th ed. Rockville, MD: United States Pharmacopeial Convention; 1994:11.

9. American Society of Hospital Pharmacists. ASHP technical assistance bulletin on handling cytotoxic and hazardous drugs. *Am J Hosp Pharm*. 1990; 47:1033–49.

Chapter 6
Environmental Monitoring

Philip J. Schneider

To reduce the potential for contamination, sterile products must be manipulated and stored in an appropriate environment. The maintenance of such an environment requires constant monitoring of numerous factors.

ENVIRONMENTAL REQUIREMENTS

Most standards on sterile product preparation describe two types of environments:

1. The *controlled area,* where unsterilized products, inprocess materials, and containers are handled.[1]
2. The *critical area,* where sterile products, containers, and closures are exposed to their surroundings.[1]

For both of these areas, environmental requirements have been defined by the Food and Drug Administration,[1] National Aeronautics and Space Administration,[2] and U.S. Air Force.[3] Their specifications are summarized in the following sections for seven parameters:

- ❏ Temperature.
- ❏ Relative humidity.
- ❏ Air exchange (airflow).
- ❏ Percentage of fresh air.
- ❏ Pressure differential.
- ❏ Particulates.
- ❏ Microbial organisms.

Controlled Areas

Table 6-1 summarizes the environmental requirements for controlled areas. Temperature should be 72 ± 5° F, while relative humidity should be in the 30–50% range. Moreover, the volume of air in a controlled area should be exchanged 20 times/hr. The percentage of fresh air can vary from 5 to 20%.

To avoid transfer of particulates and contaminants into controlled areas, a positive air pressure (i.e., 0.05 in of water) must be maintained relative to adjacent, less clean areas.

Air quality, the most recognized measurement of environmental conditions, involves two components: nonviable particulates and

Table 6-1. *Environmental Requirements for Controlled Areas (Class 100,000)[3]*

Parameter	Requirement
Temperature	72 ± 5° F
Relative humidity	30–50%
Air exchange	20/hr
Percentage fresh air	5–20%
Pressure differential	0.05 in of water
Air quality	
Particulates	≤100,000 of ≥0.5 µm/cu ft
Microbial organisms	≤2.5/cu ft

Table 6-3. *Environmental Requirements for Critical Areas (Class 100)[3]*

Parameter	Requirement
Temperature	72 ± 5° F
Relative humidity	30–50%
Airflow	90 ft/min ± 20%
Air quality	
Particulates	≤100 of ≥0.5 µm/cu ft
Microbial organisms	≤0.1/cu ft

microbial organisms. Class numbers (e.g., Class 100) are commonly used to describe air quality and refer to the number of particles 0.5 µm or larger per cubic foot of air. Controlled areas are usually Class 10,000 or 100,000, meaning that the air has no more than 10,000 or 100,000 particles 0.5 µm or larger per cubic foot, respectively (see Table 6-2).

These class categories also specify the maximum number of microbes per cubic foot of air. In a Class 10,000 environment, the number is 0.5/cu ft. For Class 100,000 air, the requirement is no more than 2.5 organisms/cu ft.

Critical Areas

Table 6-3 summarizes the environmental requirements for critical areas. Because sterile components are manipulated there to produce final sterile products, the requirements are more stringent than those for controlled areas. For example, airflow velocity across the entire work surface should be maintained at 90 ft/min (±20%). Air particle counts are Class 100 conditions—no more than 100 particles 0.5 µm or larger per cubic foot. Moreover, there should be no more than 0.1 microbial organism/cu ft. To

ensure these conditions, work should not take place until 15 min after the laminar-airflow unit is operational.

MONITORING DEVICES

The seven aspects of the environment can be monitored to determine its quality.

Temperature and Relative Humidity

Temperature and relative humidity can be measured using inexpensive thermometers and hygrometers, respectively. They are readily available from cleanroom suppliers. More expensive devices offer printing capabilities for documenting environmental requirements.

Air Exchange, Percentage of Fresh Air, and Pressure Differential

Air exchange, percentage of fresh air, and pressure differential are usually measured by environmental engineers. Such testing is often performed for operating rooms and other isolated areas but can also be done for the pharmacy. To measure positive differential pressures continuously across adjacent walls, magnahelic gauges can be placed permanently across them.

Table 6-2. *Class Limits[a] in Particles per Cubic Foot (Size Equal to or Greater than Particle Sizes Shown)[b]*

Class	Measured Particle Size, µm				
	0.1	0.2	0.3	0.5	5
1	35	7.5	3	1	NA[c]
10	350	75	30	10	NA
100	NA	750	300	100	NA
1,000	NA	NA	NA	1,000	7
10,000	NA	NA	NA	10,000	70
100,000	NA	NA	NA	100,000	700

[a]These class limit particle concentrations are for definition only and do not necessarily represent the size distribution found in any particular situation.
[b]Reproduced, with permission, from Federal Standard 209E. Washington, DC: U.S. General Services Administration; Sept 11, 1992.
[c]NA = not applicable.

Particulates

Particulates can be measured using one of two techniques: an electronic particle counter or the dioctylphthalate (DOP) aerosol challenge test. Particle counters can evaluate air quality in rooms with Class 10,000 or 100,000 air but are not acceptable for Class 100 conditions (e.g., laminar-airflow hoods).

For Class 100 environments, the DOP aerosol challenge test should be used. The DOP aerosol is introduced upstream of the high-efficiency particulate air (HEPA) filter in a concentration of 80–100 µg/L of air. A photometer probe then scans the entire filter face and frame from about 1.2 in away. A single probe reading equivalent to 0.01% of the upstream challenge indicates a significant leak in the HEPA filter and does not meet Class 100 particulate requirements.

Particulate counters are available at a reasonable cost from cleanroom suppliers. Most pharmacists have their laminar-airflow hoods tested by a vendor who can perform the DOP aerosol test.

Microbial Organisms

Airborne microbes

Microbes in the environment can be measured by either passive or active air sampling. Both of these approaches have a role in monitoring where sterile products are prepared.

For passive air sampling, settling plates—petri dishes with a growth medium (e.g., solid nutrient agar)—are placed in strategic areas. All microorganisms that settle and grow on the plates should be sent to the laboratory for identification.

For active air sampling, a large volume of air is drawn over the growth medium. Three different devices can be used.

Reuter centrifugal sampler. This device draws up to 40 L/min of air through rotary blades, forcing particles against a nutrient agar strip by centrifugal force. It is the most convenient and least expensive of the three devices and is readily available.

Slit-to-agar impaction sampler. This device employs a revolving plate containing the growth medium under a fixed-slot orifice. Air is drawn through the slot over the medium by vacuum. With this device, a concentration–time relationship can be established.

Liquid impingement. With this device, air is drawn into the unit by vacuum. The volume of air is determined by the orifice size. Particles and microorganisms are "impinged" onto the liquid, which is then filtered. The filters are placed on nutrient media and monitored for microbial growth.

Surface microbes

Surfaces used for aseptic processing should also be monitored for microbes. Three techniques are used.

Contact (Rodac) plates. These plates are prepared with an appropriate medium (e.g., solid nutrient agar) whose surface is higher than the sides of the plate. This medium surface is then applied to a smooth, flat test surface and the plate is incubated. This device is suitable for monitoring flat surfaces such as laminar-airflow hoods, floors, and walls.

Swabs. By aseptic technique, swabs are rubbed over a test surface and immersed in a liquid medium. If the surface is contaminated, there will be growth in the medium. Swabs are suited to irregular surfaces, and results are more qualitative than with contact plates.

Agar overlay. A representative surface material is mounted in or near the preparation area and then immersed in a suitable medium. Although this technique is cumbersome, it provides an accurate, quantitative evaluation of residual effects of surface sanitizers.

Surface testing materials may be obtained from the microbiology laboratory or infection surveillance department of most hospitals. Alternatively, these supplies are available from cleanroom vendors.

RECOMMENDED ENVIRONMENTAL TESTING PROGRAM

All Class 100 environments should be certified using the DOP test every 6 months, and documentation of these tests should be maintained. For controlled areas of Class 10,000 or 100,000, particle counters should be used. Particle counts should be measured once per shift, and these records also should be kept.

The United States Pharmacopeial Convention has recommended a microbial monitoring program using passive and active air sampling and surface testing.[4] The recommended program includes a floor plan (see Figure 6-1) and a chart of monitoring devices, typical baseline contamination, and action levels (see Table 6-4). These practical recommendations can be implemented by most pharmacists.

SUMMARY

Current standards of practice warrant a comprehensive environmental monitoring program that exceeds hood certification. The technology to monitor particulates and microbes is simple enough and sufficiently inexpensive to be applicable to current pharmacy practice. Air quality

Table 6-4. *Environmental Microbial Monitoring Program*[4]

Site	Baseline Colony-Forming Units	Low-Risk Action Level	High-Risk Action Level
Settling plates[a]			
A	0,1	3	2
D	2,3	6	4
E	4,5	10	6
J	5	10	7
L	8	15	10
Contact plates			
D	2,3	6	4
E	4,6	10	7
J	6	12	8
L	8	15	10
Slit-to-agar impaction sampler[b]			
A	0,1	3	2
E	5	10	7
H	8	15	10

[a]Based on 3-hr exposure, except 1 hr for A. See Figure 6-1 for site locations.
[b]Based on 10-cu ft samples.

and surface testing should be part of any contemporary sterile products program.

REFERENCES

1. Center for Drugs and Biologics. Guideline on sterile drug products produced by aseptic processing. Rockville, MD: Food and Drug Administration; June 10, 1987.

2. Standards for cleanroom and work status for microbially controlled environments. NHB5340.02. Washington, DC: National Aeronautics and Space Administration; 1967.

3. Lee JY. Environmental requirements for clean rooms. *BioPharm.* 1988; 1 (6):40–3.

4. Sterile drug products for home use. In: United States pharmacopeia, 23rd rev./national formulary, 18th ed. Rockville, MD: United States Pharmacopeial Convention; 1994:1963–75.

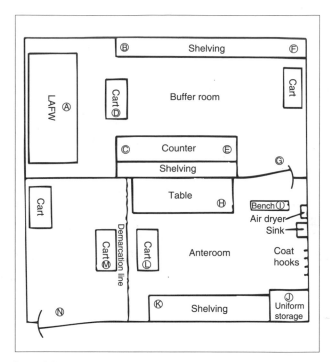

figure 6-1. *Cleanroom floor plan. (Reproduced, with permission, from Reference 4.)*

Chapter 7
Use of Aseptic Technique

Douglas J. Scheckelhoff

The preparation of sterile products requires an "aseptic technique" to maintain sterility. Although this term could describe sterile techniques used in other areas (e.g., surgery and various medical procedures), this chapter only addresses aseptic techniques used in the pharmacy.

While the importance of sterility was first recognized in the late 1800s, the concept of aseptic technique was not described until years later.[1,2] The need to sterilize solutions and equipment became accepted in the 1920s and 1930s.[3–5] Moreover, the development of sterile and pyrogen-free products and their applications continues today.

In the late 1960s, improperly prepared solutions caused a rash of complications in patients receiving IV solutions.[6–11] Following these incidents, the National Coordinating Committee on Large Volume Parenterals (NCCLVP) published recommendations on sterile product techniques for pharmacists and other health professionals.[12–18]

A training manual for IV admixture personnel, largely intended for pharmacy technicians who prepare sterile products, was first published in 1972. This manual was most recently revised in 1990.[19]

The American Society of Health-System Pharmacists [formerly the American Society of Hospital Pharmacists (ASHP)] published a videotape and study guide on aseptic technique in 1985.[20] This combination product was the first comprehensive aseptic guide with practical application to many pharmacy settings. More recently, ASHP and the United States Pharmacopeial Convention (USP) published guidelines regarding aseptic technique and further established practice standards for sterile products (see Appendices 6 and 7).[21,22] ASHP's *Manual for Pharmacy Technicians* also includes a chapter on technician training as it relates to aseptic technique and sterile product preparation.[23] In 1994, ASHP released an updated version of its original videotape and workbook.[24]

PROPER ASEPTIC TECHNIQUE

Aseptic technique describes the methods used to manipulate sterile products so that they remain sterile. Technique is a separate element in the preparation of sterile products, independent from equipment and environment. However, proper technique does not obviate the need for good equipment and proper environment. Conversely, good equipment and an ideal environment do not change the need for a good technique.

Equipment and Environment

In this chapter, the laminar-airflow hood is considered critical equipment for good aseptic technique. Issues related to handling and preparing cytotoxic agents as well as using a biological safety cabinet are not addressed here, but they will be covered in Chapter 9. This chapter generally refers to techniques used in a horizontal versus vertical laminar-airflow hood. Although these hoods are similar, the source and direction of the airflow differ. Vertical flow hoods will be addressed in Chapter 9.

The critical principle to remember in the use of laminar-airflow hoods is that nothing should interrupt the airflow between the high-efficiency particulate air (HEPA) filter and the sterile object. This aseptic compounding space is referred to as the "critical area," and any foreign object can increase wind turbulence within this area. Moreover, contaminants from the foreign object may be blown or carried onto the sterile injection port, needle, or syringe. Large materials placed within the laminar-airflow hood also can disturb the patterned flow of air from the HEPA filter. This "zone of turbulence" created behind an object could extend outside the hood, pulling or allowing contaminated room air into the aseptic environment (see Figure 7-1).

When laminar airflow is accessible to all sides of an object, the zone of turbulence extends approximately three times the diameter of that object. When airflow is not accessible on all sides (e.g., adjacent to a vertical wall), a zone of turbulence may extend six times the diameter of an object. For these reasons, objects should be at least 6 in from the sides and front edge of the hood, without blocking air vents and without obstructing airflow. Hands also should not block airflow.

The following are general principles for proper operation of laminar-airflow hoods:

1. All aseptic manipulations should be performed at least 6 in within the hood. This distance prevents reflected contamination from the worker's body and "backwash" contamination from turbulent air patterns developing at the laminar-airflow hood–room air interface.

2. A laminar-airflow hood should operate continuously. If the hood is turned off, it should not be used for a specified time when reactivated, depending on the manufacturer's recommendations (e.g., 30 min). This downtime allows all room air to be purged from the critical area.

3. Before use, all interior working surfaces of the hood should be cleaned with 70% isopropyl alcohol or another disinfecting agent and a clean, lint-free (nonshedding) cloth. Cleaning should be performed from back to front, so that contaminants are moved away from the HEPA filter. Throughout the compounding period, the hood should be cleaned often. Some materials are not soluble in alcohol and may initially require water for removal. To avoid damage, Plexiglas sides should be cleaned with warm, soapy water rather than alcohol.

4. Nothing should touch the HEPA filter, including cleaning solution, aspirate from syringes, and glass from ampuls. Ampuls should not be broken directly toward the filter.

5. A laminar-airflow hood should be positioned away from excess traffic, doors, air vents, fans, and air currents capable of introducing con-

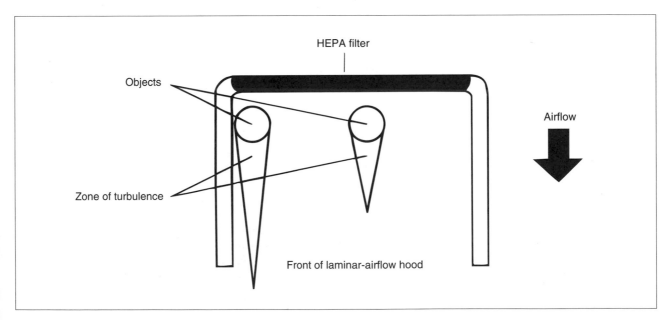

Figure 7-1. *Zones of turbulence.*

taminants.

6. Hand and wrist jewelry should not be worn; jewelry may introduce bacteria or particles.
7. Actions such as talking and coughing should be directed away from the critical area, and any unnecessary motion should be avoided to minimize airflow turbulence.
8. Only objects that are essential to product preparation should be placed in the hood—no paper, pens, labels, and trays.
9. Laminar-airflow hoods should be tested and certified by qualified personnel every 6 months, whenever the hood is moved, and if filter damage is suspected. Tests can certify airflow velocity and HEPA filter integrity.
10. Food and drink should not be permitted within the aseptic preparation area.

Although the laminar-airflow hood provides a sterile environment, strict aseptic technique must be used to ensure product sterility. The two most critical aspects of aseptic technique are proper hand washing and use and manipulation of syringes, needles, vials, and ampuls.

Hand Washing

Touch is the most common means of contaminating a pharmacy-prepared sterile product. Since the fingers harbor countless bacterial contaminants, hands should be washed properly. Before aseptic manipulations are performed, the hands, nails, wrists, and forearms should be scrubbed vigorously for at least 10–15 sec (longer if visibly soiled) with a brush, warm water, and bactericidal soap.[25]

Hand-washing agents should be selected based on their ability to kill microorganisms on the hands at the time of washing and also to provide a residual effect. A solution of 4% chlorhexidine gluconate is one of the best agents for initially reducing resident flora and transient microorganisms and also providing great residual effects.[26–28]

Results vary with isopropyl alcohol products for initial reduction of microorganisms, but these products clearly have little residual effect. Since most alcohol products are solutions, gels, or foams, they serve as hand disinfectants rather than hand-washing agents. Therefore, hand washing with soap before application of these agents sometimes is recommended. However, this additional step might lower compliance.

Povidone-iodine products have a slightly lower initial reduction in microorganisms and less residual effect compared to chlorhexidine, but they are acceptable as an overall agent. However, these products may cause more irritation and allergic reactions than other agents. Triclosan products and hexachlorophene provide poor initial reduction in microorganisms but have a good residual

effect. Furthermore, use of hexachlorophene over large surfaces of the body has been associated with absorption and related toxicity.

Rotation of hand-washing agents may reduce the development of resistant organisms. However, this theory has not been studied and reported in the literature.

Hands should be washed frequently, especially when the compounding area is reentered, to reduce contamination. Many institutions recommend sterile gloves. However, these gloves are only sterile as long as the wearer does not touch a product or other surface that is not sterile.

In addition to hand washing, aseptic preparation requires the correct use and handling of sterile equipment and supplies, including syringes and needles.

Syringes

Syringes are made of either glass or plastic. Glass syringes are used when medication is to be stored for an extended period and when drug stability is important. Disposable plastic syringes cost less and are used when the contact time is short, minimizing the potential for incompatibility with the plastic. Glass syringes made for reuse have virtually been replaced by disposables. These disposables cost less, eliminate the risk of transmitting blood-borne pathogens, and do not break.

Syringes are composed of a barrel and plunger (see Figure 7-2). The plunger, which fits inside the barrel, has a flat disk or lip at one end and a rubber piston at the other. The top collar of the barrel prevents the syringe from slipping during manipulation, while the tip is where the needle attaches. Many syringes have a locking mechanism (e.g., Luer-lok) at the tip, which secures the needle within a threaded ring. In other cases, the needle is held only by friction.

Syringes are available in numerous sizes, with volumes ranging from 0.5 to 60 ml. Graduation marks represent different increments, depending on the size of the syringe. If the syringe capacity is large, the intervals between graduation lines usually are large. For example, each line on 10-ml syringes represents 0.2 ml; on a 30-ml syringe, each line represents 1 ml.

To maximize accuracy, the smallest syringe that can hold a desired amount of solution should be used. Syringes are accurate to one-half of the smallest increment marking on the barrel. For example, a 10-ml syringe with 0.2-ml markings is accurate to 0.1 ml and can be used to measure a volume of 3.1 ml accurately. A 30-ml syringe with 1-ml markings, however, is accurate to 0.5 ml and should not be used to measure a volume of 3.1 ml.

When measuring with a syringe, the user should line up the final edge of the plunger piston to the desired graduation mark on the barrel (see Figure 7-3). To maintain sterility, two parts of a syringe cannot be touched: the tip and plunger.

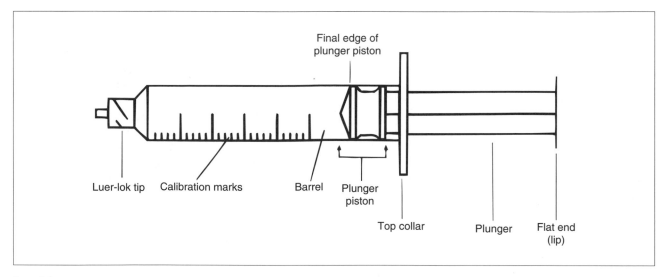

figure 7-2. *Parts of a syringe.*

Syringes are sent from the manufacturer already assembled and individually packaged in paper overwraps or plastic covers. The sterility of the contents is guaranteed as long as the outer package remains intact. Therefore, these packages should be inspected for holes or tears and discarded if damaged. The syringe package should be opened within the laminar-airflow hood to maintain sterility. To minimize contamination, however, the discarded packaging should not be laid on any surface within the hood.

Most syringes also are packaged with a protector over the tip. This protector should be left in place until needle attachment. When needles are attached to Luer-lok-type syringes, a quarter turn should secure them.

Needles

Like syringes, needles are commercially available in many sizes. These sizes are described by two numbers, gauge and length. The gauge of the needle corresponds to the diameter of its bore. The smallest needles have a gauge of 27, while the largest needles have a gauge of 13. The length of a needle shaft usually ranges from $3/8$ to $3\frac{1}{2}$ in.

The components of a simple needle are the shaft and the hub (see Figure 7-4). The hub attaches the needle to the syringe and often is color coded for a specific gauge size. The tip of the needle shaft is slanted to form a point; this slant is called the bevel, and the point is the bevel tip. The opposite end of the slant is the bevel heel.

figure 7-3. *Syringe markings on the barrel with 1.5 ml withdrawn.*

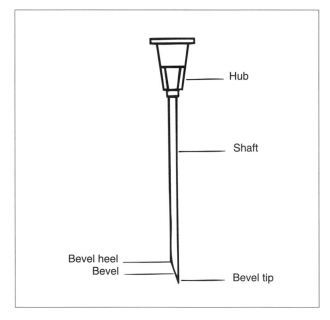

figure 7-4. *Parts of a needle.*

Needles are sent from the manufacturer individually packaged in paper and plastic overwraps. Sterility is guaranteed as long as the package remains intact. Therefore, damaged packages should be discarded. The hub of the needle should not be touched when removing the overwrap.

A needle shaft usually is metal and is lubricated with a sterile silicone coating for smooth, easy access into latex vial tops. Therefore, needles should never be swabbed with alcohol or touched. They should be handled by their protective covers only, and these covers should be left in place until the needles or syringes are used.

Vials

Injectable medications usually are supplied in vials or ampuls, each requiring different techniques for withdrawal of the medication. A vial is a plastic or glass container with a rubber stopper secured to its top by a metal ring. Unlike single-dose vials, multidose vials contain preservatives that allow their contents to be used after the rubber stopper is punctured. This stopper usually is protected by a flip-top cap or metal cover, but most caps do not guarantee sterility of the rubber closure. Therefore, all vials should be swabbed with 70% isopropyl alcohol before entry and left to dry. The correct technique is several firm strokes in the same direction over the rubber closure, using a clean, unused portion of a swab on each pass. The swabbing is effective in two ways:

- ❑ The alcohol acts as a disinfecting agent.
- ❑ The physical act of swabbing in one direction removes particles from the vial diaphragm.

Bottles or trays of isopropyl alcohol should not be used. Because alcohol may harbor resistant spores, repeated use of a nonsterile tray or bottle could promote this problem. Individually packaged swabs are sterile from the manufacturer.

When vials are pierced with needles, cores or fragments of the rubber closure can form. To prevent this problem, the needle should be inserted so that the rubber closure is penetrated at the same point with both the tip and heel of the bevel. This noncoring technique is accomplished by first piercing the rubber closure with the bevel tip and then applying lateral (away from the bevel) and downward pressure to insert the needle (see Figure 7-5).

Vials are closed-system containers, since air or fluid cannot pass freely in or out of them. Therefore, the volume of fluid to be removed from a vial should be replaced with an equal volume of air to minimize a vacuum. But this technique should not be used with drugs that produce gas when they are reconstituted (e.g., ceftazidime).

If the drug within a vial is in a powdered form, reconstitution must be performed first. The desired volume of the diluting solution or "diluent" (e.g., sterile water for

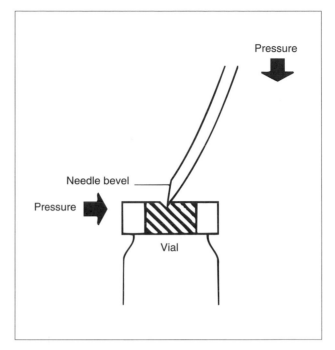

Figure 7-5. *A noncoring method of piercing a vial with a needle.*

injection) is injected into the vial. As the diluent is added, an equal volume of air must be removed to prevent a positive pressure from developing inside the vial. This procedure may be accomplished by allowing air to flow into the syringe before removing the needle from the vial. Although most drugs dissolve rapidly when shaken, personnel must be sure that a drug is completely dissolved before proceeding.

Ampuls

Unlike vials, ampuls are composed entirely of glass. Once ampuls are broken, they become open-system, single-use containers. Since air or fluid may now pass freely in and out of them, the volume of fluid removed does not have to be replaced with air.

Before an ampul is opened, any solution visible in the top portion (head) should be moved to the bottom (body) by one of the following methods:

- ❑ Swirling the ampul in an upright position.
- ❑ Tapping the head with one's finger.
- ❑ Inverting the ampul and then quickly swinging it into an upright position.

To open an ampul properly, its neck should be cleansed with an alcohol swab and the swab should be left in place. This swab can prevent accidental cuts to the fingers as well as spraying of glass particles and aerosolized drug. The head of the ampul should be held between the thumb and index finger of one hand, and the body should be held with the thumb and index finger of the other hand.

Pressure should be exerted on both thumbs, pushing away from oneself in a quick motion to "snap" the ampul open at the neck. Ampuls should not be opened toward the HEPA filter of the laminar-airflow hood or toward other sterile products within the hood. Extreme pressure may result in crushing the head between the thumb and index finger. Therefore, if the ampul does not open easily, it should be rotated so that pressure on the neck is at a different angle.

To withdraw medication from an ampul, it should be tilted and the bevel of the needle placed in the corner space (or shoulder) near the opening. Surface tension should keep the solution from spilling out of the tilted ampul. The syringe plunger is then pulled back to withdraw the solution.

The use of a filter needle (e.g., a needle with a 5-μm filter in the hub) eliminates glass or paint chips that may have fallen into a solution from being drawn up into the syringe. Sometimes, a medication (e.g., a suspension) may need to be withdrawn from an ampul with a regular needle; a filter needle should then be used to push the drug out of the syringe. In all cases, the same filter needle should not be used for both withdrawing and injecting, since it will nullify the filtering effort.

PREPARATION OF A STERILE DOSAGE FORM

Sterile dosage forms may be prepared in various final containers, including flexible plastic bags, glass bottles, semirigid plastic containers, and syringes, or as the drug vial itself. Flexible plastic bags made of polyvinyl chloride (PVC) or polyolefin usually allow easy storage and, compared to glass bottles, decreased breakage and elimination of the need for venting.

PVC bags are available in several sizes and numerous solutions. These bags are supplied in plastic overwraps, which limit fluid loss. Once this overwrap is removed, the remaining solution should be used as soon as possible. The injection port of a PVC bag, covered by a protective rubber tip, should be positioned toward the HEPA filter when an IV admixture is prepared. This positioning minimizes air turbulence in the critical area.

Before compounding, all materials should be assembled. Moreover, vials, ampuls, and IV solution containers should be inspected for cloudiness, particulate matter, cracks or punctures, expiration dates, and any indications of defects. Only necessary materials should be placed within the laminar-airflow hood.

Next, all injection surfaces should be disinfected. Drug fluid should be withdrawn from its container in the amount needed, using the syringe size just larger than the volume to be injected. To obtain an accurate measurement, air bubbles should be removed by the following method:

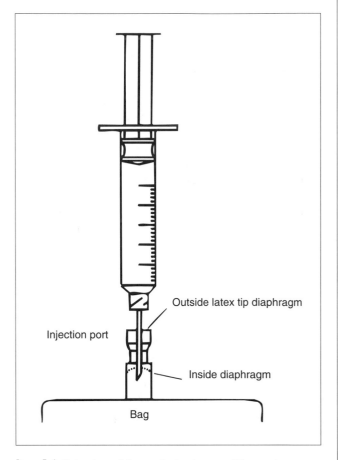

Figure 7-6. *Injection of drug solution into an IV container.*

1. Pulling back slightly on the plunger to remove any fluid trapped in the needle.
2. Tapping the syringe.
3. Depressing the plunger.

The instillation of drug into a PVC bag requires insertion of a needle into the alcohol-swabbed injection port and injection of the appropriate volume of fluid. The injection port has two diaphragms that must be pierced (see Figure 7-6):

❏ Outside latex tip.
❏ Plastic diaphragm about ³/₈ in inside the injection port.

To ensure fluid transfer into the IV bag, a needle longer than ³/₈ in should be used.

The admixture of medication to a glass infusion container begins with removal of the protective cap from the IV bottle. A drug additive then is injected through the alcohol-swabbed rubber stopper or latex diaphragm. Needles should be inserted through rubber stoppers using the noncoring technique previously described for vials. Following admixture, a protective seal is placed over the stopper of a glass container before it is removed from the laminar-airflow hood.

If the final dosage form is a syringe, the needle should be removed and discarded. Moreover, the syringe should be capped with a sterile tip. A small volume of air or overfill may be left in the syringe to allow priming of the needle or tubing prior to administration. The syringe should be placed in a plastic bag or other container for transport, which minimizes the potential for plunger depression and/or leakage.

Syringes and needles used in the preparation of a sterile dosage form should be discarded according to institutional policy. These syringes and needles (uncapped to prevent accidental needlestick) usually should be placed into a puncture-resistant, sealable container for disposal (usually incineration).

Once the sterile product is compounded, it should be properly labeled and inspected for cores and particulates. Furthermore, all drug and IV solution containers should be checked by a pharmacist to verify that the technician added the proper amount of the correct drug to the correct IV solution and affixed the correct label.

SUMMARY

Aseptic technique is a means of manipulating sterile products without contaminating them. Proper use of the laminar-airflow hood, strict aseptic technique, and conscientious work habits are the most important factors in preventing contamination. To ensure accuracy and completeness, the label and final product must be validated by a registered pharmacist before use.

REFERENCES†

1. Griffenhagan GB. The history of parenteral medication. *Bull Parenter Drug Assoc.* 1962; 16:12–9.
2. Howard-Jones N. The origins of hypodermic medication. *Sci Am.* 1971; 224:96–102.
3. Seibert FB. Fever producing substances found in distilled water. *Am J Physiol.* 1923; 67:90–104.
4. Masson AH. The early days of intravenous saline. *Pharm J.* 1976; 217:571–80.
5. Dudrick SJ. Rational intravenous therapy. *Am J Hosp Pharm.* 1971; 28:82–91.
6. Maki DG, Goldmnan DA, Rhame FS. Infection control in intravenous therapy. *Ann Intern Med.* 1973, 79:867–87.
7. Deeb EN, Natsios GA. Contamination of intravenous fluids by bacteria and fungi during preparation and administration. *Am J Hosp Pharm.* 1971; 28:764–7.
8. Letcher K. In use contamination of intravenous solutions in flexible plastic containers. *Am J Hosp Pharm.* 1972; 29:673–7.
9. Curry CR, Quie PG. Fungal septicemia in patients receiving parenteral hyperalimentation. *N Engl J Med.* 1971; 285:1221–5.
10. McGowan JE. Six guidelines for reducing infections associated with IV therapy. *Am Surg.* 1976; 42:713–5.
11. Duma RJ, Latta T. What have we done—the hazards of intravenous therapy. *N Engl J Med.* 1976; 294:1178–80.
12. National Coordinating Committee on Large Volume Parenterals. Recommended methods for compounding intravenous admixtures in hospitals. *Am J Hosp Pharm.* 1975; 32:261–70.
13. National Coordinating Committee on Large Volume Parenterals. Recommended system for surveillance and reporting of problems with large-volume parenterals in hospitals. *Am J Hosp Pharm.* 1975; 32:1251–3.
14. National Coordinating Committee on Large Volume Parenterals. Recommendations for the labeling of large volume parenterals. *Am J Hosp Pharm.* 1978; 35:49–51.
15. National Coordinating Committee on Large Volume Parenterals. Recommended procedures for in-use testing of large volume parenterals suspected of contamination or of producing a reaction in a patient. *Am J Hosp Pharm.* 1978; 35:678–82.
16. National Coordinating Committee on Large Volume Parenterals. Recommended guidelines for quality assurance in hospital centralized intravenous admixture services. *Am J Hosp Pharm.* 1980; 37:645–55.
17. National Coordinating Committee on Large Volume Parenterals. Recommended standards of practice, policies, and procedures for intravenous therapy. *Am J Hosp Pharm.* 1980; 37:660–3.
18. Barker KN, ed. Recommendations of the NCCLVP for the compounding and administration of intravenous solutions. Bethesda, MD: American Society of Hospital Pharmacists; 1981.
19. Hunt ML Jr. Training manual for intravenous admixture personnel, 4th ed. Chicago, IL: Baxter Healthcare Corp.; 1990.
20. American Society of Hospital Pharmacists. Aseptic preparation of parenteral products. Bethesda, MD: American Society of Hospital Pharmacists; 1985. Videotape and study guide.
21. American Society of Hospital Pharmacists. ASHP technical assistance bulletin on quality assurance for pharmacy-prepared sterile products. *Am J Hosp Pharm.* 1993; 50:2386–98.
22. Sterile drug products for home use. In: United States pharmacopeia, 23rd rev./national formulary, 18th ed.

Rockville, MD: United States Pharmacopeial Convention; 1994:1963–75.

23. American Society of Hospital Pharmacists. Manual for pharmacy technicians. Bethesda, MD: American Society of Hospital Pharmacists; 1993.

24. American Society of Hospital Pharmacists. Quality assurance of pharmacy-prepared sterile products. Bethesda, MD: American Society of Hospital Pharmacists; 1994. Videotape and workbook.

25. Garner JS, Favero MS. CDC guidelines for the prevention and control of nosocomial infections. Guideline for handwashing and hospital environmental control, 1985. *Am J Infect Control.* 1986; 14 (3):110–29.

26. Ayliffe GAJ, Babb JR, Davies JG, et al. Hand disinfection: a comparison of various agents in laboratory and ward studies. *J Hosp Infect.* 1988; 11:226–43.

27. Reybrouck G. Handwashing and hand disinfection. *J Hosp Infect.* 1986; 8:5–23.

28. Doebbeling BN, Stanley GL, Sheetz CT, et al. Comparative efficacy of alternative hand-washing agents in reducing nosocomial infections in intensive care units. *N Engl J Med.* 1992; 327:88–93.

---

†*This chapter was partially adapted from References 20 and 23 (Chapter 9).*

Chapter 8
Personnel Behavior and Garb Use

Barbara T. McKinnon

By itself, strict adherence to aseptic technique cannot prevent microbial contamination during the compounding of sterile products. Personnel behavior and proper garb use are also critical factors.

PERSONNEL PREPARATION

Proper preparation for performing assigned responsibilities includes personal dress and grooming. Prior to entering the aseptic compounding area, personnel should remove outer laboratory jackets and cover both their head and facial hair. Cosmetics that are likely to flake, such as powder and mascara, also should be removed. Similarly, hair spray, perfume, and other scented cosmetics should not be used. Furthermore, finger and wrist jewelry should be minimized or eliminated.[1]

Health Status

Employees involved in compounding should be free of infectious diseases that can be transmitted through contaminated products. Especially harmful to the compounding environment are individuals with respiratory ailments accompanied by fluid discharge, sneezing, or excessive perspiration. Similarly, conditions that cause shedding of skin particles, such as rashes and sunburn, increase the risk of contamination. While severely afflicted, the employee should be excluded from aseptic compounding activities.[2]

Hand Washing

Hand washing can prevent personnel-transmitted infections.[3] Before compounding, personnel should scrub hands and arms to the elbows with an appropriate cleanser. Although the Centers for Disease Control and Prevention[4] (CDC) and the United States Pharmacopeial Convention[2] (USP) recommend the use of plain soap and water, the American Society of Health-System Pharmacists (ASHP) suggests an antimicrobial skin cleanser.[1] Plain soap and water may not provide enough protection in high-risk situations.

Antimicrobial cleansing products

Five antimicrobial ingredients currently are available as hand-washing products:

❑ Alcohols.

❏ Chlorhexidine gluconate.
❏ Iodophors.
❏ Parachlorometaxylenol.
❏ Triclosan.

Hexachlorophene was widely used in the 1970s but is no longer recommended because of its limited coverage and potential toxicity.[3]

Although alcohols effectively disinfect skin, they may cause drying and discomfort. Newer emollient-containing preparations may be more acceptable. Alcohol rinses or foams, however, may be helpful for periodically disinfecting hands during work activities.

Chlorhexidine gluconate also is an effective disinfectant but is slower acting than alcohol. Moreover, several applications may be required to reduce flora significantly. Chlorhexidine has some residual antimicrobial activity, and it is better tolerated than alcohol during frequent washings.

Iodophors, commonly used for surgical scrubbing, are excellent antibacterials. Their relative harshness to the skin and staining properties, however, limit their routine use.

Triclosan and parachlorometaxylenol, although less effective than the other agents, are mild and produce some sustained residual activity.[3]

When a hand-washing product is chosen, safety, efficacy, cost, comfort, and the concentration of the active ingredient are the most important considerations. Alcohols and chlorhexidine are most effective at concentrations of 60–90% and 2–4%, respectively. Iodophors generally contain 7.5% free iodine, although lower concentrations may be effective.[5] Triclosan and parachlorometaxylenol are active at 1% and higher.[3] Once an agent is selected, it may be cost effective to use it throughout the health care facility.

Duration, frequency, and preparation

The duration, frequency, and technique of hand washing are all important factors. To ensure that the topical antimicrobial has the desired effect, an adequate amount must be used for at least 10 sec.[4] In one study, bacterial counts dropped significantly on hands of persons who used 3–5 ml of antimicrobial soap compared with persons using only 1 ml.[6]

Hand washing more than eight times per day with an antimicrobial product has been reported to reduce bacterial counts.[7] However, neither increasing the volume of product or the frequency of washing provided further benefits when plain soap was used.

Finally, the prewashing preparation is important. Since most microbes come from beneath the fingernails, nails should be trimmed short and scrubbed carefully. Rings should not be worn because they increase bacterial counts on the hands,[8] interfere with washing, and may tear gloves.

Other factors that discourage effective hand washing, such as artificial nails and nail polish, also should be avoided.[3]

Hand washing is sometimes incorrectly omitted when gloves are worn, the assumption being that they provide enough protection. In fact, microorganisms multiply rapidly inside warm moist gloves and then can leak through them. The leakage rate is more than 50% when gloves are stressed during use.[9] For this reason, the CDC has stated that gloving does not replace hand washing and that hand washing is imperative after gloves are removed.[10]

GLOVES AND GLOVING

Gloves—of various materials and thicknesses—are available in powdered, nonpowdered, sterile, and nonsterile versions. Controversy exists as to whether operators should use sterile gloves during aseptic compounding. A primary disadvantage of these gloves is that wearers may believe that the gloves remain sterile during operations when they do not. They contain bacteria-laden particles that may be shed, even from properly scrubbed hands.[1] Actually, the gloves are not sterile once they contact the air outside the laminar-airflow hood, supplies, work counters, and other surfaces that are clean but not sterile.

Some authorities believe that, instead of wearing gloves, personnel should work with clean, scrubbed, and disinfected hands and develop manipulation techniques that keep the fingers and hands away from critical sites. In this situation, hands should be wiped with foam alcohol or another suitable disinfectant periodically. Sterile latex gloves are recommended, however, if the drugs being handled are allergenic or hazardous.[11]

When gloves are used, their selection should be based on the type of compounding to be performed as well as on the material's durability, reliability, comfort, and protection from bacteria or hazardous drug penetration. Glove composition significantly impacts performance. In one study, latex and vinyl gloves from five manufacturers were compared. Disposable gloves (often vinyl) had a substantially greater rate of visible defects, bacterial penetration, and failure in use than did surgical gloves. Latex surgical gloves performed much better under normal use.[9]

Glove Recommendations

Sterile versus nonsterile gloves

Sterile gloves are recommended for Risk Levels 2 and 3 compounding activities[1] and for compounding sterile products for home use.[2] Nonsterile gloves, wiped with a disinfectant, may be acceptable for low-risk compounding or to protect hands during cleaning activities and while handling nonsterile supplies or equipment. During sterile product preparation, all gloves should be rinsed thoroughly with a disinfectant (e.g., sterile 70% isopropyl alcohol) and changed if punctured, torn, or contaminated.[1]

Sterile gloves are available packaged in individual pairs or in bulk and in hand-specific or ambidextrous styles. Hand-specific gloves fit more comfortably for long periods, but ambidextrous gloves are cheaper. Individually packaged glove pairs provide better assurance of sterility but at the cost of increased particulates when the paper packaging is opened. Some new products come in polyethylene bags to minimize particulate shedding.

Powdered versus nonpowdered gloves

Powdered gloves increase the particulate level of filtered air within laminar-airflow hoods or other high-efficiency particulate air (HEPA) filtered work stations. A powder residue also can be deposited on supplies, products, and hands. Therefore, powdered gloves should be avoided. If only powdered gloves are available, all powder should be washed off the outside of the glove before work is started, and hands should be washed once gloves are removed.[12]

Protective Value

Because of less than perfect technique, spills, and container breakage, appropriate gloves are necessary to protect workers from hazardous drugs.[12] Gloves provide some protection against skin contact with irritants, vesicants, and drugs, including cyclophosphamide, that are systemically absorbed through the skin.[13]

Various glove materials have been evaluated for drug penetration. Permeability varies with the drug, contact time, and material. No glove material is impervious to all drugs or even statistically superior.

Glove thickness

Gloves come in various thicknesses:

- ❑ 3 mils—light weight.
- ❑ 5 mils—normal weight.
- ❑ 6.5 mils or more—heavy weight.

A thick glove material is optimal.[14–17] A lightweight glove can tear and compromise both the worker's and the product's safety. Fingertips of special chemotherapy gloves may be up to 18 mils thick, and double gloving is not necessary with them.

Hazardous use

Workers should wear powder-free, disposable, surgical latex gloves when preparing hazardous drugs.[12] The practice of double gloving is also recommended, but wearing single gloves that are sufficiently protective is acceptable. For double gloving, surgical latex gloves may fit best and have adequate elasticity while allowing tactile sensation for aseptic manipulations.[12] Fresh gloves should be worn when beginning any task involving hazardous drugs.

When double gloving, personnel should place one glove under the gown cuff and one over it. The glove and gown should completely cover all skin on the arm and wrist. The outer glove should be changed immediately if contaminated. Both gloves should be changed when the outer glove is torn, punctured, or overtly contaminated with drug (as in a spill) or every hour during continuous operations.

When gloves are removed, the contaminated glove fingers should not touch the inside of the glove or the skin. To limit transfer of contamination from the biological safety cabinet (BSC) to the work area, outer gloves should be removed and placed in a sealable container for disposal.[12]

GARMENTS

When garments are selected, the products to be prepared, type of compounding facility, and cost all must be considered. To be most efficient, garments should be appropriate for the majority of products compounded, with only minor revisions (e.g., donning of double gloves for chemotherapy compounds).

Coats

Laboratory coats made of a low-particulate material (e.g., polyester) are adequate for compounding low-risk products (lab coats worn elsewhere in the facility are not acceptable for compounding areas). Because of particulate shedding, sleeves should be fitted with elastic cuffs—not ribbed knit fabric.

Sleeve covers are an alternative to lab coats for compounding in a laminar-airflow hood or BSC. To minimize particulate contamination from clothing, sleeve covers often are worn with clean uniforms ("scrubs").

Gowns and Coveralls

Gowns and coveralls should be made of a low-particulate material that protects against bacterial passage and drug permeability. The fabric must act as a filter, removing particles and fibers released from the wearer's clothing. The tighter the fabric weave, the more particles are removed. However, the tighter the weave, the harder it usually is for the garment to breathe, making the wearer feel warmer.[18]

Tyvek has been the standard for nonpermeable garments. It provides excellent protection against bacterial penetration (99.9% filtered). Special gowns for chemotherapy compounding are coated with an impervious material (e.g., Saranex-laminated Tyvek or polyethylene-coated Tyvek) to increase their protection against drug penetration.[19]

Newer washable, reusable gowning materials, such

as multifilament high-density polyester taffeta, provide comparable bacterial filtration to Tyvek with improved appearance. The breathability of such fabrics allows the evaporation of perspiration, enhancing worker comfort. These garments can be laundered—withstanding high temperatures and chlorine—and are steam autoclave, ethylene oxide, and gamma radiation compatible for sterilization.[20]

Shoe Covers

Shoe covers should be put on before the feet touch the floor on the "clean" side of a bench or line of demarcation. Most pharmacists use slip-on shoe covers; for high-risk compounding, however, some pharmacists prefer ankle-high booties for complete coverage between pant cuffs and shoes.

Masks

Masks should be donned just prior to work at a horizontal laminar-airflow workbench because normal talking, sneezing, or coughing generates air velocities that exceed the velocity of air from the workbench. Masks are optional in a vertical flow BSC where a solid transparent shield establishes a physical barrier between the operator's face and workspace.[2] A tightly fitting surgical mask provides some barrier protection against bacteria, but its protective properties are reduced when wet. Masks should be changed each time personnel leave the compounding area and whenever their integrity is compromised.

Surgical masks provide no protection against the inhaling of powdered or aerosolized hazardous drugs.[12]

When such agents are handled outside a BSC (e.g., during a spill cleanup), an approved[21] air-purifying half-mask respirator and eye protection should be worn.

GOWNING PROCEDURES

Garb and Garment Selection

Recommendations for aseptic compounding garb are found in Table 8-1. Selection of appropriate garments is based on the risk level (see Chapter 1) of the products to be prepared[1] as well as the cleanliness level required in the compounding area.

Risk Level 1 garb

Low-risk products often are compounded in a Class 100 laminar-airflow hood in a limited-access area. Clean clothing, low in particulates, should be worn. Clothing that produces lint, such as fuzzy sweaters, should be avoided. Some practitioners choose to wear uniforms (e.g., scrub suits), because typical clothing may carry a substantial particulate load after contact with environmental pollutants, cigarette smoke, pets, etc.

For compounding activities, a clean gown or closed coat with elastic sleeve cuffs is recommended.[1] Masks and hair coverings, including beard covers if necessary, should be worn. Hands and arms should be scrubbed to the elbows with an appropriate antimicrobial skin cleanser.[1] Workers in the anteroom or other limited-access area, who are not actually compounding products, may wear clean low-particulate clothing and hair covers.

Table 8-1. *Recommendations for Aseptic Compounding Garb*

Activity	Clean, Low-Particulate Clothing	Gown or Coat with Elastic Cuffs	Hair Cover	Mask	Gloves	Double Gloves	Shoe Covers	Coverall	Approved Respirator	Goggles
Risk Level 1 product preparation	✔	✔	✔	✔						
Risk Level 2 product preparation	✔	✔	✔	✔	✔		✔			
Risk Level 3 product preparation	✔		✔	✔	✔		✔	✔		
Chemotherapy compounding	✔	✔ᵃ				✔				✔
Chemotherapy spill handling		✔ᵇ			✔		✔	✔ᵇ	✔	✔

ᵃDisplosable.

ᵇEither gown or coverall is acceptable.

Risk Level 2 garb

For Risk Level 2 compounding, all requirements for Risk Level 1 should be met. Gloves, gowns or closed coats, hair covers, and masks should be worn. Shoe covers also are recommended to help maintain cleanliness of controlled areas.[1]

Risk Level 3 garb

For Risk Level 3 compounding, full cleanroom garb is necessary. Attire should consist of a low-shedding coverall, head cover, face mask, and shoe covers as well as sterile gloves. If personnel leave the controlled or support area during processing, they should regown with clean garments before reentering.

Gowning Techniques

Proper gowning techniques protect the compounding environment and allow the correct garments to perform optimally. Gowning normally takes place in an anteroom equipped for hand washing and storage of both personal clothes and cleanroom garments. To enter the gowning area, employees should walk over an adhesive mat; this mat removes loose particles from shoes. Outer personal garments are then stored, and scrubs or other uniforms are donned. Jewelry and makeup should be removed, and hands should be washed thoroughly before cleanroom garments are worn.

Gowning order

Low-risk compounding. Ideally, gowning should be performed from the head down before the compounding area is entered.

1. Hair should be covered with a bouffant head cover to confine particles released from hair and to keep hair from protruding into the compounding area.
2. A mask (and beard cover if needed) must be worn.
3. Shoe covers should be donned before a gown or closed coat to capture particles on shoes.

High-risk compounding. Typically, the order of gowning for high-risk compounding, assuming shoe covers and a hair cover are in place before the compounding area is entered, would be

1. Hood.
2. Face mask.
3. Coverall.
4. Overboots or a second pair of shoe covers.
5. Gloves.

A hood minimizes shedding of particles from the head, particularly if open reservoir mixing is planned. To wear a detachable face mask, the nose piece should be bent first to ensure a snug facial fit and then the strings should be tied on the outside of the hood or hair cover. Goggles then can be added for eye protection.

Preventing contamination

Cleanroom garments should never touch or drag on the floor—they could carry dirt and particles into the cleanroom. The garment's outside surface should be kept as clean as possible. When coveralls are donned, the hems should be turned up several inches to prevent pant legs from touching the floor. If sterile garments are used for high-risk compounding, personnel should don gloves before handling these garments to protect them from contamination by body secretions and skin flakes.

When donning shoe covers or overboots for high-risk compounding, some practitioners use a bench between clean and nonclean areas. With both feet on the nonclean side of the bench, a shoe cover is carefully placed on one foot and this leg then is transferred to the clean side. The process is repeated for the other foot.

Finally, cleanroom gloves should be donned. For the first glove, only the upper cuff area should be touched—and as little as possible. Only sterile areas of the second glove should be touched by sterile areas of the previously gloved hand. For maximum reduction of particulate shedding, the second glove should be placed over the sleeve. For maximum chemical protection, the second glove should be placed under the sleeve.

Garment Fit and Integrity

Cleanroom garments must fit properly to prevent their billowing as well as the shedding of particles through openings. Garment cuffs should form a snug seal. To check this seal, a noncontaminating pencil-sized object can be slid between the wrist and the cuff with the arm hanging straight down. A properly fitting garment will hold the object. Similarly, if the collar is too large, particles will be emitted. The collar should be snug but not uncomfortable.

The use of rewashable garments has been prompted by environmental concerns. Although scrubs and uniforms can be washed by normal laundry procedures, they should be separated from other contaminated laundry (e.g., patients' linens). Low-particulate coats or coveralls, of Tyvek or high-density polyester, may be laundered but only by a special cleanroom laundry service to avoid introduction of particulates. Normally, hair covers, masks, shoe covers, and gloves are disposed after a single use.

Reusable cleanroom garments should be inspected regularly, and any damage should be promptly repaired. Particles may leak through garment holes or from weak and broken garment fibers. Regular inspection and repair will extend a garment's life and help protect sterile products from particulates.[22]

SUMMARY

The prevention of contamination in the preparation of sterile products requires more than proper aseptic technique. Personnel must ensure appropriate grooming, hand washing, and attire.

The use of garb—gloves, gowns, hair covers, masks, and shoe covers—is critical in preventing microbial contamination. Both the garments and the gowning technique should be selected based on the risk level of the prepared products.

∽

REFERENCES

1. American Society of Hospital Pharmacists. ASHP technical assistance bulletin on quality assurance for pharmacy-prepared sterile products. *Am J Hosp Pharm.* 1993; 50:2386–98.

2. Sterile drug products for home use. In: United States pharmacopeia, 23rd rev./national formulary, 18th ed. Rockville, MD: United States Pharmacopeial Convention; 1994:1963–75.

3. Larson E. Handwashing: it's essential—even when you use gloves. *Am J Nurs.* 1989; 89:934–9.

4. Garner JS, Favero MS. CDC guidelines for the prevention and control of nosocomial infections. Guidelines for handwashing and hospital environmental control, 1985. *Am J Infect Control.* 1986; 14 (3):110–29.

5. Berkel RL. Increased bactericidal activity of dilute preparations of povidone–iodine solutions. *J Clin Microbiol.* 1982; 15:635–9.

6. Quantity of soap as a variable in handwashing. *Infect Control.* 1987; 8:371–5.

7. Larson E. Persistent carriage of gram-negative bacteria on hands. *Am J Infect Control.* 1981; 9:112–6.

8. Jacobson G. Handwashing: ring wearing and number of microorganisms. *Nurs Res.* 1985; 34:186–8.

9. Korniewicz D. Integrity of vinyl and latex procedure gloves. *Nurs Res.* 1989; 38:144–6.

10. Update: universal precautions for prevention of transmission of human immunodeficiency virus, hepatitis B virus, and other bloodborne pathogens in health-care settings. *MMWR.* 1988; 37 (Jun 24): 377–82, 387–8.

11. Avis KE, Akers MJ. Sterile preparation for the hospital pharmacist. Ann Arbor, MI: Ann Arbor Science Publishers; 1981:4.

12. American Society of Hospital Pharmacists. ASHP technical assistance bulletin on handling cytotoxic and hazardous drugs. *Am J Hosp Pharm.* 1990; 47:1033–49.

13. Hirst M, Tse S, Mills DG, et al. Occupational exposure to cyclophosphamide. *Lancet.* 1984; 1:186–8.

14. Conner TH, Laidlaw JL, Theiss JC, et al. Permeability of latex and polyvinyl chloride gloves to carmustine. *Am J Hosp Pharm.* 1984; 41:676–9.

15. Laidlaw JL, Conner TH, Theiss JC, et al. Permeability of latex and polyvinyl chloride gloves to 20 antineoplastic drugs. *Am J Hosp Pharm.* 1984; 41:2618–23.

16. Slevin ML, Ang LM, Johnston A, et al. The efficiency of protective gloves used in the handling of cytotoxic drugs. *Cancer Chemother Pharmacol.* 1984; 12:151–3.

17. Stoikes ME, Carlson JD, Farris FF, et al. Permeability of latex and polyvinyl chloride gloves to fluorouracil and methotrexate. *Am J Hosp Pharm.* 1987; 44:1341–6.

18. Soules WJ. Considerations in garment selection. *CleanRooms.* 1993; 7:32–8.

19. Laidlaw JL, Conner TH, Theiss JC, et al. Permeability of four disposable protective-clothing materials to seven antineoplastic drugs. *Am J Hosp Pharm.* 1985; 42:2449–54.

20. Araclean Services, Inc. introduces Burlington's high density Maxima barrier fabrics. *Araclean Newsl.* 1993; Oct:1–9.

21. National Institute of Occupational Safety and Health. Respirator decision logic. NIOSH Publication 87-108. Washington, DC: U.S. Department of Health and Human Services; 1987.

22. Goldwater M. The "best-dressed" follow stringent gowning procedures. *CleanRooms.* 1994; 8:22–3.

Chapter 9

Handling, Preparation, and Disposal of Cytotoxic and Hazardous Agents

Douglas J. Scheckelhoff

Some medications, primarily those used for treating cancer, can harm individuals who touch, inhale, or ingest them. These drugs, referred to as "cytotoxic" or "hazardous," require special procedures to minimize the potential for accidental exposure. Immunosuppressants are another group of agents that also may warrant these special procedures.[1,2]

Concerns about the effects of exposure to hazardous agents heightened in the late 1970s and early 1980s, and procedures for proper handling began to be established.[3-7] Articles continue to be published on this subject.[1,8,9]

Direct contact with some antineoplastic agents can cause immediate reactions.[10] For example, nitrogen mustard can irritate mucous membranes, eyes, and skin.[11] Spills of doxorubicin onto abraded skin can result in necrosis and sloughing of tissue.[12] Moreover, exposure to antineoplastics in unventilated areas can result in dizziness, nausea, headache, and allergic reactions.[13,14] Studies also suggest that repeated exposure to small amounts of these drugs may cause organ or chromosome damage, impaired fertility, and cancer.[15-18]

Special procedures used in the handling, preparation, and disposal of cytotoxic and other hazardous agents will be covered in this chapter. The ASHP Technical Assistance Bulletin on Handling Cytotoxic and Hazardous Drugs is a comprehensive source of current information.[19]

HANDLING OF HAZARDOUS DRUGS

Labeling

Steps for preventing accidental exposure begin as soon as hazardous drugs enter a facility. These drugs should be identified by distinctive labels that indicate special handling requirements. The labels should be attached to drug packages as well as their storage shelves, bins, and areas. Access to these areas should be limited to trained, authorized personnel. Separation of the inventory also reduces the potential for errors (e.g., pulling a look-a-like vial from an adjacent drug bin). While prevention of these errors is always important, the ramifications of wrongfully administering a cytotoxic agent warrant the separation.

Staff should be trained to recognize and handle hazardous materials in any form (e.g., intact vials, syringes, and IV bags). Material safety data sheets should be kept on file, and staff should know their location and use.[19]

Storage and Transport

Storage and transport equipment should be designed to minimize breakage. Shelves should have front barriers, and carts should have rims. Hazardous drugs should be kept at eye level or lower and stored in bins. Refrigerated hazardous drugs should be stored separately in individual bins.

The method of transport should prevent container leakage or breakage. All hazardous drug containers must be securely capped or sealed to protect them during transport. If leakage or breakage occurs, special procedures for spill cleanup should be followed (discussed later in this chapter). A hazardous drug should not be transported through a pneumatic tube because the mechanical stress can break the container.

Protective Apparel

The use of protective apparel also minimizes exposure to hazardous drugs. If skin or eye contact occurs, then

- ❑ First aid procedures should be followed.
- ❑ Medical attention should be sought immediately.
- ❑ The injury should be documented.

Every work area should have an eyewash fountain or sink and appropriate first aid equipment.

Several pieces of protective apparel should always be worn, with some variations based on the situation.

Coveralls or gown

The preparer should wear disposable coveralls or a disposable solid-front gown made of low-permeability, lint-free fabric.[19,20] This clothing must have long sleeves and tightly fitting elastic or knit cuffs. Moreover, it should not be worn outside of the work area and should be changed immediately if contaminated.

Gloves

Gloves are essential apparel for all hazardous drug procedures.[19,21–24] Hands should be washed thoroughly before putting on gloves and after removing them. Good quality, disposable, powder-free latex gloves can be used, but surgical latex gloves are preferred because of their fit, elasticity, and tactile sensation. If only powdered gloves are available, the powder should be washed off before work is begun.

One pair of gloves should be tucked under the gown's cuffs, and a second pair should be placed over the cuff. If an outer glove becomes contaminated, it should be changed immediately. Both the inner and outer gloves should be changed immediately if the outer glove is torn, punctured, or heavily contaminated. If only one pair is worn, as in drug administration, the glove should be tucked under or over the cuff so that skin is not exposed.

Shoe and hair covers

Shoe and hair covers should be worn to minimize the potential for particulate contamination.[25]

PREPARATION OF HAZARDOUS DRUGS

The preparation of cytotoxic and other hazardous drugs requires proper manipulative technique as well as protective equipment and materials. Institutional quality-assurance programs should require at least an annual evaluation of hazardous drug-handling skills and knowledge. All personnel, especially women who may be pregnant, should be warned about the possible dangers of repeated exposure.

Biological Safety Cabinets

An important piece of equipment for safely preparing hazardous drugs is the biological safety cabinet (BSC). A horizontal laminar-airflow hood should not be used because the airflow directs particles and aerosolized drug at the preparer.[26,27] Instead, sterile hazardous drugs should be prepared in a Class II BSC.[19,20]

The front air barrier or "curtain" that these cabinets create between the handler and the work zone guards against contamination by drug dust and aerosols. Room air is pulled into the front intake grill and then filtered through a high-efficiency particulate air (HEPA) filter. The air then passes through the work zone, the front intake and rear exhaust grills, and a HEPA filter before it is recirculated or exhausted to the outside. Objects placed on or near the front intake or rear exhaust grills may obstruct airflow and reduce the effectiveness of the cabinet.

Two types of Class II cabinets are used:

- ❑ Type A. About 30% of the air is pumped back into the room after it passes through a HEPA filter (see Figure 9-1). Airflow from the exhaust filters should not be blocked.
- ❑ Type B. Air from the work zone is sent through a HEPA filter and then to the outside of the building through an auxiliary exhaust system (see Figure 9-2). These cabinets offer greater

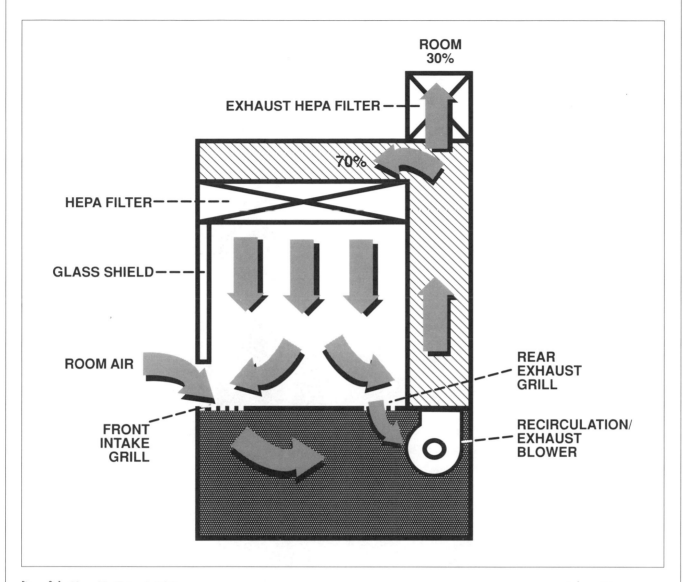

ROOM
30%

EXHAUST HEPA FILTER

70%

HEPA FILTER

GLASS SHIELD

ROOM AIR

FRONT INTAKE GRILL

REAR EXHAUST GRILL

RECIRCULATION/ EXHAUST BLOWER

figure 9-1. *Class II, Type A BSC.*

protection than Type A cabinets because the inward flow of air is faster and the filtered air is sent outside.

BSCs should be located away from traffic and other drafts.[19,25] They must be operated continuously and be inspected and certified every 6 months.[19] The manufacturer's recommendations on operation and maintenance, particularly on replacement of HEPA filters, should be followed.

A BSC should be cleaned and disinfected regularly. It should be cleaned at least after every 8 hr of use or after visible spillage. Water or a solution recommended by the cabinet manufacturer can be used on the work surface, back, and side walls. However, aerosol cleaners can damage the HEPA filters and cabinet.

Before sterile manipulations are performed, the work surface should be disinfected with 70% isopropyl alcohol or other disinfectant and allowed to dry.[25] Although alcohol may remove some substances that water would leave, alcohol is not a good cleaner. Moreover, excessive amounts of alcohol may build up vapors in the cabinet.

During cleaning and disinfection of the hood, the following items should be worn:[19]

- ❏ Gown.
- ❏ Latex gloves.
- ❏ Respirator.
- ❏ Hair cover.
- ❏ Eye protection (the front shield may need to be raised).

The blower should remain on while the hood is cleaned from the top (where contamination is least) to the bottom with heavy toweling or gauze, cleaner, and distilled deionized water. The cover over the HEPA filter should be removed and cleaned within the cabinet. To

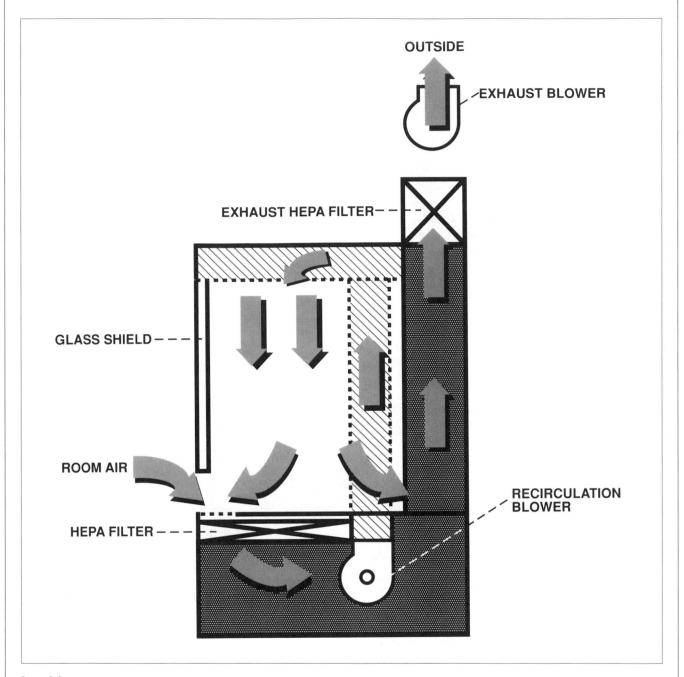

Figure 9-2. **Class II, Type B BSC.**

clean underneath the work tray, it should be leaned against the back wall. The drain spillage trough also needs a thorough scrub. Torn gloves should be changed immediately, and all contaminated waste should be discarded (e.g., cleaner and water containers, protective apparel, and cleaning materials).

Decontamination procedures of BSCs are more involved than routine cleaning and disinfection (see ASHP Technical Assistance Bulletin on Handling Cytotoxic and Hazardous Drugs[19]). BSCs should be decontaminated weekly, before the hood is serviced or moved, and immediately after a large spill.

Procedures

When preparing sterile hazardous drugs in a BSC, personnel should wash their hands and wear a gown with two pairs of latex gloves.[19] The work surface should be disinfected with alcohol. Moreover, the front shield should protect the eyes and face. Some institutions place a plastic-backed liner on the work surface. Although this liner may introduce particles into the work zone, it absorbs any small spills.

Sufficient materials should be assembled for the preparation process to avoid leaving and reentering of the work area.[25] Only necessary items should be present. These objects should not block the downward flow of air (e.g., IV bags or bottles should not be hung above sterile objects). They should be handled well inside the cabinet so as not to be contaminated by unfiltered air at the front air barrier. Air quality is lowest at the sides of the work zone, so manipulations should be performed at least 6 in away from each side wall in the horizontal plane.

If possible, IV sets should be attached to containers and primed before drug is added.[19] Syringes and IV sets with Luer-lok fittings are preferred because they are less likely to separate than friction fittings. Needles are secured to Luer-lok fittings with a quarter turn.

For drugs in vials, pressure can build up inside the vial and cause the drug to spray out around the needle. Therefore, a slight negative pressure should be maintained. Too much negative pressure, however, can cause leakage from the needle when it is withdrawn from the vial. A chemotherapy dispensing pin can help to eliminate pressure buildup. One end of this disposable device is attached to the Luer-lok fitting of the syringe, and its other end is inserted into the drug vial. This device has a venting unit that equalizes pressure, thereby eliminating any buildup.

The constitution of a drug in a vial requires a large enough syringe so that the plunger does not separate from the barrel when filled with solution.[25] After the diluent is drawn up, the needle is inserted into the vial and the plunger is pulled back (to create a slight negative pressure inside the vial) so that air is drawn into the syringe. Small amounts of diluent should be injected slowly as equal volumes of air are removed. The needle should be kept in the vial, and the contents should be swirled carefully until dissolved. With the vial inverted, the proper amount of drug solution should be gradually withdrawn while equal volumes of air are exchanged for solution. Excess drug should remain in the vial. With the vial in the upright position, a small amount of air should be drawn from it into the needle and hub before the needle is removed.

If a hazardous drug is transferred to an IV bag, care must be taken to avoid puncturing of the bag. After the drug solution is instilled into the IV bag, the IV port, container, and set should be wiped with moist gauze and labeled with a warning. For safety, the IV should be placed in a sealable bag to contain any leakage.[19]

To withdraw cytotoxic or hazardous drugs from an ampul, the neck or top portion should be gently tapped.[19] After the neck is sprayed or wiped with alcohol, a 5-μm filter needle should be attached to a syringe that is large enough to hold the drug. Then the fluid should be drawn through the filter needle and cleared from the needle and hub. After this needle is exchanged for a regular one of similar gauge and length, any air and excess drug should be ejected into a sterile vial (leaving the desired volume in the syringe). Aerosols should be avoided. Then the drug may be transferred to an IV bag or bottle. If the dose

is to be dispensed in the syringe, the plunger should be drawn back to clear fluid from the needle and hub. The needle should be replaced with a locking cap, and the syringe should be wiped with moistened gauze and labeled.

If a BSC is not available (e.g., in a low-volume clinic or home), the same preparation procedures should still be followed. The hazardous drug should be prepared in a quiet, low-traffic area, away from drafts and other personnel. A careful preparation technique is then even more critical to maintain product sterility and avoid contamination.

The drug should be prepared on a disposable, plastic-backed absorbent liner. A gown or coveralls, eye protection, double gloves, and a respirator are essential. The same procedures should be used to prevent drug dusts and aerosols. Moreover, pressure inside the vials should be equalized with the atmosphere so that drug is not sprayed. Ordinary venting needles should be avoided because fluid and powder can escape. A 0.2-μm hydrophobic filter venting unit is desirable. Lastly, contaminated equipment and apparel should be disposed of appropriately.

WASTE DISPOSAL AND SPILL CLEANUP OF HAZARDOUS DRUGS

Institutional policies and procedures should be established for the identification, containment, collection, segregation, and disposal of hazardous waste.[19] This waste should be disposed of in separate containers and handled only with uncontaminated gloves. Regular trash should not be placed in hazardous waste containers.

All glass fragments and needles (unclipped) should be placed in a puncture- and leak-resistant container. All other materials, including the outer pair of gloves, should be placed in sealable plastic bags. All waste containers should be sealed before being removed from the BSC and then disposed of in designated, labeled containers. Finally, the gown and then the inner pair of gloves should be removed and discarded. When the gloves are removed, the fingertips and the insides of the gloves should not touch the skin. Then hands should be washed.

All persons who handle hazardous drugs must be oriented and prepared to handle spills. Spills, as well as routine drug preparation and administration, generate contaminated waste. In the event of a hazardous drug spill, a "spill kit" should be used and the cleanup should follow established procedures.[19] Kits should be assembled and accessible in any area where hazardous drugs are handled.

Spill kits should contain protective gear—eye protection, respirator, utility and latex gloves, disposable gown or coveralls, and shoe covers. These kits also should contain the equipment needed to clean up the spill—disposable scoop, puncture- and leak-resistant plastic container for glass fragments, absorbent spill pads, gauze and disposable toweling, absorbent powder, and sealable, plastic disposal bags.

A warning sign should be posted in the area to alert other people of the hazard. All protective apparel should be worn (e.g., latex gloves covered by utility gloves), and all broken glass should be placed in the appropriate container. Liquids should be absorbed with disposable towels or spill pads; powders should be removed with dampened towels or gauze. The contaminated surface should be rinsed with water, washed with detergent, and then rinsed again (starting at the outside of the spill and working toward the center). All contaminated materials belong in sealable, plastic disposal bags.

Institutional policies and procedures also should be established for handling spills in carpeted areas. Absorbent powder and "hazardous drug only" vacuum cleaners should be available.

If a large spill occurs in a BSC, certain additional steps must be taken. The spill kit previously described should be used. Utility gloves are required for handling broken glass. The drain spillage trough should be thoroughly cleaned and the cabinet should be decontaminated, if necessary. All contaminated materials should be sealed in hazardous waste containers while inside the cabinet and then transferred to leak-resistant containers. The circumstances and handling of spills also must be documented.

Hazardous waste must be stored in leak-resistant containers until disposal in accordance with state and local regulations as well as institutional policy.[19,28] Unless these regulations are more restrictive, hazardous substances usually are classified as either trace- or bulk-contaminated waste. Bulk waste is defined as containers that hold more than 3% (by weight) of the total capacity of the container. These waste containers should be stored in sealed, leak-proof receptacles until they can be disposed of through an EPA-approved mechanism (e.g., special landfill sites and incineration). Trace-contaminated containers with 3% or less waste (e.g., empty drug vials and IV bags) are sent through normal trash disposal.

SUMMARY

Use of the proper technique in handling hazardous materials can greatly reduce exposure risks to health care workers. They must be trained to label, store, and transport these agents properly. They also must be familiar with proper protective apparel and BSCs. Similarly, health care workers must understand the differences in preparation, cleanup, and disposal of these agents versus other sterile products.

REFERENCES†

1. Arrington DM, McDiarmid MA. Comprehensive program for handling hazardous drugs. *Am J Hosp Pharm.* 1993; 50:1170–4.

2. McDiarmid MA, Gurley HT, Arrington D. Pharmaceuticals as hospital hazards: managing the risks. *J Occup Med.* 1991; 33:155–8.

3. Zimmerman PF, Larsen RK, Barley EW, et al. Recommendations for the safe handling of injectable antineoplastic drug products. *Am J Hosp Pharm.* 1981; 38:1693–5.

4. Wilson JP, Solimando DA. Aseptic technique as a safety precaution in the preparation of antineoplastic agents. *Hosp Pharm.* 1981; 16:575–81.

5. American Society of Hospital Pharmacists. Procedures for handling cytotoxic drugs. Bethesda, MD: American Society of Hospital Pharmacists; 1983.

6. Stolar MH, Power LA, Viele CS. Recommendations for handling cytotoxic drugs in hospitals. *Am J Hosp Pharm.* 1983; 40:1163–71.

7. U.S. Public Health Service, National Institutes of Health. Recommendations for the safe handling of parenteral antineoplastic drugs. NIH Publication 83-2621. Washington, DC: U.S. Department of Health and Human Services; 1983.

8. Power LA, Anderson RW, Coropassi R, et al. Update on safe handling of hazardous drugs: the advice of the experts. *Am J Hosp Pharm.* 1990; 47:1050–60.

9. McDiarmid MA. Medical surveillance for antineoplastic-drug handlers. *Am J Hosp Pharm.* 1990; 47:1061–6.

10. Occupational Safety and Health Administration. OSHA workplace guidelines for personnel dealing with cytotoxic (antineoplastic) drugs. *Am J Hosp Pharm.* 1986; 43:1193–204.

11. Levantine A, Almeydda J. Cutaneous reactions to cytostatic agents. *Br J Dermatol.* 1974; 90:239–42.

12. Rudolph R, Suzuki M, Luce JK. Experimental skin necrosis produced by Adriamycin. *Cancer Treat Rep.* 1979; 63:529–37.

13. Crudi CB. A compounding dilemma: I've kept the drug sterile but have I contaminated myself? *Natl Intraven Ther J.* 1980; 3:77–80.

14. Reynolds RD, Ignoffo R, Lawrence J, et al. Adverse reactions to AMSA in medical personnel. *Cancer Treat Rep.* 1982; 66:1885.

15. Bingham E. Hazards to healthcare workers from antineoplastic drugs. *N Engl J Med.* 1985; 313:1120–1.

16. Falck K, Grohn P, Sorsa M, et al. Mutagenicity in urine of nurses handling cytostatic drugs. *Lancet.* 1979; 1:1250–1.

17. Waksvik H, Klepp O, Brogger A. Chromosome analysis of nurses handling cytostatic agents. *Cancer Treat Rep.* 1981; 65:607–10.

18. Selevan SG, Lindbohm ML, Hornung RW, et al. A

study of occupational exposure to antineoplastic drugs and fetal loss in nurses. *N Engl J Med.* 1985; 313:1173–8.

19. American Society of Hospital Pharmacists. ASHP technical assistance bulletin on handling cytotoxic and hazardous drugs. *Am J Hosp Pharm.* 1990; 47:1033–49.

20. Laidlaw JL, Conner TH, Theiss JC, et al. Permeability of four disposable protective-clothing materials to seven antineoplastic drugs. *Am J Hosp Pharm.* 1985; 42:2449–54.

21. Conner TH, Laidlaw JL, Theiss JC, et al. Permeability of latex and polyvinyl chloride gloves to carmustine. *Am J Hosp Pharm.* 1984; 41:676–9.

22. Slevin ML, Ang LM, Johnston A, et al. The efficiency of protective gloves used in the handling of cytotoxic drugs. *Cancer Chemother Pharmacol.* 1984; 12:151–3.

23. Stoikes ME, Carlson JD, Farris FF, et al. Permeability of latex and polyvinyl chloride gloves to fluorouracil and methotrexate. *Am J Hosp Pharm.* 1987; 44:1341–6.

24. Laidlaw JL, Conner TH, Theiss JC, et al. Permeability of latex and polyvinyl chloride gloves to 20 antineoplastic drugs. *Am J Hosp Pharm.* 1984; 41: 2618–23.

25. American Society of Hospital Pharmacists. ASHP technical assistance bulletin on quality assurance for pharmacy-prepared sterile products. *Am J Hosp Pharm.* 1993; 50:2386–98.

26. Commissioner, Federal Supply Service, General Services Administration. Clean room and work station requirements, controlled environments. Federal Standard 209c. Washington, DC: U.S. Government Printing Office; 1988.

27. Avis KE, Levchuk JW. Special considerations in the use of vertical laminar-flow workbenches. *Am J Hosp Pharm.* 1984; 41:81–7.

28. Vaccari PL, Tonat K, DeChristoforo R, et al. Disposal of antineoplastic wastes at the National Institutes of Health. *Am J Hosp Pharm.* 1984; 41:87–93.

†*This chapter was partially adapted from: American Society of Hospital Pharmacists. Safe handling of cytotoxic and hazardous drugs study guide. Bethesda, MD: American Society of Hospital Pharmacists; 1990.*

Chapter 10
Preparation and Sterilization of Batch Compounds

Barbara T. McKinnon

The term "extemporaneous compounding" describes the preparation of drugs or solutions that have no commercially available equivalents. For sterile products, this term is associated with relatively high-risk batch compounding activities (e.g., intermediate pooling of ingredients, batch mixing in open reservoirs, and use of nonsterile ingredients or components). Examples of extemporaneous compounding include the preparation of (1) injectable morphine from nonsterile powder or tablets and an appropriate diluent and (2) nutritional solutions from nonsterile ingredients.

PREPARATION TECHNIQUES

Batch compounding is a useful technique to prepare multiple dosage units efficiently with optimal dose-to-dose uniformity. Before initiating a program, pharmacists should consider what products are needed and what method is most appropriate. Table 10-1 lists products that are typically compounded as a batch process.

Requirements for facility design, operator and process validation, garb, product testing, and the environment must be met for the product's risk level (see Chapter 1). If the pharmacy cannot comply with the requirements for high-risk compounding, an alternative approach should be considered. For example, for IV catheter flushes, commercially available prefilled syringes can be used instead of compounded batches of heparin syringes. Similarly, new preservative-free commercial morphine products, in various concentrations, may reduce the need for extemporaneously compounding morphine solutions from powdered morphine.

Various batch compounding methods are available, ranging from the preparation of a single dose of morphine from nonsterile tablets to the preparation of a 200-L batch of parenteral nutrition solution in an open tank. However, the precautions specific to each method should be recognized.

Syringe Compounding

Syringes may be used as a final dosage form for repackaged medications or as a processing step in the reconstitution of powdered ingre-

Table 10-1. **Common Batch-Prepared Products**

Antibiotic unit doses in syringes, minibags, or manufacturers' piggybacks

Standardized parenteral nutrition solutions

Injections repackaged into unit dose syringes

Repackaged respiratory therapy solutions

Ophthalmic solutions

Epidural morphine solutions

Cardioplegia solutions

dients. If syringes are used to repackage a commercially available sterile injectable solution, the solution must be compatible with the materials of the syringe and plunger. Expiration dates assigned for such products should be based on potency testing or the literature.[1]

Syringes are convenient closed containers for reconstitution of small quantities of nonsterile powdered ingredients. These reconstituted solutions must be sterilized through a 0.22-μm filter and then transferred into a sterile sealed container before dispensing. Moreover, a postuse filter integrity test should be performed for products compounded from nonsterile ingredients.

Mass Reconstitution

Reconstitution of parenteral drugs is time consuming. However, efficiency can be increased by reconstituting multiple dosages in bulk and then refrigerating or freezing them. For this technique, a reconstitution device can be used. The device consists of a spring-loaded syringe attached to one end of a two-way valve; tubing, with a spike on one end, is attached to the other end of this valve. The spike on the tubing is attached to the solution container.

As the plunger of the syringe is pulled back, solution from the container enters the syringe. As the plunger is pushed in, solution is forced out of the spring-loaded syringe and through the needle attached to the two-way valve. The plunger can be adjusted to deliver any volume of diluent and then locked to that position. Once the syringe is adjusted and the plunger is pushed in to expel the solution, the plunger automatically returns to the same place. This procedure allows the same volume of diluent to enter the syringe repeatedly.

Some advantages of mass reconstitution are accuracy, control, and speed.[2] Applications of this technique include

❑ Mass reconstitution of multiple vials of powdered drugs for injection.

❑ Dispensing of reconstituted, bulk-packaged antibiotics into multiple minibags.
❑ Reconstitution of lyophilized medications supplied as manufacturers' piggybacks.

Pharmacy compounding pumps also are useful for mass reconstitution. They make the operation both easier and more precise when properly calibrated.

Pooling

"Pooled" products are made by combining sterile ingredients in a sterile closed system, by aseptic transfer, before subdivision into patient units. These products have a higher risk level than similar products made by aseptic transfer without this intermediate pooling process. The risk is greater because contamination of the pooled product could cause contamination of multiple patient units. However, pooling may be convenient and save time.

For example, for parenteral nutrition solutions, an electrolyte pool may be made in a sterile closed container. The total quantity of each required electrolyte is multiplied by the total number of units to be compounded. Then, the total volume of all additives required for one patient unit is calculated. Incompatible additives, such as calcium and phosphate, are excluded. Base solutions of dextrose and amino acids are prepared first, and then the calculated volume of additives for each patient unit is aseptically transferred from the electrolyte pool. Calcium or phosphate is added last.

The pool process decreases the number of entries into each container and may save time. To avoid potential error, calculations should be doublechecked.

Open Reservoir Mixing

Open reservoir mixing combines multiple ingredients, either sterile or nonsterile, by using an open-system transfer or an open reservoir before terminal sterilization or subdivision into units. These products are defined as Risk Level 3 in the ASHP Technical Assistance Bulletin on Quality Assurance for Pharmacy-Prepared Sterile Products.[3]

Requirements for processes, facilities, and final product assessment are more demanding in Risk Level 3 than in Risk Levels 1 and 2. Personnel must be specially trained and thoroughly knowledgeable about Class 100 critical area technology and design. Even a sterile, commercially available product cannot be defined as sterile when it is manipulated in an open reservoir. Moreover, maintenance of a Class 100 environment and the use of specialized compounding garments do not guarantee sterility when a product is exposed to the environment.

The critical aspect of compounding that involves nonsterile components or equipment is the sterilization of the nonsterile products. This process requires more effort than simply manipulating a previously sterile product without introducing contamination. Use of an appropriate, validated sterilization process is essential for Risk Level 3 products.

BATCH STERILIZATION

Product sterility is defined as the absence of viable microorganisms. However, on a practical basis, absolute sterility cannot be demonstrated due to limitations in testing. For this reason, the term "sterility assurance" defines the probability that a lot of product is sterile. Sterility assurance can be established only by adequate sterilization and validated aseptic processing.[4]

Terminal sterilization should be used for products made with nonsterile components or equipment. Sterilization may be accomplished, in the final sealed container, by autoclaving.[4] If heat sterilization capabilities are nonexistent or if heat-labile drug products or container-closure systems preclude it, products may be sterilized by filtration and processed aseptically.[5] The suitability of sterilization procedures for a particular purpose should be validated.[5]

Sterilization by Filtration

A sterilizing filtration process should remove microorganisms from the solution. The filter must have a rated pore size of 0.22 μm or smaller.[6] The pharmacist may rely on vendor certification for commercially available, presterilized, ready-to-use filter devices. This certification indicates their appropriateness for human use in sterile pharmaceutical applications. Manufacturer certification includes microbial retention testing with *Pseudomonas diminuta*, at a minimum concentration of 10^7 organisms/cm^2, as well as testing for membrane and housing integrity, nonpyrogenicity, and extractables.[5]

When relying on vendor certification, pharmacists should ensure that the testing conditions (e.g., duration of filtration, rate, temperature, and product pH, viscosity, and osmolarity) are representative of the pharmacy's intended parameters of use. For filtration apparatus assembled in the pharmacy, validation should be established experimentally.[5]

During sterilization by filtration, microbial contamination of the filtrate should be prevented. The sterilized product should be filtered into presterilized containers under aseptic conditions. Pharmacy personnel involved in such high-risk compounding should have sufficient knowledge, training, and experience to perform their tasks correctly and safely and to ensure quality.

Filter selection

The pharmacist should select the appropriate filter size, based on the volume of solution to be filtered and the particulate load, so that a single filter can process the entire batch. Filters should not have to be replaced during the filtration process.

Filter selection should be based on the characteristics of the filter and of the solution. Filters and their housing apparatus must be physically and chemically compatible with the solution and be capable of withstanding the processing temperatures and pressures. When filters are selected, four characteristics must be considered:

- ❏ Pore size.
- ❏ Compatibility.
- ❏ Fluid volume.
- ❏ Particulate load.

Reference 7 offers a more indepth discussion of filter selection.

Pore size. Pore size determines the size of the particles retained by the sieving action of the membrane filter. Some particles smaller than the pore can be retained by entrapment within the membrane. To achieve clarification, particles that measure about 5 μm or more must be removed.

Sterilization requires a filter with a maximum rated pore size of 0.22 μm. Although this process is not absolute, it carries a certain probability of success called the sterility assurance level (SAL). The SAL for sterilizing a solution with a 0.22-μm filter is normally accepted as 1:1000. In other words, no more than 0.1% of the originally present microorganism remains.[7,8]

Compatibility. Membrane filters are compatible with most pharmaceutical solutions. In general, the polymers are inert and contain few additives. The inherent charge on some filters can lead to loss by adsorption of susceptible molecules, such as proteins and polypeptides. Therefore, great care must be exercised when choosing filters for biological products. Moreover, solvents in pharmaceutical solutions—mainly alcohols, glycols, and dimethylformamide—can cause swelling and even dissolution of the polymer.[7]

Fluid volume. To provide a practical flow rate of a solution, a filter with the appropriate surface area must be used (i.e., the larger the volume of solution, the greater the amount of filter membrane surface area required). In the pharmacy, the volume of solution ranges from a few milliliters to a few liters; a disk filter of 25- or 47-mm diameter often is suitable. If many liters of a viscous solution have to be filtered, a cartridge filter with more surface area may provide an appropriate flow rate.[7]

Particulate load. Most pharmaceutical solutions are prepared under controlled conditions, and the load of particles is low. However, some preparations may have a large

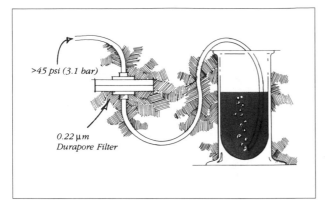

figure 10-1. *Setup for a bubble-point test. Pressure >45 psi applied through tubing to the 0.22-μm filter produces air bubbles in the water reservoir downstream from the filter. (Reproduced, with permission, from Millipore Corporation, Bedford, MA.)*

load (e.g., an impure research drug). If the filtration is intended to sterilize the filtrate, the process should be completed without changing the filter. Some preliminary experimentation may be needed to determine the rate of clogging. When the particulate load is high, one or more prefilters (e.g., depth filters) are used upstream of the sterilizing filter to remove most particulates. This process may be completed in two or more individual steps with sterile, disposable filter units. If the particulate load is relatively low (e.g., glass particles in a sterile solution after an ampul is opened), a 5-μm membrane filter may be used.[7]

Filter integrity

Sterilization filters should be checked for integrity at the time of use. Integrity of commercially available, sterile, self-contained filter devices may be tested at the conclusion of filtration. Integrity testing is performed by assessing the resistance of the filter to a substance being forced through it. Greater resistance can be detected if air is forced through a wet filter membrane (the airlock principle). For a simple integrity test, an attempt should be made to force a large syringe of air through the wet filter membrane. If the membrane is intact, the air will not pass through it.

Filter integrity kits, suitable for pharmacy use, are commercially available for testing the bubble point of small disk filters. A pressure gauge

attached to a three-way stopcock quantifies the pressure held by the filter. This test must be performed with a large-caliber syringe because a small-caliber syringe, such as a tuberculin, may generate excessive pressure.[5]

Quantitative integrity testing (e.g., bubble point or pressure hold) should be performed with pharmacy-assembled filtration apparatus.[5] Bubble point is integrity testing with a more definite endpoint. When a source of nitrogen or compressed air is used to apply pressure gradually upstream of a water-wet disk membrane filter, air bubbles suddenly appear downstream in the transparent tubing or water reservoir in an open flask or other container (see Figure 10-1). The pressure that is causing bubbles is the bubble point, which is a reliable indicator of the largest pores in a membrane filter. The bubble point is approximately 50 psi for a water-wet, 0.22-μm polysulfone filter and approximately 30 psi for a 0.45-μm filter (see Figure 10-2). These values vary with the manufacturer and polymer. Specific values are available from manufacturers.[7]

The bubble point has been correlated with the retention of microorganisms by the filter. This point is related to the logarithm of the reduction value (LRV) for the microbial population in the filtrate (see Figure 10-3).[9] The LRV is an expression of the filter's efficiency at removing microbes. It is calculated as the ratio of the concentration of microorganisms in the unfiltered solution

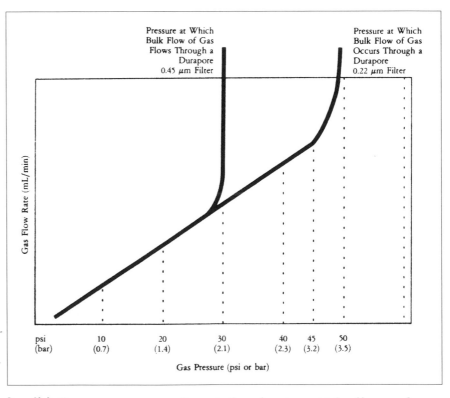

figure 10-2. *Gas pressure versus gas flow rate through water-wet polysulfone membrane filters with 0.45- or 0.22-μm pores. (Reproduced, with permission, from Millipore Corporation, Bedford, MA.)*

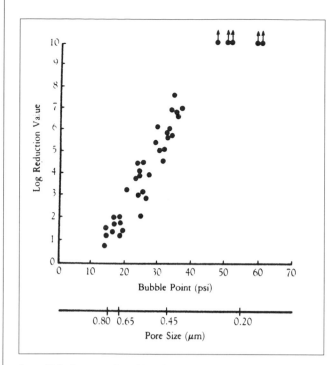

Figure 10-3. *Scatter plot of bubble point (or pore size) versus bacterial reduction. Bacterial reduction is the logarithm of the reduction in the bacterial count achieved by filtering a standardized suspension of* Pseudomonas diminuta. *(Reproduced, with permission, from Millipore Corporation, Bedford, MA.)*

to that in the filtrate, expressed as the logarithm to base 10.

As the pore size decreases, the bubble point increases so that fewer bacteria can pass through the filter. At 0.45 μm, only some smaller bacteria can pass. At 0.22 μm, or a bubble point of approximately 50 psi, bacteria are completely removed. Therefore, some microorganisms are removed when a pharmaceutical solution passes through a membrane filter larger than 0.22 μm, but sterilization is unlikely.[7] Certain drug products may lower the bubble point of the filter, resulting in air passing through it at a lower pressure than expected. If the test is questionable, the product should be resterilized. Table 10-2 describes a sample procedure for filter integrity testing of small disk filters.

The bubble-point test must be modified for cartridge filters because they have a much higher surface area than disk filters. This modification or pressure-hold test is based on air diffusion through the water in pores of the thoroughly water-wet membrane.[10] Air pressure is applied upstream of the cartridge filter until a designated pressure, usually about 80% of the bubble-point pressure, is shown on an expanded-scale gauge. This pressure is shut off. Its loss over a period is a measure of the diffusive airflow through the water in the membrane pores. The filter manufacturer states the maximum allowable loss in pressure.[7]

Table 10-2. *Procedure for Postuse Filter Integrity Testing of Small Disk Filters*

1. The following items should be assembled: filter integrity test kit containing a 10-ml syringe, three-way stopcock, and small pressure gauge (30 psi minimum); sterile 0.22-μm filter appropriate for solution to be sterilized; and sterile water for injection.
2. The product should be prepared as usual, using aseptic technique, and filtered through the presterilized filter membrane into a sterile container.
3. The filter membrane should be aseptically disconnected and connected to a syringe containing at least 10 ml of sterile water for injection. The filter membrane should be flushed with the sterile water for injection to remove traces of drug that could alter the bubble-point test.
4. The syringe should be disconnected; the three-way stopcock should be connected to the syringe tip.
5. The pressure gauge should be attached to the perpendicular connection of the three-way stopcock.
6. Then 10 ml of air should be drawn up in the syringe, and the filter should be reconnected to the three-way stopcock.
7. Pressure should be applied (about 50 psi for a 0.22-μm filter) with the syringe plunger and held for 15 sec. The expected bubble point of each filter membrane is available from the manufacturer.
8. Integrity of the filter housing and membrane is proven by retention of air and steady pressure in the syringe. Failure of integrity is indicated by airflow through the filter.
9. If failure occurs, connections should be checked for leaks and the above steps should be repeated. With any filtration failure, the product should not be released for patient use. It must be resterilized and packaged in a new container, and the filter integrity test must be repeated. When this test is repeated, the volume of sterile water for injection flush should be increased to remove all traces of drug.

Sterilization by Heat

By using saturated steam under pressure, thermal sterilization is carried out in a chamber called an autoclave. Products or components are terminally sterilized when they are processed in the autoclave to achieve a 10^{-6} microbial survivor probability. This probability assures only one chance in a million that viable microorganisms are still present in the sterilized article. With heat-stable items, the approach often is to "overkill"—to exceed the critical time necessary to achieve the 10^{-6} microbial survivor probability. However, for articles that may be damaged by excessive heat exposure, the development of sterilization cycles depends on knowledge of the microbial burden of the product.

The D value is the time in minutes required to reduce the microbial population of a specific solution by 90% or one log cycle at a specific temperature. For example, if the D value of a biologic indicator (e.g., *Bacillus stereothermophilus* spores) is 1.5 min at 121° F, its lethality can be described as 8D when treated for 12 min. This D value can be applied to products with a known initial bioburden. If the microbial burden of a product before sterilization is 10^2, a lethality input of 8D is needed to achieve a probability of 10^{-6}.[4]

Sterilization cycles should be validated to ensure that the survival of the most resistant microorganisms is no greater than 10^{-6} under specified operating conditions and parameters (e.g., sterilization time and temperature, size and nature of load, and chamber loading configuration). The validation and monitoring of heat sterilization should be in writing along with specific critical parameters, such as necessary temperatures, pressures, and use of commercially available biologic indicators. Monitoring data from each cycle should be recorded to ensure that the processes are performed properly and that all critical parameters are within specified limits during processing.[5] Autoclaving must be reserved for items that can be penetrated by water vapor. Therefore, dry sealed containers, oils, and waxes may not be suitable for sterilization via autoclaving.

Sterilization by Gas

Gas sterilization may replace heat when the material to be sterilized cannot withstand high temperatures or moisture. The active ingredient used in gas sterilization is ethylene oxide. Disadvantages of this agent are its highly flammable nature (unless mixed with suitable inert gases), its mutagenic properties, and the possibility of toxic residues in treated materials, particularly those containing chloride ions.

Materials to be sterilized must be dry because moisture may inactivate ethylene oxide. Items that might dissolve and retain ethylene oxide, such as oils and waxes, should not be sterilized using this method. Generally, gas sterilization is carried out in a pressurized chamber similar to a steam autoclave. Facilities using ethylene oxide should provide adequate poststerilization degassing to (1) enable microbial survivor monitoring and (2) minimize exposure of operators to the potentially harmful gas.

Validation of this sterilization procedure requires monitoring of temperature, humidity, vacuum/positive pressure, and ethylene oxide concentration. All critical process parameters within the chamber must be adequate during the entire cycle. Validation generally is performed by using biologic indicators such as *Bacillus subtilis*. These indicators also should be used to monitor routine runs. Ethylene oxide is limited in its ability to diffuse gas to the innermost product areas that require sterilization. Package design and chamber loading patterns must provide minimal resistance to gas diffusion.[4]

Sterilization by Radiation

The proliferation of heat-sensitive medical devices and concerns about ethylene oxide safety have resulted in numerous applications of radiation sterilization.[4] It can be used for drug substances and final dosage forms. The advantages of this sterilization include low chemical reactivity, low measurable residues, and fewer variables to control.

The two types of ionizing radiation are radioisotope decay (gamma radiation) and electron beam. In both types, the radiation dose should be established to yield the required degree of sterility assurance (within the range of minimum and maximum doses set) so that the properties of the article being sterilized are acceptable. Validation of this sterilization procedure includes

- ❏ Establishing compatibility of the materials to be sterilized.
- ❏ Establishing a product loading pattern and completion of dose mapping in the sterilization container (including identification of minimum and maximum dose zones).
- ❏ Demonstrating delivery of the required sterilization dose.

For electron-beam irradiation, validation also must include online control of the voltage, current, conveyor speed, and electron-beam scan.[4]

SUMMARY

Batch preparation can be used for products such as antibiotic minibags or syringes, parenteral nutrition solutions, and epidural morphine solutions. Processes classified as batch preparation include syringe repackaging, mass reconstitution, pooling of multiple ingredients, and open reservoir mixing. Each method requires a high level of quality assurance, because these products may be used as multiple doses for one patient or as single doses for numerous patients.

Quality assurance also should guarantee the sterility of these batch-prepared products. Depending on the product characteristics, sterilization can be performed by filtration, by heat or chemical means, or by radiation.

REFERENCES

1.   Trissel LA. Handbook on injectable drugs, 8th ed. Bethesda, MD: American Society of Hospital Phar-

macists; 1994.

2. Hunt ML Jr. Training manual for intravenous admixture personnel, 4th ed. Chicago, IL: Baxter Healthcare Corp.; 1990.

3. American Society of Hospital Pharmacists. ASHP technical assistance bulletin on quality assurance for pharmacy-prepared sterile products. *Am J Hosp Pharm.* 1993; 50:2386–98.

4. Sterilization and sterility assurance of compendial articles. In: United States pharmacopeia, 23rd rev./national formulary, 18th ed. Rockville, MD: United States Pharmacopeial Convention; 1994:1976–81.

5. Sterile drug products for home use. In: United States pharmacopeia, 23rd rev./national formulary, 18th ed. Rockville, MD: United States Pharmacopeial Convention; 1994:1963–75.

6. Leahy TJ, Sullivan MJ. Validation of bacterial-re-
tention capabilities of membrane filters. *Pharm Technol.* 1978; 2 (Nov):65–75.

7. McKinnon BT, Avis KE. Membrane filtration of pharmaceutical solutions. *Am J Hosp Pharm.* 1993; 50:1921–36.

8. Office of Compliance, Division of Manufacturing and Product Quality. Guidelines on sterile drug products produced by aseptic processing. Rockville, MD: Food and Drug Administration; 1987.

9. Fifield CW, Leahy TJ. Sterilization filtration. In: Block SS, ed. Disinfection, sterilization, and preservation. Philadelphia, PA: Lea & Febiger; 1983: 147–8.

10. Emory SF. Principles of integrity-testing hydrophilic microporous membrane filters, part II. *Pharm Technol.* 1989; 13 (Oct):36–46.

Chapter 11
Batch Preparation Documentation

Barbara T. McKinnon

Batch preparation involves the compounding of multiple sterile product units, in a single discrete process, by the same individuals during one limited period.[1] The term "batch preparation" often has been associated with preparation of units for multiple patients, but a batch also may be prepared for one patient. For example, hospital pharmacists may prepare a batch of identical cardioplegic solutions for multiple patients, while home care practitioners may prepare a batch of parenteral nutrition solutions for a single patient's use over several days. Careful documentation of raw materials, preparative processes, product evaluations, and environmental tests is necessary to maintain control of a batch's quality.

Batch production can be an efficient method of preparing commonly used sterile products. Advantages include

- ❏ Cost savings in labor, drugs, and supplies.
- ❏ Savings in resources and time.
- ❏ More consistent and reliable service to patients and customers.
- ❏ Finished product testing and other quality-control monitoring.

However, if batch preparation is not properly managed, the health and safety of numerous patients can be threatened.

Master work sheets and batch preparation records can help to establish and maintain a quality-assurance program for batch-processed sterile products.

MASTER WORK SHEETS

A standardized record of preparation or "master work sheet" should be developed for routinely compounded products. To keep consecutive batches nearly identical, all compounding activities should be reproduced uniformly by following this master work sheet. It includes the[2]

- ❏ Master formula.
- ❏ Records of quality checks of components.
- ❏ Specifications for necessary equipment and supplies.
- ❏ Checks of preparative procedures.

❏ Compounding directions.
❏ Sample of the product labeling.
❏ Results of inprocess testing.
❏ Result of end-product evaluations.

Each time the product is made, a batch record is generated to document its manufacture, control, and distribution. The master work sheet is the permanent record of the production and control of all batches of one particular product.[2]

Although a sheet is not needed for all compounded sterile products, it should be developed for batch-prepared sterile products and all Risk Level 3 products (see Chapter 1).[1] For example, master work sheets should be established for (1) standardized parenteral nutrition solutions compounded as a batch in anticipation of orders, (2) cardioplegic solutions, and (3) batches of ophthalmic solutions used by multiple patients.

Master Formula

A specific formula must be developed to address desired product attributes (e.g., final concentrations of ingredients, final pH, and osmolarity). The required diluents, preservatives, and other excipients—antioxidants, chelating agents, and buffers—also should be addressed. The formula should be reviewed by a pharmacist to determine if the product meets formulation and stability requirements as well as physiologic norms for solution osmolarity and pH appropriate for the intended route of administration.

Master formulas should list all products clearly by name, concentration, and total quantity (weight or volume required). A complete listing of names and quantities of all batch ingredients, including excipients, is necessary. An identifying code for each product (e.g., NDC code number) can minimize errors.

All calculations required in compounding should be specified in the master formula. For example, the method for increasing the volume of a formula to allow for overfill should be indicated. An overfill factor may be specified so that calculations of required excess amounts are handled consistently for each ingredient. Similarly, directions should specify how to handle existing overfill when product additives are measured.

The *theoretical* yield of the master formula, in either weight or volume (as appropriate), should be specified for Risk Level 3 products.[1] The acceptable *actual* yield also should be set; if it is not met, the cause should be investigated.

Component Quality Checks

Commercially available sterile products

When commercially available sterile components are used (e.g., drug products, ready-to-use containers, and devices), they should be routinely inspected. If they are expired, defective, unsuitable for the intended use, or inappropriately stored, these products should not be used. Defective products should be promptly reported to the Food and Drug Administration[3] and identified by name, lot number, and expiration date. Ingredients used to compound sterile products should be stable, compatible, and appropriate, according to the manufacturer, United States Pharmacopeial (USP) guidelines, or relevant scientific references.[1]

Nonsterile components

When nonsterile drug components are utilized, they should meet USP standards. Certificates of analysis, from reputable manufacturers of bulk drug substances, can establish that each lot received by the pharmacy meets specifications.[4] If the material is USP, National Formulary, or reagent grade, the minimum assay of the manufacturer may be assumed. Specifications can include color, appearance, assay requirements, purity, and heavy metal content.[5]

After receiving each lot of bulk drug substance, the pharmacy should inspect the lot and document any visual evidence of deterioration, unacceptable quality, and wrong identity. Documentation also should verify that components have been assayed by the manufacturer to meet specifications (see Figure 11-1).

Bulk drug substances that are stored properly in the pharmacy should retain their quality until the manufacturer's labeled expiration date. Substances without a labeled expiration date should be

❏ Dated on receipt.
❏ Stored properly.
❏ Dated when the container is opened.
❏ Used within a reasonable time (based on available references).
❏ Visually inspected by the pharmacist when used.

The conditions under which containers of bulk drug substances are opened and the technique of content withdrawal should be strictly controlled. Additionally, the devices used for withdrawal should be clean to avoid contamination of the remaining contents. The pharmacy may repackage bulk drug substances into smaller, suitable, and properly sealed containers (e.g., shrink-seal or zip-closure plastic bags) to minimize contamination.[4]

Raw materials

When raw materials are received without a certificate of analysis from the manufacturer, they must be quarantined to prevent use until testing is completed. Each lot represents a single batch of raw materials, in one or more containers, represented by a single manufacturer's control number. Records (see Figure 11-2) should be kept of the

Lot # (Pharmacy)	Name of Chemical	Grade	Date received	Mfg.	Lot # Exp. Date	Quantity received	Remarks	Approval date
UM601	Sodium chloride, cryst	USP	7-7-94	xyz Chem	000726 None	2 x 100lbs	Fiber drums	JAP 7-8-94
UM602	Alcohol 95%	USP	7-8-94	USChem	TI3366 None	1 x 54 Gal.	Metal drum	7-8-94 AR
UM603	Dextrose, Anhydrous	USP	7-10-94	Starch Prod.	MBKX None	5 x 100 lbs.	Bags	PMJ 7-12-94

figure 11-1. *Component inventory record for nonsterile components with manufacturers' certificates of analysis. (Adapted, with permission, from Reference 5.)*

❏ Chemical name.
❏ Grade.
❏ Quantity received.
❏ Date received.
❏ Manufacturer.
❏ Manufacturer's lot number.
❏ Expiration date.
❏ Results of tests for identity and purity.

If the raw materials are not graded, an assay report should be obtained from the manufacturer. A decision can then be made about whether the material meets the desired specifications. Assays usually are performed on labile chemicals, such as calcium chloride (anhydrous) and magnesium sulfate, which readily gain or lose moisture. Purity and identification can be tested by various methods. Usually, several chemical and physical tests can identify the material and ascertain its purity. For example, a mixed melting point or optical rotation determination may suffice for purity tests. To identify the drug, a simple chemical color reaction, chemical color change reaction, characteristic odor, taste, or physical appearance may suffice.[5] If the pharmacy cannot perform these tests, the material should be sent to another laboratory.

Inhouse-prepared components

Sterile injectable products that are prepared inhouse but used as components of other sterile injectables deserve special attention. Lack of quality (e.g., purity, potency, and sterility) of the component solution adversely affects the quality of the resulting solution. All nonsterile ingredients used to prepare sterile component solutions should be inspected; the final product also must be tested to ensure that it meets all specifications. An analytical request and results form (see Figure 11-3) should be sent to the laboratory along with the test solution. Figure 11-4 illustrates the process used to review analytical results from testing and to approve release of component solutions.

Equipment and Supplies Specifications

The master work sheet should specify all equipment, containers, and supplies needed for compounding. The brand name and model or item number of equipment and supplies should be listed as well as any applicable performance characteristics (e.g., weight limits for scales). Specification of all details, such as lengths and diameters of tubing, ensures that the same items can be reordered if equipment malfunctions or supplies become depleted (see Figure 11-5). For complicated equipment setups, a diagram can illustrate the proper sequence of assembly.

The preparation of equipment and supplies also should be part of the master work sheet. For example, a procedure should be established to calibrate or verify the accuracy of automated compounding devices used in aseptic processing.[1] If products are dispensed by weight, the

Pharmacy Lot #	Description	Identification	Solubility	Specific Rotation	Acidity	Color of solution	Heavy metals	Soluble starch	Approval	Analyst date
UM603	passes	passes	passes	passes	passes	passes	0.0005 %	passes	approved	PMJ 7/12/94

figure 11-2. *Raw materials testing record. (Adapted, with permission, from Reference 5.)*

PHARMACY - ANALYTICAL REQUEST & RESULTS

Product: _____Dextrose 50% USP_____ Lot No._____

Testing Bottles Submitted: _____

Anticipated Q.C. Release Date for this Lot: _____

Analyses Requested By:_____ Date of Request: _____

Analyses Requested	Procedure	Production Specification	Laboratory Results					
			Bott.	P/F	Bott.	P/F	Bott.	P/F
pH	2-1-001-85	3.5-6.5						
Specific Gravity	2-1-126-85	1.100 - 1.200						
Dext. Hyd.	2-1-004-82	47.5 - 52.5 g%						
Nitrogen	2-1-006-82							
Acetate	2-1-163-82							
Chloride	2-1-032-82							
Sodium	2-1-013-82							
Potassium	2-1-211-82							
Phosphate	2-1-250-82							
Magnesium	2-1-252-82							
Calcium	2-1-251-82							
Vitamin K_1	2-1-397-82							

Chemistry No. _____ , _____ , _____ By: _____ Checked: _____

Date Received: _____ Date Initiated: _____ Date Completed: _____

Particulate Count	Bottle 2-2-080-	Not >50 p/ml = to 10μm				Particle Description		
		Not >5 p/ml = to 25μm						

Sterility (Membrane Filtration)	2-2-113-82	Must Pass	Bottle No.	7 Day Incubation				B &F	
				FTM		SCD			
				+	-	+	-	Pass	Fail	Pass	Fail

Microbiology No. _____ , _____ , _____ By: _____ Checked: _____

Date Received: _____ Date Initiated: _____ Date Completed: _____

Analyses Requested	Procedure	Production Specification	Bottle No.	Basal Temp.	T_1	T2	T3	ΔT	Pass	Fail
USP XX Pyrogens	2-3-001-85	Must Pass								
1.										

Biology No. _____ , _____ , _____ By: _____ Checked: _____

Date Received: _____ Date Initiated: _____ Date Completed: _____

Figure 11-3. *Analytical testing request and results form for component solutions.*

HOSPITAL PHARMACY

QUALITY CONTROL ANALYTICAL REPORT

TEST ASSAY OR PROPERTY	METHOD	SPECIFICATIONS	OBSERVATION OR RESULTS 1	2	3
COMPLETE LABEL	Visual	Check for correct formula Cat. # Lot # Exp. date			
INTACT CONTAINER	B/W Bkg Visual	No hairline cracks or Imperfections			
CLARITY	B/W Bkg Visual	No visible particulate Matter			
COLOR	Visual	Clear (No color)			
ODOR	Smell	None			
pH	pH Meter	3.5 - 6.5			
TASTE	Taste	Sweet			
WEIGHT or VOLUME	Volu-metric	1025 - 1060ml			
SPECIFIC GRAVITY	Hydro-meter	1.100 - 1.200			
STRENGTH					
Dextrose (Anhydrous)	Chem.	45 (42-46) g%			
PARTICULATE MATTER	Visual	(Yes - No) Inspect Black/White for presence of particular matter			
STORAGE PROCEDURE	Room Temp	Yes - No			

Raw Material — ND: 0264-1128-00 — No. Containers — Catalog # 51280

In-Process — Manufacturer Lot Number — No. Containers

End Product — Manufacturer — No. Containers — Sample Date

Product: DEXTROSE 50% USP — Strength — Manufacturer: McGAW — Date of Manufacture — Lot Number

FINAL APPROVAL OF MATERIAL OR PRODUCT FOR USE

▼

	Incomp.	Complete
PHARMACEUTICAL BULK COMPOUNDING MASTER WORKSHEET		
BIOLOGICAL TESTS WORKSHEET		

COMMENTS:

APPROVED: ☐

CONDITIONALLY APPROVED: ☐
EXPLAIN:

REJECTED: ☐
EXPLAIN:

_____ RPh _____ RPh
Analyst   Date   Released By   Date

figure 11-4. *Form for final approval and release of component solutions.*

83

EQUIPMENT RECORD

1. Perma-San stainless steel mixing tank and cover (100 gallon)
2. P-35S 1" stainless steel flush valve
3. MixMor G-14 stainless steel electric mixer and stand
4. Stainless steel calibration strip A
5. Climet 411 printer
6. Climet CI-4100 particle counter

ASSEMBLY AND POOLING EQUIPMENT (STERILE)

	Equipment Code Number	
1. Plastic paddle	No. _____	No. _____
2. Beaker 4000 ml	No. _____	No. _____
3. Cylindrical graduate	No. _____	No. _____

FILLING

1. XX2504700 6-Place manifold	No. _____	No. _____
2. XX2504705 1/4" NPTM to 3/8' I.D. Hose (6)	No. _____	No. _____
3. XX6700101 1/4" tee	No. _____	No. _____
4. XX6700L11 1/4" NPT to tubing adapter (6)	No. _____	No. _____
5. YY2004040 2" T.C. clamp assembly	No. _____	No. _____
6. Tubing, latex surgical, 1/4" x 3/32" wall	No. _____	No. _____
7. XX6700030 1/4" quick release coupling and nipple (7)	No. _____	No. _____
8. BD needle adapter (6)	No. _____	No. _____
9. 18 gauge 1-1/2" needles	No. _____	No. _____
10. YY1301009 1/4' pipe plug	No. _____	No. _____
11. YY1412229 1/2" T.C. to 1/4" NPT adapter	No. _____	No. _____
12. Pressure tubing 3/8" I.D. PVC	No. _____	No. _____
13. 7549 Masterflex variable speed peristaltic pump	No. _____	No. _____
14. 6408-73 tygon tubing	No. _____	No. _____
15. YY1301015 1/4" Pressure gauge, 0-100 psi	No. _____	No. _____
16. XX6700111 1/4" NPTF Coupling	No. _____	No. _____
17. No. 12122, 0.2 micrometer Gelman Capsule	No. _____	No. _____

Figure 11-5. *Equipment record.*

type of weighing device and the product's specific gravity should be documented.

The pharmacy should ensure that equipment, apparatus, and devices used in compounding operate properly and are within acceptable tolerance limits. Records of equipment calibration, testing, maintenance, and cleaning should be kept on file and be easily retrieved. Moreover, routine maintenance checks should be performed as necessary. Before operating the equipment, personnel should receive training and experience. They also should be able to determine whether their equipment is operating properly or malfunctioning.[4]

The master work sheet generally includes requirements for cleaning and disinfecting the compounding area before work is begun. Sterilization procedures for any equipment heat sterilized by the pharmacy should include review of a biologic indicator to validate that sterilization occurred prior to product use.[4]

All nonsterile equipment (e.g., tubings, filters, and containers) that contacts the sterilized final product should be properly cleaned and sterilized before entering the controlled area. The sterilization process should be monitored and documented. Equipment that does not contact the finished product should be properly cleaned, rinsed, and disinfected. Large equipment (e.g., tanks, carts, and tables) kept in the controlled area or cleanroom should be made of a material, such as stainless steel, that can be easily cleaned and disinfected.[1]

Furthermore, requirements for packaging of products (e.g., types of containers and methods of closure) should be included in the master work sheet. The final container for the sterile product should maintain its integrity (i.e., identity, strength, quality, and purity) throughout the shelf life. Presterilized containers from licensed manufacturers should be used when possible. In an aseptic filling operation, the container should be sterile at the time of the operation; if nonsterile containers are used, methods for sterilization should be established.[1]

Preparation Procedure Checks

The methods for preparing sterile products and the use of process controls should ensure that finished products have the required identity, strength, quality, and purity. Any deviation from established methods should be documented and appropriately justified.[1]

Procedures should be written clearly and be easily understood so that personnel who follow the master work sheet can compound the product uniformly. The order of addition of products also should be specified if a certain sequence is required (e.g., calcium and phosphate or amino acids, dextrose, and lipids). A step-by-step procedure

should be developed for all preparation activities, including inprocess tests (e.g., pH checks).

Furthermore, conditions suitable for product preparation should be documented. For example, Risk Level 3 products must be prepared in a Class 100 certified laminar-airflow hood within a Class 10,000 controlled area or in a properly maintained and monitored Class 100 cleanroom.[1] Other required operating conditions, such as cleaning and disinfection of work surfaces, also should be included.

Compounding Directions

Compounding procedures should be checked and double checked. Technicians should be adequately supervised by a licensed pharmacist in the compounding area. The pharmacist should check that correct ingredients are selected and that correct volumes or weights are added. Finally, the pharmacist must verify that the volume of the final container is correct and check the labeled product.

Data entered into an automated compounding device should be verified by a pharmacist before compounding is begun, and end-product checks should verify the accuracy of ingredient delivery. These checks may include weighing (see Figure 11-6) and visually inspecting the final product. The expected weight, based on the specific gravities of the ingredients and their respective volumes, can be documented on the batch record, dated, and initialed by a pharmacist. Once compounding is completed, each final product can be weighed and compared with the expected weight. The product's actual weight should fall within an established threshold for variance.[7]

To verify a product visually, the beginning level of each bulk container should be marked before the start of

---

COMPOUNDED BY: __S E__

PHARMACIST: __Coronado__

500.00 ml X _____ O.F. X __1.07__ S.G. = __535__ Grams

UNIT#	WEIGHT	UNIT#	WEIGHT	UNIT#	WEIGHT	UNIT#	WEIGHT	UNIT#	WEIGHT	UNIT#	WEIGHT
1	535	9	536	17		25		33			
2	540	10	535	18		26		34			
3	539	11	540	19		27		35			
4	538	12	539	20		28		36			
5	537	13	538	21		29		37			
6	536	14	537	22		30		38			
7	535	15		23		31		39			
8	540	16		24		32		40			

figure 11-6. *Weight record. (Reproduced, with permission, from PharmaThera, Memphis, TN.)*

the automated mixing process. Then the container should be checked after completion of the mixing to determine whether the final levels are reasonable compared to expected volumes. The operator should periodically observe the automated compounding device during mixing to ensure its proper operation.[8]

Additional quality controls may be needed when multiple sterile ingredients are combined into a single sterile or nonsterile reservoir for subdivision into multiple units. Associated calculations should be verified by a second pharmacist and documented.[1] Methods of sterilization and end-product testing for sterility are discussed in Chapters 10 and 17, respectively. If there are doubts about whether a product has been properly prepared or sterilized, it should not be used.

Sample Label

A sample label should be part of the master work sheet. Standardized label text should be developed for each commonly prepared batch product to ensure consistency among batches. If products are prepared in advance, stored, and then issued to individual patients, both a product label and a final patient-specific label are required.

When the patient-specific label is affixed, the original product lot number and assigned expiration date must still be visible. The issuing and use as well as destruction of any unused or damaged preprinted labels should be documented. Product labeling is discussed further in Chapter 13.

Inprocess Testing

Inprocess testing verifies that the compounding environment and the actual product meet established criteria. No sterile products should be prepared in a controlled area that fails to meet these criteria. Environmental checks might include

- ❑ Counting of airborne particles with a calibrated particle counter.
- ❑ Monitoring of the positive pressure of the compounding room relative to other areas.
- ❑ Microbial sampling of the air and surfaces.

This monitoring may be performed routinely (e.g., weekly) or before or during compounding, depending on the risk level of the product. Techniques for environmental monitoring are discussed in Chapter 6.

When the environment does not meet established criteria, sterile product processing should immediately cease and corrective action should be taken. The preparation of Risk Level 3 sterile products is especially critical. Written policies and procedures should delineate alternative preparation methods to enable timely fulfillment of prescription orders.[1] Additionally, steps taken to correct the problem and their results should be documented.

Inprocess testing may be as simple as visual inspections for physical properties (e.g., color, smell, and clarity) or as complex as detailed chemical analyses for content. Checks for pH can be easily performed with a small, hand-held meter. This meter monitors the adjustment of product pH before and after subsequent additions of acid or base (e.g., acetic acid or sodium bicarbonate). Refractive index measurements may help to verify the addition of certain ingredients.[9] For example, these measurements can approximate the concentration of dextrose in batch-compounded parenteral nutrition solutions. Similarly, specific gravity measurements can check the dextrose content of parenteral nutrition solutions.[10]

End-Product Testing and Quarantine Requirements

The master work sheet should list the appropriate checks and tests to ensure that batch-prepared sterile products are free from defects and meet all quality specifications. A sterile product should not be released until all quality specifications have been reviewed and all release requirements are met.[4] Tests should include visual inspection as well as checks for compounding accuracy and formulation integrity, including pyrogenicity and sterility.

Visual inspection

As a condition of release, each product unit should be inspected immediately after compounding against lighted white and black backgrounds for visible particulates or other foreign matter. The final product also should be inspected for proper labeling, container leaks and integrity, and solution cloudiness, color, and volume (see Figure 11-7). Defective products should be immediately discarded or marked and segregated to prevent their administration. When products are not distributed promptly after preparation, a predistribution inspection should be conducted because defects (e.g., precipitation, cloudiness, and leakage) may develop.[4]

Compounding accuracy

A pharmacist should verify that the product was compounded accurately with the correct ingredients, quantities, containers, and reservoirs. The additive containers and the syringes used to measure additives should be quarantined with the final products for a final check. Syringe plungers should be drawn back to the volume mark used for each additive if the additive volume was not checked prior to the addition.

Automated pump settings should be verified just prior to or just after pumping and mixing. In addition, the volumes of each pumped ingredient should be checked to establish that the automated pump is within the accuracy limits set by the manufacturer. All drug product units

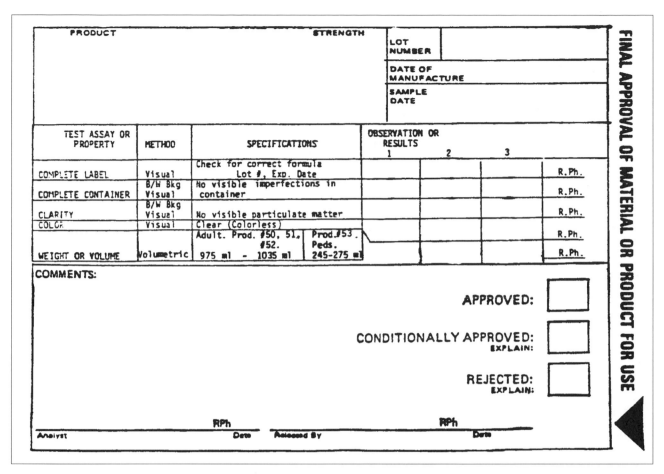

PRODUCT			STRENGTH			
			LOT NUMBER			
			DATE OF MANUFACTURE			
			SAMPLE DATE			

TEST ASSAY OR PROPERTY	METHOD	SPECIFICATIONS	OBSERVATION OR RESULTS 1	2	3	
COMPLETE LABEL	Visual	Check for correct formula Lot #, Exp. Date				R.Ph.
COMPLETE CONTAINER	B/W Bkg Visual	No visible imperfections in container				R.Ph.
CLARITY	B/W Bkg Visual	No visible particulate matter				R.Ph.
COLOR	Visual	Clear (Colorless)				R.Ph.
WEIGHT OR VOLUME	Volumetric	Adult. Prod. #50, 51, #52. 975 ml - 1035 ml / Prod.#53. Peds. 245-275 ml				R.Ph.

COMMENTS:

APPROVED: ☐

CONDITIONALLY APPROVED: ☐
EXPLAIN:

REJECTED: ☐
EXPLAIN:

Analyst ___ RPh ___ Date ___ Released By ___ RPh ___ Date ___

figure 11-7. *Final product release record.*

used should be accounted for according to written procedures.[4] Other methods (e.g., observation during compounding, calculation checks, and documented records) also may be used for end-product verification.[1]

Formulation integrity

Formulations involving nonsterile ingredients require additional evaluations to ensure that the final product meets desired specifications for potency, purity, identity, and quality. Quality-control tests demonstrate the unique properties of parenteral dosage forms (e.g., sterility and freedom from pyrogens and visible particulate contamination). (See Figure 11-8.)

Sterility tests evaluate the product's contamination with microbiological impurities. Sterility tests should be performed on Risk Level 3 products at the completion of preparation. This test, including the sampling scheme, should be conducted according to a USP method. The USP methods estimate the probable—not actual—sterility of numerous articles. After a few batch samples are tested for sterility, they are assumed to be representative of every article from the batch. However, these samples can be inadvertently contaminated during the testing procedure. Despite these limitations, some end-product test-

ing must be performed to protect consumers from contaminated products. Although the sterility of every article is not guaranteed, the sterility test indicates that a representative sample of a lot or batch is uncontaminated. End-product testing also checks the sterility of products sterilized in the pharmacy, such as those prepared by a filtration process.[11]

Pyrogen tests evaluate the capability of the product to form a gel in the presence of limulus amoebocyte lysate. The prevention of pyrogens is preferred over their removal in parenteral products. Pyrogenic contamination can be prevented by the use of ingredients, packaging materials, and processing equipment that have been initially depyrogenated. Then, correct and proper procedures must be used during compounding to minimize pyrogen development.

Pyrogen testing should be performed on all products compounded from a nonsterile drug component or with nonsterile equipment.[11] The limulus amoebocyte lysate test is convenient and offers results rapidly (generally within 1 hr). The product should not be released until it has been determined that the specified endotoxin limit has not been exceeded; pyrogen testing is not required for ophthalmic or topical solutions.[4]

Clarity tests check for visible particulate contami-

PHARMACY - ANALYTICAL REQUEST & RESULTS

Product: _____ TROPHAMINE 2% w DEXTROSE 15% 1000 ML _____ Lot No. __57__

Testing Bottles Submitted: __#3, 5, 6, 10, 20, 30, 40, 50, 60, 70, 80, 90, 96, & 97__ _____

Anticipated Q.C. Release Date for this Lot: _____

Analyses Requested By: _____ Date of Request: _____

Analyses Requested	Procedure	Production Specification	Laboratory Results					
			Bott.	P/F	Bott.	P/F	Bott.	P/F
pH	2-1-001-85	5.0-7.0						
Specific Gravity	2-1-126-85	1.0 - 1.2						
Dext. Hyd.	2-1-004-82	13.3 - 16.5 gm%						
Nitrogen	2-1-006-82	2.79 - 3.41 g/L						
Acetate	2-1-163-82	17.4 - 21.4 mEq/L						
Chloride	2-1-032-82	18 - 22 mEq/L						
Sodium	2-1-013-82	4.5 - 5.5 mEq/L						
Potassium	2-1-211-82	21 - 27 mEq/L						
Phosphate	2-1-250-82	5.4 - 6.6 mEq/L						
Magnesium	2-1-252-82	4.5 - 5.5 mEq/L						
Calcium	2-1-251-82	4.1 - 5.1 mEq/L						
Vitamin K_1	2-1-397-82	1.0 mg/L Yes-No						

Chemistry No. _____ , _____ , _____ By: _____ Checked: _____

Date Received: _____ Date Initiated: _____ Date Completed: _____

Particulate Count	Bottle # 6 2-2-080-85	Not >50 p/ml = to 10μm	
		Not >5 p/ml = to 25μm	

Sterility (Membrane Filtration)	2-2-302-85	Bottle No.		7 Day Incubation		B & F	
		10, 20, 30, 40, 50, 60, 70, 80, 90, & 97		Pass	Fail	Pass	Fail

Microbiology No. _____ , _____ , _____ By: _____ Checked: _____

Date Received: _____ Date Initiated: _____ Date Completed: _____

Analyses Requested	Procedure	Bottle No.	Basal Temp.	T_1	T2	T3	Δ T	Pass	Fail
USP PYROGEN	2-3-001-85	# 5							
USP PYROGEN	2-3-001-85	# 96							

Biology No. _____ , _____ , _____ By: _____ Checked: _____

Date Received: _____ Date Initiated: _____ Date Completed: _____

Figure 11-8. *Analytical testing request and results form for finished product.*

nation, and particulate analytical tests quantitate the number and size of the particulates. Package integrity tests are performed, for glass-sealed ampuls and other parenteral packaging systems, to check the potential for ingress of microbiological contamination.[10]

Sterility and pyrogen testing typically requires product quarantine until the results are available. If products prepared from nonsterile components must be dispensed before end-product testing is completed, a procedure must allow for their immediate recall.[1] End-product evaluations and procedures for product quarantine are discussed further in Chapter 17.

BATCH PREPARATION RECORDS

The master work sheet is the recipe for preparation of multiple, identical batches of a given product. The batch record, however, documents the preparation of a *single* batch product. Typically, master work sheets are only needed for commonly produced batches or for high-risk products. However, the batch record may be helpful for compounding directions and documentation of any product prepared as a batch.

Each time a product is produced, the batch record documents its preparation, control, and distribution. To save time, batch records can be standardized, computerized, and reprinted whenever a product is compounded. When compounding is begun, the batch record is filled out with the following items:

- ❏ Date.
- ❏ Number of units compounded.
- ❏ Component quantities.
- ❏ Lot numbers and expiration dates of components.
- ❏ Initials of personnel who check each step of the process.
- ❏ Results of inprocess and end-product evaluations.
- ❏ Lot number assigned to the batch.
- ❏ Expiration date assigned to the batch.
- ❏ Names of personnel directly involved in compounding.

A batch record offers several advantages. It helps to ensure that all subsequent refills are compounded in exactly the same manner, using the same brands of products and the same diluents. The batch record provides a clear list for gathering the necessary drugs, solutions, and supplies from storage areas. It provides precise directions for compounding, which may be particularly helpful for technicians. Errors also can be minimized by using the

```
5/15/95  Location:D-416        Volume:1257ml  IV#:  1
       * * *  S O L U T I O N   F O R M U L A  * * *
__ Additive _____ ml _____  Additive _____ ml __
   Aminosyn II 10%  600.00      MgSO4 50% .....    2.40
   Dextrose 70% ..  428.57      M.T.E.-5 ......    3.60
   NaCl 2.5mEq ...   24.00      M.V.I.-12 .....   12.00
   KCl 2mEq ......   24.00      Albumin 25% ...  120.00
   K Phosphate 3mM    8.00      Selepen .......    1.50
   Ca Gluconate ..   25.81      Ranitidine inj    7.20


    5/15/95  Location:D-416        Volume:1257ml  IV#:   1

   Ion  Conc. delivered     Ion  Conc. delivered
   Na    69.69 mEq/L         Zn    2.86 mg/L
   K     66.19 mEq/L         Cu    1.15 mg/L
   Ca     9.55 mEq/L         Mn    0.29 mg/L
   Mg     7.64 mEq/L         Cr   11.46 mcg/L
   PO4   19.09 mM/L          Se  105.01 mcg/L
   Ace   34.37 mEq/L         I     0.00 mcg/L
   Cl    85.92 mEq/L
```

Figure 11-9. *Batch preparation record for a Risk Level 1 parenteral nutrition solution. (Reproduced, with permission, from PharmaThera, Memphis, TN.)*

documented system of checks. Additionally, a record of lot numbers and expiration dates of product components can help in the event of a product recall.

For low-risk products, completion of a batch record may not be time consuming. Some pharmacy software programs automatically generate simple batch records along with product labels (see Figure 11-9). These records typically document the product, strength, and volume to be added for each ingredient. To save cost and time, one extra product label can be generated to document the exact products, strengths, and volumes used for compounding. This batch record can then be attached to the prescription or medication order to document the compounding process.

For high-risk products, a more thorough batch record is required (see Figure 11-10). Because these products may be stored or administered over prolonged periods or given to multiple patients, records should be maintained of product lot numbers and expiration dates. These records are invaluable if a component is recalled, if the product fails an end-product test (e.g., sterility or pyrogen), or if the product's sterility or potency is questioned.

Products prepared for multiple patients may be given a lot number for easy identification and retrieval in case of defects. Simple strategies can be devised for assigning a lot number. For example, a sequential number may be assigned to each batch of a particular product. Or numbers representing the month, date, year, and batch prepared in a day can be used (e.g., 112295-6 for the sixth batch

PRX525-2   COMPOUNDING RECORD CHECK AND LOT NUMBER RECORD   05/15/95   10:19

| | | Initial Master Approved | R.Ph. sign/date |
| | | Final Product Approval | R.Ph. sign/date |

Patient:
Nbr:
Rx Nbr:
Physician:
Date Compounded:
Patient Order is for containers   100 through   128
Total Number of Units   29

Hood Nbr:
F.G. List-IC: 999910-51
A96700 Approximate Container Volume: 1350   ml

Pharmacist's initials each drug. This check is for containers:

Drug Item	Order Qty	List - Size Cd	Lot Number Rcrd Mult Lots	Original Drug Conc	Amount per Container	Per Cont Final Conc
1. TRAVASOL 10% 1000ML	17	629-04	exp.	10.00%	552.00 ml	4.09%
2. DEXTROSE 70% 1000ML	21	1519-05	exp.	70.00%	699.00 ml	36.26%
3. SODIUM CHLORIDE 2.5MEQ/ML 250ML	2	4219-02	exp.	2.5 meq/ml	12.00 ml	30.00mEq
4. SODIUM ACETATE 2MEQ/ML 100ML	5	3299-06	exp.	2.0 meq/ml	15.00 ml	30.00mEq
5. POTASSIUM CHLORIDE 2MEQ/ML 250ML	1	1513-02	exp.	2.0 meq/ml	5.00 ml	10.00mEq
6. CALCIUM GLUCONATE 10% 4.65MEQ/10ML 100ML	4	6524-00	exp.	0.46 meq/ml	10.86 ml	5.00mEq
7. MAGNESIUM SULFATE 50% 4.06MEQ/ML 50ML	5	2168-03	exp.	4.1 meq/ml	7.38 ml	30.00mEq
8. MULTI TRACE (MTE-4) 10ML SDV	9	8100-30	exp.		3.00 ml	3.00ml
9. SELEPEN 40MCG/ML 10ML	3	8820-30	exp.	40.0 mcg/ml	1.00 ml	40.00mcg
10. STERILE WATER FOR INJ 2000ML	2	7118-07	exp.		98.00 ml	98.00ml
11. EMPTY IV BAG 2000ML		113610-25				1.35
12.						
13.						
14.						
15.						

*Lot Nbr - Record Responsibility

1) Tech. or R.Ph. responsible for compounding.............. sign
2) Second Tech. or R.Ph. responsible for compounding..............

Check not required when R.Ph. compounding

Pharmacists Performing Check:

(Signature/Date)   (Signature/Date)   (Signature/Date)

Figure 11-10. *Batch preparation record for a high-risk product. (Reproduced, with permission, from PharmaThera, Memphis, TN.)*

prepared on November 22, 1995). A batch log is useful to track products easily by lot number and to avoid the assignment of the same sequential number to two products compounded at approximately the same time. If separate compounding areas exist, an identifying letter can be used with the lot number to determine the compounding area.

To assign responsibility for the process and the product, the involvement of all personnel must be documented. For short or uncomplicated procedures (e.g., combination of two solutions), the signatures should appear at the end of the document. By signing, these individuals attest that all information is accurate and that they are responsible for the product. For products requiring several components or several compounding steps, each step must bear the signature or initials of the persons responsible. However, a pharmacist must still take responsibility for the finished product.

Criteria for the release and use of the product must be established in advance and adhered to from batch to batch. Release data may include end-product laboratory analysis, physical and visual inspection, and results of other parameters (e.g., environmental testing, proper labeling, accurate weight or volume, and container/closure integrity). Then, the finished product is compared to established specifications. If the product meets these criteria, it is released for use. If the criteria are not strictly met, the product may be conditionally released, pending results of further investigation. However, this occurrence is rare, and the decision for conditional release should be made only after careful analysis.

If the product fails any major specification, it must be rejected. Rejected products may be reprocessed, depending on the reason for failure, or destroyed. A pharmacist who is trained and knowledgeable in sterile product preparation and analysis must be responsible for the product's release. Two pharmacists probably should review all results. Regardless of the outcome, the pharmacists must document their decision in the batch record and sign the release document (see Figure 11-11).

As in the master work sheet, batch preparation records may contain the following:

- ❏ A component test record for nonsterile ingredients, with manufacturers' certificates of analysis to document their acceptability (see Figure 11-1).
- ❏ A raw materials testing record (see Figure 11-2).
- ❏ An analytical request and results form for testing components of inhouse-prepared sterile solutions (see Figure 11-3).
- ❏ A final approval and release form for components of inhouse-prepared sterile solutions (see Figure 11-4).
- ❏ An equipment form to record the supplies used

for compounding and, if necessary, the checks of calibration, filter integrity, etc. (see Figure 11-5).
- ❏ Records of component lot numbers and expiration dates as well as quantities used (see Figure 11-10).
- ❏ Inprocess test records, including product weight (see Figure 11-6) and various other tests.
- ❏ A final release form for the product, including results of tests and release from quarantine (see Figure 11-11).

Finally, a sample label for each lot number is affixed to the batch record, and the batch is visually checked for container integrity, clarity, color, and weight or volume before any product is released (see Figure 11-7). A separate document is not necessary for each type of record. One form usually can be used for components, equipment, and results of tests (see Figure 11-12). Then, the label is affixed to the back of the form.

SUMMARY

Batch preparation of multiple sterile product units, if performed correctly, can produce cost savings in labor, drugs, and materials. However, this process requires strict adherence to procedure. Any failure in the process can lead to significant waste and/or pose a threat to patient safety.

Master work sheets and batch processing records can establish a uniform approach to the preparation process. The work sheet provides exact directions on the standard preparation of the batch product. The batch record then records the completion of these tasks and identifies that each process has been followed.

REFERENCES

1. American Society of Hospital Pharmacists. ASHP technical assistance bulletin on quality assurance for pharmacy-prepared sterile products. *Am J Hosp Pharm.* 1993; 50:2386–98.
2. Avis KE, Lachman L, Lieberman HA, eds. Pharmaceutical dosage forms: parenteral medications, vol 1. New York: Marcel Dekker; 1984.
3. Kessler DA. MedWatch: the new FDA medical products reporting program. *Am J Hosp Pharm.* 1993; 50:1921–36.
4. Sterile drug products for home use. In: United States pharmacopeia, 23rd rev./national formulary, 18th ed. Rockville, MD: United States Pharmacopeial Convention; 1994:1963–75.

TPN QC SUMMARY/ RELEASE

TPN: 4.25% Amino Acids / 20% Dextrose   Date:_____

Formula No. : _____HP20 1L_____   Lot No. : _____

<table>
<tr><td colspan="2">

BACTERIOLOGY

Sterility:_____ Pass _____ Fail
Lab Test No. _____

Pyrogen:_____ Pass _____ Fail
Lab Test No. _____

</td><td colspan="2">

STERILITY RETEST

Reason for Retest:_____
Number of Bags Sent:_____
Date Samples Sent:_____

RESULTS: _____ Pass _____ Fail
Lab Test No. _____

</td></tr>
</table>

INGREDIENT	Labeled Content	Test Result	Satisfactory	Discrepant
Amino Acid	4.25 %			
Dextrose	20.00 %			
Sodium	35.00 mEq/L			
potassium	30.00 mEq/L			
magnesium	10.00 mEq/L			
chloride	35.00 mEq/L			
acetate	64.60 mEq/L			
calcium	5.00 mEq/L			
phosphorous	10.00 mM/L			
copper	1.00 mg/L			
zinc	2.00 mg/L			
selenium	40.00 µg/L	N/A		

<table>
<tr><td>

PRODUCT RELEASE

Pharmacist: _____

Date:_____

</td><td>

PRODUCT REJECTED

Reason: _____
Date: _____
Discarded Date:_____
Pharmacist: _____

</td></tr>
</table>

Figure 11-11. *Final product quality-control summary/release.*

CARDIOPLEGIA SOLUTION, TYPE "C"
LOG SHEET

Date:_____

Quantity of bags to be made, Type "C" _____

Prepared by: _____   Checked by: _____
             (print name)   (print name)

Assigned Lot # _____   Expiration Date: _____

SOLUTIONS USED:	MFG:	VOLUME:	LOT#	EXPIRATION
Sterile Water for Inj.	(Baxter)	2000 ml		_____
Anticoagulant CPD Soln.	(Abbott)	500 ml		_____
Tham 0.3 Molar Soln.	(Abbott)	500 ml		_____
Potassium Chloride 2mEq/ml	(_____)	200 ml		_____
Dextrose 50% in Water	(_____)	50 ml		_____
Glutamate-Aspartate Sol.	(UIH)	30 ml		_____
Viaflex Automix Bag	(Baxter)	1000 ml		_____

PHASE I

New Transfer Set Used?   YES / NO : _____ (R.Ph. Initials)

Automix Calibrated?   YES / NO : _____ (R.Ph. Initials)

Automix Set-up Checked
and Verified for Base
Solution Compounding?   YES / NO : _____ (R.Ph. Initials)

PHASE II

Additive Set-up Checked
and Verified?   YES / NO : _____ (R.Ph. Initials)

Compounding Process Completed: _____ (R.Ph. Signature)

END PRODUCT TESTING

End Product Testing Done? YES / NO : _____ (R.Ph. Initials)

Microbial Testing Results? POS. / NEG. : _____ (R.Ph. Initials)

Potassium Chloride Conc., Type "C" Sample: _____ mEq/ml
                        (0.034 mEq/ml)

Release Date / Pharmacist: _____ / _____

figure 11-12. *Batch preparation record of components, equipment, and test results.*

5. Patel JA. Quality control and standards. In: Brown TR, Smith MC, eds. Handbook of institutional pharmacy practice, 2nd ed. Baltimore, MD: Williams & Wilkins; 1986:402–11.

6. Neidich RL. Selection of containers and closure systems for injectable products. *Am J Hosp Pharm.* 1983; 40:1924–7.

7. Murphy C. Ensuring accuracy in the use of automatic compounders. *Am J Hosp Pharm.* 1993; 50:60. Letter.

8. Brushwood DB. Hospital liable for defect in cardio-plegia solution. *Am J Hosp Pharm.* 1992; 49:1174–6.

9. Bardas SL, Ferraresi VF, Lieberman SF. Refractometric screening of controlled substances used in operating rooms. *Am J Hosp Pharm.* 1992; 49:2779–81.

10. Silverberg JM, Webb B, Pawlak R. Specific gravity-based determination of dextrose content of total parenteral nutrient solutions for neonates. *Am J Hosp Pharm.* 1993; 50:2090–1.

11. Akers MJ. Parenteral quality control. New York: Marcel Dekker; 1985.

Chapter 12
Factors Influencing Expiration Dates

Barbara T. McKinnon

A product's expiration date or shelf life indicates the period when at least 90% of the drug is available for delivery.[1] These dates are applied to intact formulations from the manufacturer. Typically, shorter use times are assigned to drugs that have been reconstituted and diluted for administration. These products should bear labels that specify their storage requirements, expiration dates, and latest time of day for use (when appropriate).[2,3] However, expiration dates can be affected by physical, chemical, and delivery system-related incompatibility or instability as well as sterility considerations.[4]

Incompatibility refers to physicochemical phenomena, such as concentration-dependent precipitation and acid–base reactions.[2] When incompatibilities result in visible changes (e.g., precipitation, cloudiness or haziness, color change, viscosity, and effervescence), the term "physical" or "visual" incompatibility is used.

Instability usually refers to chemical reactions that are continuous and irreversible and that result in different chemical entities (degradation products). These entities can be therapeutically inactive and still exhibit toxicity. Examples include hydrolysis and oxidative reactions.[5]

Common incompatibilities or instabilities often are classified as "physical" or "chemical," even though all incompatibilities have a chemical basis. Moreover, physical incompatibilities may be related to solubility changes or container interactions rather than to molecular changes in the drug itself.[4]

PHYSICAL INCOMPATIBILITIES

Solubility

Drugs can be maintained in aqueous solution as long as their concentrations are less than saturation solubility.[4] If a solution is supersaturated, precipitation may begin. Drugs with poor water solubility are often formulated with water-miscible cosolvents (e.g., ethanol, propylene glycol, and polyethylene glycol). One such formulation is diazepam injection. Dilution of its dosage form may result in precipitation at some concentrations,[6–8] while further dilution (below the saturation solubility point) results in a physically stable admixture.

Other examples of drug formulations using a cosolvent include digoxin, phenytoin, trimethoprim–sulfamethoxazole, etoposide, and teniposide.[4]

pH effect on solubility

Solubility is related to pH for drugs that are weak acids or bases. Because many of these drugs are insoluble in aqueous diluents, they are made into salts to increase their solubility. Weak acids usually are made into salts of weak acids and strong bases (e.g., penicillin G potassium and pentobarbital sodium), while weak bases are made into salts of weak bases and strong acids (e.g., morphine sulfate and tetracycline hydrochloride). Generally, salts of weak acids and strong bases cause physical and chemical incompatibilities with salts of weak bases and strong acids.

In addition, both the stability and solubility of such salts may be affected by the pH of the diluting or reconstituting solution. For example, salts of weak acids and strong bases (e.g., ampicillin sodium) may be less stable in acidic IV solutions such as dextrose 5%, which has a pH of 4.5–5.5. Moreover, drugs that are placed in nonaqueous diluents to increase their solubility and stability may undergo a change of solvent or pH effect in 100% aqueous IV solutions. This change may result in precipitation or chemical instability. Examples include diazepam, digoxin, and phenytoin sodium injection.

Insolubility of parenteral nutrition solutions

The problem of precipitation due to the formation of relatively insoluble salts has been widely publicized by the Food and Drug Administration (FDA). A safety alert was issued by the FDA to focus attention on the hazards of precipitation associated with parenteral nutrition.[9] Furthermore, the phenomenon of calcium and phosphate solubility is complex. The potential for formation of insoluble compounds is further complicated by the various components (e.g., amino acids, dextrose, fat emulsion, electrolyte salts, trace minerals, and vitamins) in a typical parenteral nutrition solution.

pH-related precipitation. Precipitation can occur due to the formation of a dibasic calcium phosphate salt. Although this salt is nearly insoluble in water, monobasic calcium phosphate is relatively soluble. The pKa is 7.2 for the equilibrium between dibasic and monobasic phosphate ions. Raising the pH increases the amount of phosphate in the dibasic form, increasing the probability of calcium phosphate precipitation. Highly reactive salts (e.g., sodium bicarbonate and calcium chloride) should be avoided, because they also might contribute to precipitate formation.[10]

Temperature-related precipitation. Calcium phosphate precipitation also may be related to temperature. As temperature rises, particle movement increases. Therefore, the probability increases of a collision between free calcium and dibasic phosphate ions. This effect may explain the reported occurrence of calcium phosphate precipitation within both the lumen of central venous catheters[11] and the parenteral nutrition solution tubing for infants in incubators.[10]

Other causes of precipitation. Enhanced precipitate formation usually results from high concentrations of calcium and phosphate, increases in solution pH, decreases in amino acid concentrations, and increases in temperature. Other factors may include the addition of calcium before phosphate, lengthy time delays or slow infusion rates that increase exposure of the product to room temperature conditions, and use of the chloride salt of calcium.[4,12]

Increase in solubility of parenteral nutrition solutions

Factors leading to greater calcium/phosphorus stability include

❐ Increased amino acid concentration, which buffers the solution.
❐ Lower pH, which reduces the dibasic phosphate salt available for precipitation with calcium.
❐ Lower storage and administration temperature, which reduces the risk of precipitation.
❐ More stable form of calcium gluconate or acetate rather than calcium chloride.

2-in-1 solutions. If the calcium concentration is maintained at less than 10 mEq/L and the phosphorus concentration is less than 30 mM/L, the risk of precipitation in a 2-in-1 solution is relatively low. Moreover, solubility of the added calcium should be based on the volume when calcium is added—not on the final solution volume. For automated compounding devices, the manufacturer's protocol for additives must be followed. Medical personnel as well as patients or caregivers who administer parenteral nutrition solutions should be trained to agitate the solution and visually inspect for precipitation.[9]

3-in-1 solutions. Total nutrient admixtures (TNAs) or 3-in-1 solutions—when dextrose, amino acids, and lipid emulsions are combined in one container—have complicated stability considerations. The mixing order is critical. Although numerous combinations are acceptable, lipid emulsion should not be combined directly with dextrose without amino acid solutions.

If automated compounding devices are used, the manufacturer's protocol for the order of additives must be followed. A final pH greater than 5 is needed for stability, limiting the use of TNAs with pediatric parenteral nutrition solutions containing a cysteine additive.[13] Concentrations of divalent cations, such as calcium and magnesium, should be limited to avoid destabilizing the emulsion. Because no foolproof method has been found to predict TNA stability, expiration dates should be conservative.

Solubility of large organic ions

Large organic anions and cations also may form precipitates or insoluble complexes.[4] For example, heparin (a large anionic complex) may precipitate with cationic drugs such as aminoglycosides.[14] Such precipitation depends on whether the solubility product of the heparin salt of the cationic drug is exceeded. Therefore, precipitation may occur at high concentrations but not if the drugs are sufficiently diluted.[4]

Sorption

Sorption occurs when drug is lost (from the solution to be administered) by adsorption to the surface or absorption into the matrix of the container material, administration set, or filter.[4] Drugs that exhibit sorption include nitroglycerin, diazepam, warfarin, vitamin A, dactinomycin, and insulin.

Adsorption

For drugs administered in small quantities or low concentrations, adsorption is important because a clinically relevant amount may be removed from the solution. Drugs given in larger quantities lose a smaller percentage of the total dose because of saturation of binding sites on the container surface.[4]

Absorption

Absorption into the matrix of plastic containers and administration sets, especially ones made of polyvinyl chloride (PVC), is a source of loss for lipid-soluble drugs (e.g., vitamin A).[15–17] Phthalate plasticizers are used to make the plastic soft and flexible, but lipid-soluble drugs diffuse into them. However, plastics that contain little or no phthalate plasticizers (e.g., polyethylene and polypropylene) do not readily absorb lipid-soluble drugs.[18] Because of this difference in absorption potential, specialized administration sets may be needed for some solutions (e.g., nitroglycerin). To minimize sorption, short tubing and small tubing diameters also may be helpful.

The opposite effect—leaching of phthalate plasticizers into the solution—also may occur. Concerns have been expressed about the extraction of the plasticizer d-2-ethylhexylphthalate (DEHP) by lipid emulsions.[19]

Other Physical Incompatibilities

Other physical incompatibilities include

- ❑ "Salting out" or precipitation of organic drugs in the presence of strong electrolytes.
- ❑ Complexation phenomena such as the formation of chelates of tetracycline with aluminum, calcium, iron, and magnesium.
- ❑ Color changes from chemical degradation to a colored decomposition product and gas evolution (evident in reconstitution of ceftazidime).[4]

CHEMICAL DEGRADATION

Drugs may undergo degradation by various chemical reactions. Although a few reactions produce visible changes, such as color and gas evolution, most chemical incompatibilities are not visually observable.[4]

Hydrolysis, Oxidation, and Reduction

Hydrolysis reactions involve the attack of labile bonds, by water, in dissolved drug molecules with resultant molecular changes. However, oxidation and reduction reactions involve exchange of electrons and valence changes in the drug molecules. To control oxidation reactions in parenteral products, manufacturers evacuate oxygen from glass containers and fill any head space with nitrogen. They also may adjust pH, add chelating agents such as ethylenediaminetetraacetic acid (EDTA), or add antioxidants such as sodium bisulfate.[4]

To avoid the formation of toxic hydroperoxides,[20] lipid emulsions should be packaged in glass containers only. Repackaging them in plastic IV bags, which are relatively permeable to oxygen, should be avoided. TNAs can be packaged in plastic because the antioxidant from the amino acid product also protects the lipid emulsion; however, non-DEHP-containing bags are preferred. PVC bags that utilize alternative plasticizers or ethylene vinyl acetate bags are available.

Photolysis

Photodegradation or photolysis is the catalysis of degradation reactions by light. Although various decomposition mechanisms may occur, energy is always generated to cause change at a chemical bond and rearrange to a new chemical entity.[4] The more intense a light source is and the closer the photolabile drugs are to it, the greater is the rate of photodegradation.[5] Additionally, ultraviolet light is more harmful than visible light, and daylight is more harmful than fluorescent light.[4]

To administer photolabile drugs, light must be excluded from the container. Furthermore, tubing should be wrapped with foil (if necessary). Protection of the product should continue from preparation until use or conclusion of administration.[2]

STABILITY RELATED TO DRUG DELIVERY SYSTEMS

When an expiration date is assigned to a drug admixture,

the delivery system also should be considered. Important points include the type of system and its environmental temperature. Different environments have different temperatures that may affect storage conditions and, therefore, stability and expiration dating.

Delivery Systems

Large volume parenterals

Large volume parenteral admixtures are often used to administer one or more drugs or electrolytes continuously. Parenteral nutrition solutions present a worst case scenario because numerous components (including nutrients, electrolytes, vitamins, minerals, and drugs) are coinfused in the same container. Due to the long contact time and exposure to ambient temperature and light conditions, the potential for drug stability and compatibility problems increases.[2]

Syringes

When syringes are used for drug administration, more concentrated drug solutions frequently are used than is common for other infusions. The same principle is true for reservoirs of concentrated drugs used for home administration via ambulatory electronic pumps. If more than one concentrated drug is combined in a syringe or reservoir, the potential for an incompatibility is increased due to high concentrations and prolonged contact time.

Y-site administration

When drug administration is required for a patient on parenteral nutrition without another venous access, a Y-site technique may be preferred. Y-site or piggyback drug delivery helps to minimize problems with drug incompatibility by decreasing the contact time of multiple solutions to about 15 min.[14] Few combinations of drugs are so chemically unstable that Y-site administration is precluded.[4]

Environmental Temperatures

Clinical setting

The effects of temperature on drug delivery in the clinical setting should be considered. Drugs may be refrigerated or frozen, but warming to room temperature typically takes place during preparation for administration. Administration of drugs may require prolonged exposure to ambient temperatures. Additionally, portable pumps—either ambulatory electronic pumps or disposable elastomeric devices—may expose drugs to 30–32° C temperatures. With implantable pumps, drugs are maintained at about 37° C. The stability of the drug at its expected delivery temperature must be assessed to ensure adequate stability throughout the labeled period of use.[3,4]

Pharmacists also should consider the effect of cumulative room temperature storage on a product's stability. For example, sterile products may be removed from the refrigerator, warmed to room temperature, and then—if not used immediately—returned to the refrigerator. The original expiration date could easily be invalidated under these circumstances. Therefore, the pharmacist should determine the expected stability of the product under actual storage conditions and then appraise whether it is still appropriate for use. The product's manufacturer or other credible reference[21] source also should be consulted.

Home setting

In the home setting, the growing use of IV products has increased the need for extended drug stability. Home care practice demands that the pharmacist assign a maximum expiration date that is still within appropriate stability limits. This maximum date helps to minimize additional delivery costs and reduce waste.

A common problem is the use of drugs with limited room temperature stability. For drugs to be administered via an ambulatory infusion device, at least 24-hr stability at room temperature or warmer is typically required. For drugs with limited room temperature stability, the device used should combine them with the diluent immediately before administration.

STERILITY LIMITATIONS

Even under the best aseptic processing conditions, microorganisms might inadvertently contaminate sterile products. Therefore, sterile products not intended for prompt use should be stored at no more than 4° C to inhibit microbial growth. Products intended for prompt administration after compounding may be retained at room temperature.[2,21]

When the sterility-associated risk is evaluated, a product's ability to support microbial growth must be considered. Although clinical infections related to microbial contamination of infusion solutions occur less frequently than other causes of infusion-related infections (e.g., catheter related), solution contamination can lead to epidemic infections.[22]

In clinical practice, reported rates of infusate-related contamination are

- ❑ 0.39–3.8% for standard IV fluids.[23–25]
- ❑ 0–0.91% for crystalline amino acid and dextrose solutions.[23,26–28]
- ❑ 2–4% for TNAs.[29,30]
- ❑ 3% for in-use bottles of lipid emulsion.[31]

The variability of these contamination rates depends on the capability of differing solutions to support microbial growth.

Isotonic Solutions

Isotonic solutions, such as dextrose 5% and normal saline, provide an adequate media for the survival of microorganisms. Septicemia has been associated with intrinsically contaminated IV fluids (during the manufacturing process).[32,33] Extrinsic contamination (during handling and use) during solution manipulations in pharmacies has been reported.[34] In a recent report, however, normal saline did not support bacterial or yeast growth over a 7-day study period when incubated at 3, 25, or 37° C, presumably because of a lack of nutrients.[35]

Parenteral Nutrition Solutions

After reports of protein hydrolysate contamination with both bacteria and fungi, parenteral nutrition solutions gained a reputation of being prone to contamination.[36–38] Actually, the crystalline amino acid solutions currently in use are a poor growth media for bacteria. Most strains either die or show minimal growth.[37,38]

Poor bacterial survival has been attributed to the low pH and hypertonicity of amino acid and dextrose solutions. However, *Pseudomonas aeruginosa* and *Escherichia coli* can withstand the pH and osmolarity of central vein parenteral nutrition formulations. Moreover, dilution of the dextrose (as in peripheral vein formulations) improves survival of *Staphylococcus aureus*, *Streptococcus faecalis*, and *P. aeruginosa*.[37,39]

Fungi, particularly *Candida albicans*, proliferate in standard crystalline amino acid-based solutions.[37,38] Numerous cases of fungal sepsis associated with parenteral nutrition have been reported.[40–43]

Because of the potential for fungal proliferation within a brief period (24 hr), parenteral nutrition solutions should be refrigerated immediately after admixture.[22] Prolonged storage (7 days–12 weeks) has been reported with no bacterial contamination.[37,44–46] However, a validated compounding process should ensure that no bacterial proliferation occurs in purportedly sterile solutions. For these solutions, stability of components may be a more important consideration for expiration dating. Significant losses of tryptophan and other amino acids have been reported.[44] Additionally, end-product sterility testing is recommended for prolonged storage of solutions.[44]

TNAs

In certain patient groups, TNAs that combine fat emulsion with dextrose and amino acids may be clinically useful. The risk of microbial contamination may be reduced because of fewer manipulations of the hyperalimentation fluid and tubing. However, these admixtures may provide better growth media for pathogenic microorganisms.[47]

Because TNAs cannot be filtered through a bacterial-retentive 0.22-μm filter,[48] growth of even a few microorganisms could harm the patient. *Staphylococcus*
epidermidis, *C. albicans*, and *E. coli* can survive in TNAs. A 1.2-μm filter removes *C. albicans* but not *S. epidermidis* and *E. coli*.

Growth of most microorganisms was significantly better in TNAs than in standard parenteral nutrition solutions without lipid emulsion.[39] However, with inoculum sizes approximating touch contamination, bacterial and fungal growth were limited to less than 1 log/24 hr. About 48 hr was required to reach stationary phase growth in TNAs.[49] Therefore, maximum infusion times of 24 hr at room temperature are recommended.[49,50]

Lipid Emulsions

Lipid emulsions (given separately or as a Y-site infusion) have the potential for contamination. They provide an excellent media for the growth of gram-positive, gram-negative, and fungal species at room temperature[51] and after refrigeration. In one report, lipid emulsions supported bacterial and fungal growth at the same level as trypticase soy broth.[52]

In 1981, the Centers for Disease Control recommended a 12-hr hang time for lipid emulsions because of concerns about infection.[22] One study found no differences in microbial contamination in a clinical setting between bottles left hanging for less than or greater than 12 hr and no increase in infection complications with a hang time of 24 hr.[31] Therefore, a hang time of 24 hr has become accepted in clinical practice.

IV Immune Globulins

IV immune globulins (IVIGs) are expensive biological substances. Although their solutions remain chemically stable for 1 month at 37° C,[53] package directions recommend administration as soon as possible to maintain product sterility rather than stability. However, a recent report stated that IVIG preparations cannot support bacterial and fungal growth at refrigerated, room, or body temperatures. Therefore, expiration dates should be reconsidered.[35]

Ganciclovir

The manufacturer of ganciclovir recommends immediate use of the drug (within 24 hr after reconstitution),[54] but several studies document its stability (reconstituted with dextrose 5% or normal saline) at 5[55]–35 days.[56,57] Stability is relevant to home care practitioners because (1) ganciclovir may be continued for several years and (2) many patients prefer to receive it at home. However, a 24-hr expiration date is not practical because daily preparation and delivery would be required. Furthermore, the patient or caregiver should not be allowed to mix each dose in the home immediately before use since ganciclovir has both mutagenic and carcinogenic potential.[54] Ideally, it should be prepared as an antineoplastic agent by using a biological safety cabinet and appropriate safety garments.

In December 1993, Syntex reported that crystals were occasionally observed in reconstituted vials during quality testing of ganciclovir.[58] These crystals were identified as an antioxidant or component of the rubber stoppers on the vials. For this reason, the manufacturer recommends use of an inline filter (preferably 0.22 µm) during infusion of ganciclovir solutions.[58]

Portable Pumps

Sterility often is a concern for drugs used in portable pumps that may be exposed to warmer than room temperatures for up to a week. In one study, Baxter PCA infusors containing standard morphine solutions (1 and 5 mg/ml preserved with chlorobutanol) were inoculated with microorganisms. These solutions were bacteriocidal for most organisms at most storage conditions. Only relatively high inocula (104 organisms) of *P. aeruginosa* or *Klebsiella pneumoniae* survived in an "in-use" temperature of about 30° for 8 days.[59] In another study, 15 patients receiving epidural morphine from an external pump had no clinical infections. Although 0.6% of the drug reservoirs had bacteria, the epidural filters were free from growth.[60]

Multidose Vials

Time limits on using multidose vials after opening them have been investigated. The primary concern is that contamination of the vials could lead to nosocomial sources of infection.[61] After examining vials used in a hospital for 3 months, one study found a relatively low risk of contamination. The study's proposed guidelines would require multidose vials to be dated when opened and discarded[62]

- ❑ When empty.
- ❑ After the manufacturer's expiration date.
- ❑ At the end of 3 months.
- ❑ When contamination is suspected.

Additionally, reports state that heavy bacterial contamination of the rubber septum or use of a contaminated needle is required to produce consistently positive cultures.[63] Other reports confirm that some physicians reenter a vial with the same needle used in another patient.[64]

Preservatives help to maintain the sterility of multidose vials, but guidelines for their use do not apply to single-use vials. Aseptic technique should be practiced, including the wiping of the rubber septum of vials with 70% isopropyl alcohol and use of sterile syringe-needle units for each entry.

DETERMINATION OF EXPIRATION DATES

When possible, expiration dates should be in accordance with the product's approved labeling. However, reliable, published stability information is sometimes lacking. Also, information about long-term stability of drugs for home use often is unavailable or absent from the labeling.

Manufacturer Information

A pharmacist may be unable to comply with a product's approved labeling and guidelines. For example, a higher concentration of drug may be prescribed, a different diluent may be required, or a patient may require a product for longer periods (e.g., home delivery).

Ideally, pharmacists should consult with the manufacturer to establish an expiration date. They also should communicate the deviations from the package insert when requesting stability information. The exact strength, diluent, fill volume, and container type (e.g., PVC bag, plastic syringe, and elastomeric infusion device) should be included. Moreover, pharmacists should obtain a letter from the manufacturer certifying the expiration date.[2] However, time constraints and immediate needs for drug products may preclude advice from the manufacturer.

Published Stability Information

Published stability information, if carefully applied, can help to determine a theoretical expiration date for a given product. References on drug stability include the *Handbook on Injectable Drugs*,[2] *Remington's Pharmaceutical Sciences*,[21] and other reliable published research.

Applying published stability data can introduce inaccuracies if the characteristics of the product to be compounded differ greatly from the characteristics of the reported products. Differing characteristics (e.g., composition, concentrations of ingredients, fill volume, and container type and material) should not be assumed to be equivalent. Additionally, conditions during inhome use (e.g., homes without air conditioning in a hot climate) must be considered.

When informational resources are used to establish an expiration date, the pharmacist should ensure that they have undergone critical evaluation. Expiration dates predicted from these resources should not extend beyond the realistic and practical patient care needs of the pharmacy.

Pharmacists should maintain a record of resources used for establishing expiration dates[3] and develop policies and procedures for their appropriate assignment.[2] A table or chart of accepted expiration dates for commonly prepared products may be helpful. In addition to saving time, this procedure can ensure that assigned expiration dates are both consistent and appropriate.

Product-Specific Experimental Studies

For the prediction of expiration dating, the only valid evidence of stability is from product-specific experimental studies. The greater one's doubt about the accuracy of the dating, the greater is the need to determine dating periods experimentally. For example, failure of one product to support bacterial and fungal growth under specific conditions should not be extrapolated to other products unless specific and reliable data are available. Experimental studies should be considered for sterile products prepared from nonsterile bulk active ingredients that have therapeutic activity (especially when compounded routinely).

Semiquantitative procedures, such as thin-layer chromatography, may be acceptable for some products. However, quantitative stability-indicating assays (e.g., high-performance liquid chromatography) are more appropriate for critical products. Examples include drugs with

1. A narrow therapeutic range.
2. Minimal supporting evidence of an appropriate expiration dating period.
3. A significant margin of safety that cannot be verified for the proposed theoretical period.

Expiration dates not specifically referenced in the product's approved labeling should be limited to 30 days.[2]

SUMMARY

In this cost containment era, expiration dating has important implications. Products with longer dates may allow more efficient batch preparation in pharmacies, less frequent deliveries for home care practitioners, and recycling of unused products in hospitals.

Expiration dates for admixture preparations must be based on stability and sterility considerations. Both physical and chemical breakdowns are possible. Solubility-related problems may occur from changes in pH, temperature, and drug structure. In addition, drug adsorption to and absorption within product containers must be considered. Chemical degradation due to hydrolysis, oxidation, reduction, or photolysis also can quickly deteriorate a product. Moreover, the method and environment of drug administration can affect stability.

Sterility is separate from but as important as stability. Although a product may be stable for an extended period, its sterility also must be a factor in assigning an expiration date. The potential for bacterial growth has been widely studied and verified. With an increased use of TPN, TNA, IVIG, and ganciclovir in the home setting (requiring extended usage and administration time), this issue becomes even more important.

After considering physical, chemical, and delivery system effects, a pharmacist may still have to limit expiration dating. Some manufacturers or published studies can offer information regarding extended expirations, but a pharmacist may have to conduct separate product-specific experimental studies.

REFERENCES

1. Stella VJ. Chemical and physical bases determining the instability and incompatibility of formulated injectable drugs. *J Parenter Sci Technol*. 1986; 40:2142–63.
2. Trissel LA. Handbook on injectable drugs, 8th ed. Bethesda, MD: American Society of Hospital Pharmacists; 1994.
3. American Society of Hospital Pharmacists. ASHP technical assistance bulletin on quality assurance for pharmacy-prepared sterile products. *Am J Hosp Pharm*. 1993; 50:2386–98.
4. Sterile drug products for home use. In: United States pharmacopeia, 23rd rev./national formulary, 18th ed. Rockville, MD: United States Pharmacopeial Convention; 1994:1963–75.
5. Newton DW. Physicochemical determinants of incompatibility and instability of drugs for injection and infusion. *Am J Hosp Pharm*. 1978; 35:1213–22.
6. Newton DW, Driscoll DF, Goudreau JL, et al. Solubility characteristics of diazepam in aqueous admixture solutions: theory and practice. *Am J Hosp Pharm*. 1981; 38:179–82.
7. Mason NA, Cline S, Hyneck ML, et al. Factors affecting diazepam infusion: solubility, administration-set composition, and flow rate. *Am J Hosp Pharm*. 1981; 38:1449–54.
8. Morris ME. Compatibility and stability of diazepam injection following dilution from intravenous fluids. *Am J Hosp Pharm*. 1978; 35:669–72.
9. Food and Drug Administration. Safety alert: Hazards of precipitation associated with parenteral nutrition. *Am J Hosp Pharm*. 1994; 51:1427–8.
10. Driscoll DF, Newton DW, Bistrian BR. Precipitation of calcium phosphate from parenteral nutrient fluids. *Am J Hosp Pharm*. 1994; 51:2834–6.
11. Robinson LA, Wright BT. Central venous catheter occlusion caused by body-heat mediated calcium phosphate precipitation. *Am J Hosp Pharm*. 1982; 39:120–1.
12. Niemiec PW, Vanderveen TW. Compatibility considerations in parenteral nutrient solutions. *Am J Hosp Pharm*. 1984; 41:893–911.
13. Wells P. A guide to total nutrient admixtures. Chicago, IL: Precept Press; 1992.
14. Leissing NC, Story KO, Zaske D. Inline fluid dynamics in piggyback and manifold drug delivery systems. *Am J Hosp Pharm*. 1989; 46:89–97.
15. Niemiec PW, Waler JZ. Vitamin A availability from parenteral solution delivery systems. *Nutr Supp Serv*. 1983; 3:53, 56.
16. Gillis J, Jones G, Peuchanz P. Delivery of vitamins A, D, and E in total parenteral nutrition solutions. *J Parenter Enter Nutr*. 1983; 7:11–4.

17. Riggle MA, Brandt RB. Decrease of available vitamin A in parenteral nutrition solutions. *J Parenter Enter Nutr*. 1986; 10:388–92.

18. Kwaluk EA, Roberts MS, Polack AE. Interactions between drugs and intravenous delivery systems. *Am J Hosp Pharm*. 1982; 39:460–7.

19. Pelham LD. Rational use of intravenous fat emulsions. *Am J Hosp Pharm*. 1981; 38:198–208.

20. Helback HJ, Moltehnik DA, Ames BN. Toxic hydroperoxides in intravenous lipid emulsions used in preterm infants. *Pediatrics*. 1993; 91:83–7.

21. Remington's Pharmaceutical Sciences, 18th ed. Easton, PA: Mack Publishing Company; 1990.

22. Simmons BP. Guidelines for prevention of intravascular infections. Atlanta, GA: Centers for Disease Control; 1981.

23. Bozzetti F, Bonfanti G, Regalie E, et al. Catheter sepsis from infusate contamination. *Nutr Clin Pract*. 1990; 5:156–9.

24. Band JD, Maki DG. Safety of changing intravenous delivery systems at longer than 24 hour intervals. *Ann Intern Med*. 1979; 91:173–8.

25. Miller WA, Smith GL, Latiolais CJ, et al. A comparative evaluation of compounding costs and contamination rates of intravenous admixture systems. *Drug Intell Clin Pharm*. 1971; 5:51–60.

26. DeCicco M, Chiaradia V, Veronese A, et al. Source and route of microbial colonization of parenteral nutrition catheters. *Lancet*. 1989; 2:1258–61.

27. Takagi J, Kalidi N, Wolk RA, et al. Sterility of total parenteral nutrition solutions stored at room temperature for seven days. *Am J Hosp Pharm*. 1989; 46:973–7.

28. Bronson MH, Stennett DJ, Egging PK. Sterility testing of home and inpatient parenteral nutrition solutions. *J Parenter Enter Nutr*. 1988; 12:25–8.

29. Dolvin BJ, Davis PD, Holland TA. Contamination rates of 3-in-1 total parenteral nutrition in a clinical setting. *J Parenter Enter Nutr*. 1987; 1:413–5.

30. Sitges-Serra A, Jaurrieta E, Pallares R, et al. Clinical experience with fat containing TPN solutions. In: Johnson I, ed. Advances in clinical nutrition. Boston, MA: MTP Press; 1983:207–12.

31. Ebbert ML, Farraj M, Hwang LT. The incidence and clinical significance of intravenous fat emulsion contamination during infusion. *J Parenter Enter Nutr*. 1987; 11:42–5.

32. Centers for Disease Control. Nosocomial bacteremias associated with intravenous fluid therapy—USA. *MMWR*. 1971; 20:special suppl to no. 9.

33. Centers for Disease Control. Septicemias associated with contaminated intravenous fluids—Wisconsin, Ohio. *MMWR*. 1973; 22:99.

34. Miller WA, Smith GL, Latiolais CJ. A comparative evaluation of compounding costs and contamina-

35. Pfeifer RW, Siegel J, Ayers LA. Assessment of microbial growth in intravenous immune globulin preparations. *Am J Hosp Pharm*. 1994; 51:1676–9.

36. Freeman JB, Lemire A, MacLean LD. Intravenous alimentation and septicemia. *Surg Gynecol Obstet*. 1972; 135:708–12.

37. Goldmann DA, Martin WT, Worthington JW. Growth of bacteria and fungi in total parenteral nutrition solutions. *Am J Surg*. 1973; 126:314–8.

38. Rowlands DA, Wilkinson WR, Yoshimura N. Storage stability of mixed hyperalimentation solutions. *Am J Hosp Pharm*. 1973; 30:436–8.

39. Scheckelhoff DJ, Mirtallo JM, Ayers LW, et al. Growth of bacteria and fungi in total nutrient admixtures. *Am J Hosp Pharm*. 1986; 43:73–7.

40. Meunier-Carpentier F, Kiehn TE, Armstrong D. Fungemia in the immunocompromised host. *Am J Med*. 1981; 71:363–70.

41. Henderson DK, Edwards JE, Montgomerie JZ. Hematogenous *Candida* endophthalmitic in patients receiving parenteral hyperalimentation fluids. *J Infect Dis*. 1981; 143:655–61.

42. Klein JJ, Watanakunakorn C. Hospital-acquired fungemia. *Am J Med*. 1979; 67:51–8.

43. Montgomerie JZ, Edwards JE. Association of infection due to *Candida albicans* with intravenous hyperalimentation. *J Infect Dis*. 1978; 137:197–201.

44. Parr MD, Bertch KE, Rapp PR. Amino acid stability and microbial growth in total parenteral nutrition solutions. *Am J Hosp Pharm*. 1985; 42:2688–91.

45. Jurgens RW, Henry RS, Welco A. Amino acid stability in a mixed parenteral nutrition solution. *Am J Hosp Pharm*. 1981; 38:1358–9.

46. Laegeler WL, Tio JM, Blake MI. Stability of certain amino acids in a parenteral nutrition solution. *Am J Hosp Pharm*. 1974; 31:776–9.

47. Thompson B, Robinson LA. Infection control of parenteral nutrition solutions. *Nutr Clin Pract*. 1991; 6:49–54.

48. McKinnon BT, Avis KE. Membrane filtration of pharmaceutical solutions. *Am J Hosp Pharm*. 1993; 50:1921–36.

49. Gilbert M, Gallagher SC, Eads M, et al. Microbial growth patterns in a total parenteral nutrition formulation containing lipid emulsion. *J Parenter Enter Nutr*. 1986; 10:494–7.

50. Brown DH, Simkover RA. Maximum hang times for IV fat emulsions. *Am J Hosp Pharm*. 1987; 44:282–4.

51. Melly MA, Mend HC, Schaffer W. Microbial growth in lipid emulsions used in parenteral nutrition. *Arch Surg*. 1975; 110:1479–81.

52. Kim Ch, Lewis DE, Kumar A. Bacterial and fungal growth in intravenous fat emulsions. *Am J Hosp Pharm*. 1983; 40:2159–61.

53. Freidi HR. Methodology and safety considerations in the production of an intravenous immune globulin preparation. *Pharmacotherapy*. 1987; 7(2):36–40S.

54. Syntex Laboratories, Inc. Cytovene package insert. Palo Alto, CA; 1992 September.

55. Visor GC, Lin LH, Jackson SE, et al. Stability of ganciclovir sodium (DHPG sodium) in 5% dextrose or 0.9% sodium chloride injections. *Am J Hosp Pharm*. 1986; 43:2810–2.

56. Silvestri AP, Mitrano FP, Baptista RJ, et al. Stability and compatibility of ganciclovir sodium in 5% dextrose injection over 35 days. *Am J Hosp Pharm*. 1991; 48:2641–3.

57. Parasrampuria J, Li LC, Stelmach AH, et al. Stability of ganciclovir sodium in 5% dextrose injection and in 0.9% sodium chloride injection over 35 days. *Am J Hosp Pharm*. 1992; 49:116–8.

58. Syntex Laboratories, Inc. New information on administration of Cytovene. Palo Alto, CA; 1993 December.

59. Harrow AG, Wakabongo M, Pesko LJ, et al. Loss of viability of four common pathogens in morphine injection stored in a PCA infusor. *Hosp Pharm*. 1993; 28:325–6.

60. Ohlsson L, Rydbert T, Edlen T, et al. Cancer pain relief by continuous administration of epidural morphine in a hospital setting and at home. *Pain*. 1992; 48:349–53.

61. Moi S, Thornton JP. Time limit on multidose vials after initial entry. *Hosp Pharm*. 1991; 26:805–6.

62. DeSilva MI, Hood E, Tisdel E, et al. Multidosage medication vials: a study of sterility, use patterns, and cost-effectiveness. *Am J Infect Control*. 1986; 14:135–8.

63. Sheth NK, Post GT, Wisniewski TR, et al. Multidose vials vs. single-dose vials: a study in sterility and cost-effectiveness. *J Clin Microbiol*. 1983; 17:377–9.

64. Carter C, ed. California facility eliminates multidose vials in response to litigation. *Drug Util Rev*. 1989; 5:155–6.

Chapter 13
Labeling of Sterile Products

Douglas J. Scheckelhoff

Once a sterile product is prepared, it should be properly labeled to ensure its appropriate use. Terminology should be descriptive but still appropriate to the knowledge of the user. Moreover, the label should be affixed so that it can be read both before and during administration. If a container is to be hung, for example, the label must be positioned upside down so that it is right side up during administration. Light-resistant bags, for photosensitive drugs, and other overwraps should not limit the accessibility to the label.

Small products may require unique methods of affixing the label. For medium-sized syringes, labels often are "flagged" so that syringe markings are not covered or obstructed. Very small syringes can be sealed in a larger bag or overwrap, which is then labeled. If the syringe might be removed from the bag some time before administration, a second, smaller label on the syringe should give key information (e.g., drug name, concentration, and expiration date).

The information on a label varies based on the product type and the patient's location. General label content is similar, but slight variations exist[1,2] in institutional and home care settings as well as for batch preparations.

LABELS IN INSTITUTIONAL SETTINGS

Figure 13-1 illustrates a sample label used in an institutional setting. The parts of this label are described below; the numbers in parentheses correspond to information on the label.

Required Labeling

Patient name and identification number (1)

A patient name on a label defines the dose as patient specific. Exclusion of a name may indicate that the product can be used on other patients and may lead to errors. Moreover, both the first and last names of the patient should be identified. A middle initial can be helpful if two patients have the same first and last names. A medical record number also identifies the patient in most hospital computer systems. However, this number is not critical to drug administration.

Patient location (2)

Location information ensures that the drug gets to the correct pa-

```
John Doe (1)        565656565 (1)     742 W (2)
#23 (12)                              12N 4/1/95 (6)


Cefazolin (3)                         1 GM (3)
in 5% Dextrose in Water (4)           50 ml (5)


Infuse intravenously (11) over 30 min (8)
Use before 12N 4/2/95 (7)
Prepared by: DS (9)
Keep refrigerated (10)
```

figure 13-1. *Sample label in an institutional setting.*

tient. Transfer or discharge of patients also should be tracked so that label information is updated. If the data are not relayed or used, delays in therapy and unnecessary or duplicate preparation could result.

Name and amount of drug added (3)

The name of the drug, preferably generic, should be clearly stated. The trade name can be included if the product is known to be consistent. The trade name should be used if it can reduce the potential for error. Moreover, the amount and units of measure should be standard and easily understood.

Name of admixture solution (4)

Identification of the admixture solution makes the label more complete. Although the amount of dextrose or sodium chloride usually is unimportant in the patient's therapy, it may be a consideration in certain clinical settings. Admixture solution information often is not listed on small volume syringes, especially when the diluent is sterile water for injection.

Approximate final total volume of admixture solution (5)

This measurement tracks the patient's total IV fluid load. If the volume of the admixture solution is not significantly different from the total volume, these measurements are used interchangeably (e.g., antibiotic solutions). For larger volume solutions with multiple additives, the actual or calculated total volume should be used (e.g., TPN solutions). For smaller volumes, such as syringes, the total volume may be listed as a concentration rather than a separate measurement.

Time and date of scheduled administration (6)

This information notifies the nursing staff of the administration schedule maintained in the pharmacy. Nurses usually have their own schedules. However, if both pharmacy and nursing schedules are the same, errors will be minimized.

If nurses follow the scheduled administration time and date printed on the label, admixtures will not be used out of sequence. When admixtures are in improper sequence, the "oldest" one (with the soonest expiration) may not be administered; its expiration date may then be passed, creating waste. Standardized administration times also reduce confusion and waste and prevent omitted doses.

Expiration date (7)

The expiration date assigned to a product can be the actual time that it is deemed unusable or a standard time in which it should be returned to the pharmacy (e.g., 24 hr). After its return, the pharmacist can determine if the product should be recycled or discarded. Methods used to assign actual expiration dates are addressed in Chapter 12.

Administration instructions (8)

For intermittent doses, administration instructions should include the duration and, sometimes, rate of administration. For continuous infusions, administration instructions generally include the rate and possibly a stop time. The rate should not be included for a continuous infusion if the drug is being titrated because the rate may change without the pharmacy's knowledge and without a notation on the label. This situation could result in a medication error or, at least, confusion. In these cases, "infuse as directed" may be more appropriate.

Initials of persons who prepare and check IV admixture (9)

The identity of the preparer and/or pharmacist who releases the product should be noted on the label or in a dispensing record in the pharmacy. State boards of pharmacy often require the initials to be on the label. This information is helpful when questions arise about product preparation.

Storage conditions (10)

Storage instructions can be put on the label or added as an auxiliary label. This information, for example, can remind nurses or other staff to refrigerate a product. Conversely, if a product should not be refrigerated, that information also should be noted. In fact, since refrigeration usually is the standard, this information should be highlighted for emphasis.

Route of administration (11)

The route of administration may be implied by the dosage form (e.g., IV bag implies IV administration unless labeled otherwise). But when a container is used outside the normal pattern or a dosage form has multiple uses, the route must be clearly stated to prevent medication errors. Often, drugs can be given only by certain routes or the amount/concentration is route specific and, therefore, may be lethal otherwise. Products used for irrigation, cardioplegia, intrathecal and epidural injections, and peritoneal dialysis should be clearly marked and distinctively labeled (by size, shape, and color).

Syringes should be clearly labeled with the intended route of administration (e.g., IV via push, pump or gravity, epidural or intrathecal, or intramuscular). In some cases, the ramifications of giving a particular drug or dose by an unintended route can be fatal (e.g., IV dose given intrathecally). Patient-controlled analgesia (PCA) containers also should be clearly marked since they may be the same for IV and epidural PCA, but the concentration of drug differs.

Auxiliary Labeling

Auxiliary labeling provides supplemental instructions and/or precautions, without the space limitations of computerized labels. Auxiliary labels have an added advantage of highlighting the information since the label looks different.

The same auxiliary labels should be used each time a particular product is dispensed; otherwise, the user may question the importance or validity of the information. Auxiliary labels often are used for information about

- ❏ Light protection.
- ❏ Final filters.
- ❏ Rate precautions.
- ❏ Storage conditions.
- ❏ Drug concentration.
- ❏ Routes of administration.

Optional Labeling

Time and date of preparation

The time and date of preparation are needed to determine actual expiration times for recycling products. This information may be contained on the required label, even if it is not stated clearly. For example, the scheduled administration time may indicate when a drug was prepared based on that batch period. Or, the expiration date may be established at 24 hr after preparation as an institutional standard.

Bottle or bag sequence number (12)

The sequence number of the container may be important, depending on the type of drug

or number of doses ordered. The total doses given also should be tracked by the nurse who administers the drug since bags might be given out of sequence or doses might be lost.

LABELS IN HOME CARE SETTINGS

Labels used in home care are similar to those used in institutions but have some unique requirements. Because the product is an outpatient prescription, it must meet state board of pharmacy requirements. Moreover, the label must be understood by the lay person since the user may be the patient, a family member, or other caregiver. The label also should contain few abbreviations or other confusing terminology.

Figure 13-2 illustrates a sample label used in the home care setting. The parts of this label are described below; the numbers in parentheses correspond to information on the label.

Required Labeling

Prescription number, date, and prescribing physician (1)

This information typically is required by state boards of pharmacy, but it also is used by the dispensing pharmacy to verify the original order.

Patient name and address (2)

The patient's name should be printed as part of the prescription label. Although the address is optional, it may simplify delivery procedures.

```
Rx: 1234567(1)              Date: 5/5/95(1)
Patient: Jane A. Doe(2)     Physician: J.R. Smith(1)
         110 S. Elm St.
         Anywhere, MD(2)


Directions: Infuse nafcillin 2 GM (24 ml) over 1
hour every 4 hours for 10 days via CADD-plus
pump. Infuse at 0.2 ml/hr between doses. Change
drug cassette every 24 hours. Keep cassettes
refrigerated and warm to room temperature prior
to infusion.(3)


Contains:
NAFCILLIN(4)                2 GM(4)
in sterile water(5)         24 ml(5)


Use before 12N 5/12/95(6)
Prepared by: DS(7)
```

Figure 13-2. *Sample label in a home care setting.*

Directions for use (3)

Directions should be easy to understand. They should include rate of administration, frequency of administration, and any special handling or storage requirements.

Name and amount of drug added (4)

This section is similar to item (3) on the institutional label; however, the admixture may contain more than one dose. In this situation, the label should indicate the amount of drug in one dose and the appropriate volume for that amount.

Name and volume of admixture solution (5)

This section is similar to item (4) on the institutional label; however, the admixture may contain more than one dose. In this situation, the volume listed should be equivalent to one dose of the drug.

Expiration date (6)

This date usually is the actual expiration date established for the product. Expiration dates often are maximized for practical reasons, such as the patient's distance from the pharmacy. Since patients typically are more stable at home than in an institution, their medications are less likely to change, requiring return to the pharmacy. Furthermore, these products will not be recycled even if returned unused because they are compounded outpatient prescriptions and were stored at home.

Initials of persons who prepare and check IV admixture (7)

Similar to the institutional setting, state boards of pharmacy often require that this information appear on the label. Furthermore, this information is helpful when questions arise about product preparation.

Auxiliary Labeling

Federal transfer labeling must be included, as with any outpatient prescription, and must be easily understood by the user.

Optional Labeling

As in the institutional setting, the bottle or bag sequence number can help to track the specific number of doses ordered and/or the total number of doses administered.

BATCH PREPARATION LABELS

Labels for batch-prepared products (not patient specific) provide information for a much longer time than other labels. Figure 13-3 illustrates a sample label used for batch-

```
Neomycin Sulfate Irrigation Solution[1]


Neomycin Sulfate[2]              1 GM[2]
in 0.9% Sodium Chloride[3]
Total Volume[4]                 1000 ml[4]

FOR IRRIGATION ONLY[5]

Refrigerate after opening[6]

Lot Number: 95051222[7]
Expires: 12/1/95[8]
```

figure 13-3. *Sample label for batch-prepared products.*

prepared products. The parts of this label are described below; the numbers in parentheses correspond to information on the label.

Required Labeling

Name of product (1)

The commonly known name of a product is useful, especially for one with multiple ingredients, so that it can be readily identified.

Name and amount of drug added (2)

The names and amounts of drugs added to a solution should be all inclusive. Additives, such as preservatives and buffering agents, also should be listed.

Diluent used (3)

Diluents, such as normal saline and 5% dextrose, may affect how a final product is used. An exception is a product with a small volume (e.g., syringe). If no diluent is listed, sterile water for injection probably was used.

Total volume of solution (4)

For syringes, the total volume may be stated as a concentration that includes both the amount of drug and the total volume in which it is contained. For other products, the concentration per milliliter or other common volume of measurement also may be helpful.

Route of administration (5)

Route of administration can be specific (e.g., "for irrigation") or general (e.g., "for injection") if the product can be used safely for more than one route.

Storage conditions (6)

Storage requirements should reflect preferred conditions before and/or after the product is opened.

Lot number (7)

A lot number tracks a product back to its production or manufacturing sheet (see Chapter 11). These numbers usually are generated internally, based on some logic, and should be readily traceable to information on how the product was made and tested. The date of preparation usually is included in the numbering logic.

Expiration date (8)

Expiration dating should be based on known stability and sterility results and should be consistent with the ASHP Technical Assistance Bulletin on Quality Assurance for Pharmacy-Prepared Sterile Products (see Appendix 6).[1] If the expiration dating is based on storage conditions other than room temperature, they also should be listed (e.g., refrigeration and freezing).

Auxiliary and Optional Labeling

Since batch-prepared products are relabeled prior to dispensing, auxiliary labels should not be used. Any auxiliary or optional information should be incorporated into the batch label. Use of auxiliary labels may lead to errors if old labels are not removed prior to dispensing of the relabeled product.

SUMMARY

The proper labeling of sterile products is critical to quality assurance. The information on the label must be accurate, easy to understand, uniform, and appropriately displayed. Minor differences exist in the label information for institutional and home care settings as well as for batch preparations. The information should include, but not be limited to

- ❏ Patient name and identification number.
- ❏ Patient location.
- ❏ Name and amount of drug added.
- ❏ Name of admixture solution.
- ❏ Approximate volume of admixture.
- ❏ Time and date of scheduled administration.
- ❏ Expiration date.
- ❏ Administration instructions.
- ❏ Personnel initials.
- ❏ Storage conditions.
- ❏ Route of administration.

REFERENCES

1. American Society of Hospital Pharmacists. ASHP technical assistance bulletin on quality assurance for pharmacy-prepared sterile products. *Am J Hosp Pharm.* 1993; 50:2386–98.
2. Brzozowski DF, Hale KM, Segal R, et al. Pharmacist opinions about compliance with recommendations for intravenous admixture practices. *Am J Hosp Pharm.* 1987; 44:2077–84.

Chapter 14
Handling of Sterile Products Within the Pharmacy

Barbara T. McKinnon

A pharmacy's responsibility for sterile products begins when components are first received and continues through product administration and waste disposal. To ensure both product quality and public safety, correct storage and handling procedures are necessary every step of the way. Specific areas of importance include

- ❑ Receipt of product components.
- ❑ United States Pharmacopeial (USP) storage conditions.
- ❑ Inventory control.
- ❑ Transport into aseptic processing areas.
- ❑ Storage of compounded products.
- ❑ Waste management.

RECEIPT OF PRODUCT COMPONENTS

Sterile Components

A procedure should specify the visual inspection of commercially available sterile drug products, sterile ready-to-use containers, and devices (e.g., syringes and needles) upon receipt in the pharmacy. All items must be free from defects, within the manufacturer's expiration dating, and otherwise suitable for their intended use. Expired, inappropriately stored, or defective products should not be used; defective drugs should be promptly reported to the Food and Drug Administration (FDA).[1]

All ingredients used to compound sterile products should be

- ❑ Identified by the product name, lot number, and expiration date.
- ❑ Determined to be stable, compatible, and appropriate[2] according to manufacturer or USP guidelines[3] or scientific references (see Chapter 12).

Nonsterile Components

Nonsterile drug components (e.g., morphine powder) should meet USP standards. Certificates of analysis from manufacturers of bulk drug substances can establish that each lot received by the pharmacy meets its specifications for[4,5]

- ❑ Identity.
- ❑ Color.
- ❑ Appearance.
- ❑ Assay specifications.
- ❑ Purity.
- ❑ Moisture content.
- ❑ Heavy metal content.

If the material is USP/NF (National Formulary) or reagent grade, the minimum manufacturer's assay may be assumed.

Upon receipt, the pharmacy should visually inspect each lot for deterioration, unacceptable quality, and wrong identity. Documentation of this inspection should then be filed (see Chapter 11).

If bulk drug substances are stored properly in the pharmacy, they should retain their quality until the manufacturer's labeled expiration date. Storage conditions may be specified for some products. Bulk drug substances without a manufacturer's expiration date should be dated when received, stored properly, dated when opened, used within compendial recommendations, and visually inspected by a pharmacist when used.

The conditions for opening bulk drug containers and the technique of contents withdrawal should be strictly controlled. Additionally, devices used for withdrawal must be clean to preclude contamination of the remaining contents. The pharmacy may repackage bulk drug substances into smaller, properly sealed containers (e.g., zip-closure plastic bags) to minimize contamination.[4]

Raw Materials

Raw materials (e.g., anhydrous dextrose powder) are not pharmaceutical grade products. If raw materials are received without a manufacturer's certificate of analysis, they must be quarantined to prevent their use until tested.

A lot of raw material, bearing a single manufacturer's control number, may be in one or more containers. Records should be kept of the

- ❑ Chemical name.
- ❑ Grade.
- ❑ Quantity received.
- ❑ Date received.
- ❑ Manufacturer.
- ❑ Manufacturer's lot number.
- ❑ Expiration date.
- ❑ Results of tests for identity and purity.

If the lot is not graded, an assay report should be obtained from the manufacturer before a decision is made as to whether the material meets the desired specifications.

Assays are usually performed on labile chemicals (e.g., calcium chloride anhydrous and magnesium sulfate), which readily gain or lose moisture.

Normally, minimum chemical and physical tests are sufficient to identify a material and ascertain its purity. For example, a simple chemical color reaction, chemical color change reaction, characteristic odor, taste, or physical appearance may identify a drug.[5] If these tests are beyond a pharmacy's capabilities, the material can be tested by a reference laboratory.

Inhouse-Prepared Components

Sterile injectable products that are prepared inhouse may be used as components of other sterile injectable products. However, if the component lacks any quality attribute (purity, potency, sterility, etc.), the final solution will be adversely affected. Therefore, although all nonsterile ingredients used in sterile component solutions must be inspected, the final product also must be tested to ensure that it conforms to specifications (see Chapter 17).

USP STORAGE CONDITIONS

Solutions, drugs, and supplies used to prepare and administer sterile products should be stored in accordance with manufacturer or USP requirements.[6] USP requirements for storage temperatures are listed in Table 14-1.

Recommended storage conditions usually are stated on a product's label and may include a specified temperature range or a designated place (e.g., "refrigerator"). Supplemental instructions (e.g., "protect from light") also should be followed carefully. If a product must be protected from light and is in a clear or translucent container enclosed in an opaque outer covering, this covering should not be removed until the contents are to be used.

In the absence of specific instructions, a product should be stored at controlled room temperature[7]—away from excessive or variable heat, cold, and light. Therefore, heating pipes and fluorescent lighting fixtures should be avoided.

Clarifying Controlled Room Temperature

Since controlled room temperature may range from 15 to 30° C, such storage may not be adequate for certain temperature-sensitive drugs.[8] Clinically important changes can result from only a 5° variation in room temperature over the shelf life of a product.[9] Alterations in temperature-related drug stability could potentially compromise a pharmacist's interpretation and assignment of expiration dates to compounded drugs. Therefore, USP has further defined controlled room temperature:[6]

> *"Controlled room temperature . . . encompasses the usual . . . working environment of 20 to 25 degrees*

Table 14-1. *USP Storage Requirements*[6]

Description	Degrees Centigrade	Degrees Fahrenheit
Frozen	−20–−10	−4–14
Cold	≤8	≤46
Cool	8–15	46–59
Room temperature	Prevailing temperature	Prevailing temperature
Controlled room temperature	15–30	59–86
Warm	30–40	86–104
Excessive heat	>40	>104

(68 to 77 F) . . . that results in a mean kinetic temperature calculated to be not more than 25 degrees; and that allows for excursions between 15 and 30 degrees (59 and 86 F) . . . in pharmacies, hospitals, and warehouses."

Monitoring Storage Conditions

To ensure that a product's potency is retained through its expiration date, pharmacists must monitor drug storage areas.[3,4] Controlled temperature areas—refrigerators, freezers, and incubators—should be monitored at least once daily and the results should be documented on a temperature log (see Chapter 6). A continuous temperature recording device or a thermometer with adequate accuracy and sensitivity may be used if properly calibrated at reasonable intervals.[4]

On each working day, pharmacy personnel should verify that the recording device is working and that temperatures are within the desired range. The temperature-detecting mechanism should be carefully placed so that it accurately reflects the area's temperature. The pharmacy also must monitor conditions that cause temperature fluctuations such as the opening of refrigerator doors.

INVENTORY CONTROL

Inventories of drugs and solutions should be inspected periodically to ensure that they are not damaged, soiled, expired, or otherwise unsuitable. Moreover, all storage areas should be monitored to ensure that temperature, light, moisture, and ventilation remain within manufacturer and compendial requirements.[3] To permit adequate floor cleaning and avoid water damage, drugs and supplies should be stored on shelves above the floor.

Temperature

Temperature may be a particular problem in large warehouse areas with garage-type doors opening to the environment. If outside temperatures are extreme, the temperature inside the warehouse may not meet USP requirements for some products. For such facilities, a tempera-

ture log may help to ensure that appropriate storage conditions are met. If temperature fluctuations exceed acceptable limits, drug supplies must be relocated.

Product Integrity

Before use, each drug, ingredient, and container should be visually inspected for damage, defects, and expiration date.[3] Products that have exceeded their expiration dates should be removed from active storage areas. A monthly physical inspection of inventory may be helpful. Organizations with computerized perpetual inventory capabilities might generate a monthly report that can be used to retrieve products about to expire.

Although "just-in-time" ordering has decreased the problem of excessive inventory and expired drugs for some organizations, little used inventory locations must still be checked carefully. For example, floor stock or emergency cart drugs must be checked monthly to ensure that drugs will be in date when needed. For home care practitioners, nurses' bags must be inventoried routinely.

Product Recall

When a product is recalled, a mechanism must be in place for tracking and retrieving it from specific patients. A batch record, with lot numbers and expiration dates, can greatly facilitate a product recall (see Chapter 11). Additionally, computerized inventory management systems may help large organizations to determine quickly whether the pharmacy has the recalled product in stock.

TRANSPORT INTO ASEPTIC PROCESSING AREAS

When products and supplies are transported from relatively uncontrolled areas (e.g., main pharmacy or warehouse) into the aseptic processing area, caution is needed to prevent its contamination. Access to the aseptic processing area should be limited to designated, qualified personnel. Furthermore, supplies, equipment, and personnel should first be decontaminated in an anteroom or similar area.

Supplies

All supplies should be removed from shipping cartons and wiped with a disinfecting agent (e.g., sterile isopropyl alcohol) while being transferred to a clean, sanitized cart for transport. Individual pouched supplies need not be wiped because the pouches can be removed when the supplies are introduced into the aseptic processing area.[4]

Although some frequently used supplies can be decontaminated and stored on shelving in the anteroom, an excessive accumulation can lead to dust collection. Objects that shed particles—pencils, cardboard boxes, paper towels, cotton items, and reference books—should not be brought into the aseptic processing area.[3,4]

Carts

Carts used to bring supplies from a storeroom should not be rolled beyond the anteroom; carts used in the aseptic processing area should not be rolled outside of it or the anteroom unless they are cleaned and disinfected before returning.[4] To maintain this segregation, carts can be designated as "clean" or "dirty."

Clean carts stay in the aseptic processing area and anteroom only, and supplies from the pharmacy or warehouse are conveyed on dirty carts. In the anteroom, a demarcation line on the floor denotes how far a dirty cart can travel. At the line, supplies are decontaminated and transferred to a clean cart. This process minimizes the ingress of particulate and microbial contamination from carts and packaging materials (see Chapter 5).

STORAGE OF COMPOUNDED PRODUCTS

Once compounded, sterile products should be refrigerated until they are used,[10] unless otherwise indicated. However, sterile products intended for administration *promptly* after compounding may be retained at room temperature.

Although there is always some risk that microorganisms may contaminate products during compounding, refrigerated storage inhibits microbial growth.[4] Since exposure to room temperatures or greater increases the risk of microbial growth, products should be placed into a risk category based on their storage requirements. Risk level categories should be considered prior to product preparation and may affect procedures. ASHP assigns products to two risk levels according to time before administration and storage temperature (see Table 14-2).

Table 14-2. *Assignment of Products to Risk Level 1 or 2 According to Time and Temperature before Completion of Administration*[2]

Risk Level	Room Temperature (15–30° C)	Days of Storage	
		Refrigerator (2–8° C)	Freezer (−20−−10° C)
1	Completely administered within 28 hr	≤7	≤30
2	Storage and administration exceed 28 hr	>7	>30

WASTE MANAGEMENT

Preparation Materials

After compounding is completed, used syringes, bottles, vials, and other supplies should be removed. Exit and re-entry into the laminar-airflow workspace should be minimized, however, to decrease the dragging of contamination into the aseptic work area.[4] Disposal of packaging materials should be performed at least daily to enhance sanitation and avoid accumulation.[2]

Needles must be disposed of carefully to prevent possible injuries. If used only for compounding sterile drug products, needles may be recapped carefully, but clipping is no longer recommended. The used needle should be placed in a puncture-resistant container that can be permanently sealed. Some practitioners prefer to discard the entire syringe and needle in the sharps container. Others carefully recap and place the needle in the sharps container but dispose of syringes with compounding waste. Either practice is acceptable.

Needles and syringes used for patient drug administration should never be recapped. They should be discarded as an intact unit, along with IV catheters or other sharp objects.

Hazardous Materials

Hazardous materials may represent an occupational hazard through inhalation of drug dusts or droplets, inadvertent ingestion, or direct skin contact.[11] Procedures should be established to handle hazardous drug wastes without spills or other exposure (see Chapter 9). Hazardous drug waste should be placed in thick, puncture-resistant, plastic bags or leakproof containers with the label

CAUTION: HAZARDOUS
CHEMICAL WASTE

These receptacles should be kept wherever the drugs are commonly used, and all—and only— hazardous drug waste should be placed in them. These waste containers should be handled with gloves; when full, they should be stored in a designated area until disposal.[11]

When hazardous drugs are compounded, excess drug should be returned to the vial whenever possible or discarded in a closed container (e.g., empty sterile vial). Placing excess drug in any open container, even while in the biological safety cabinet (BSC), is not appropriate. Moreover, excess drug should never be discarded into the drainage trough of the BSC.[11] All hazardous materials should be placed in leakproof, puncture-resistant containers within the BSC and then disposed of in larger containers outside the BSC.

To minimize aerosolization, needles should be discarded in puncture-resistant containers without being clipped.[11] Both gloves and gowns used in compounding should be discarded immediately if contaminated. Otherwise, gloves should be discarded after each use and gowns should be discarded when the aseptic compounding area is left. Hands must be washed thoroughly after hazardous drugs are handled.

Hazardous drug waste must be disposed of through a licensed contractor. To reduce disposal costs, some areas permit hazardous drug waste to be divided into trace-contaminated and bulk-contaminated materials. For example, empty IV containers and administration sets are trace waste, while half-full vials or unused final dosages are bulk waste. Bulk-contaminated materials weigh more than 3% of the capacity of the container.[12] If trace- and bulk-contaminated waste are handled separately, bulk waste should be segregated into more secure receptacles for containment and disposal as toxic material.

Hazardous waste should be held in a secure place in labeled, leakproof drums or cartons until disposal, as required by state or local regulation or by the disposal contractor. It should ultimately be disposed of in an EPA-permitted, state-licensed hazardous waste incinerator. Transport to an offsite incinerator should be done by a licensed contractor. If a licensed incinerator is not available, burial in an EPA-licensed hazardous waste dump is an acceptable alternative.[11]

Disposal of hazardous materials and toxic chemicals is only a small part of a larger controversial issue.[11] Because of past incidents of inappropriate disposal, health care facilities must now verify the license or permit status of any contractor used to remove or dispose hazardous drug waste.

Expired Drugs

Expired drugs should be segregated from other inventory so that they are not inadvertently dispensed. Certain drugs may be returned to the manufacturer for credit. Generally, expired drugs are handled in one of four ways:

1. Expired controlled substances must be removed from perpetual inventory. In some cases, they may be returned to the manufacturer. A listing

of the drugs waiting to be returned is sent to the manufacturer, who issues Drug Enforcement Agency (DEA) Form 222 to the pharmacy. This form must accompany the returned controlled drugs.

2. Open drug containers and unused finished doses are often not returnable for credit; controlled substances must be destroyed. In some states, a state board of pharmacy inspector must view this destruction of controlled substances. Alternatively, expired controlled substances may be sent to the DEA for disposal.

3. Expired hazardous drugs must be properly labeled and disposed of in punctureproof containers. These containers must be sent to a licensed hazardous waste incinerator or licensed hazardous waste dump via a licensed hazardous waste contractor.

4. Drugs other than controlled substances or hazardous materials may simply be discarded. Typically, expired large volume IV fluid containers are emptied before disposal to reduce their weight. Other intact drug containers should be bagged and disposed of with other refuse.

SUMMARY

Like the preparation and distribution of pharmacy-prepared sterile products, their storage and handling is of critical importance. Beginning with the components themselves, proper procedures for receipt, storage, and control must be established.

Once a final product has been prepared, it must be appropriately transported within and delivered from the aseptic preparation area. Furthermore, storage conditions for final products differ from those of the original components.

Finally, waste management of used supplies and drug products must be adequately defined. Strict procedures must ensure that no hazardous material contacts anyone preparing or handling this waste.

REFERENCES

1. Kessler DA. MedWatch: the new FDA medical products reporting program. *Am J Hosp Pharm.* 1993; 50:1921–36.

2. American Society of Hospital Pharmacists. ASHP technical assistance bulletin on quality assurance for pharmacy-prepared sterile products. *Am J Hosp Pharm.* 1993; 50:2386–98.

3. Official monographs. In: United States pharma-

copeia, 23rd rev./national formulary, 18th ed. Rockville, MD: United States Pharmacopeial Convention; 1994:15–1647.

4. Sterile drug products for home use. In: United States pharmacopeia, 23rd rev./national formulary, 18th ed. Rockville, MD: United States Pharmacopeial Convention; 1994:1963–75.

5. Patel JA. Quality control and standards. In: Smith MC, Brown TR, eds. Handbook of institutional pharmacy practice, 2nd ed. Baltimore, MD: Williams & Wilkins; 1986:402–11.

6. General notices. In: United States pharmacopeia, 23rd rev./national formulary, 18th ed. Rockville, MD: United States Pharmacopeial Convention; 1994:11.

7. Stability considerations in dispensing practice. In: United States pharmacopeia, 23rd rev./national formulary, 18th ed. Rockville, MD: United States Pharmacopeial Convention; 1994:1957.

8. Nahata MC. Standard room temperature needed for stability and compatibility studies. *Am J Hosp Pharm*. 1993; 50:912–3.

9. Newton DW, Miller KW. Room temperature and drug stability. *Am J Hosp Pharm*. 1994; 51:406–9.

10. Simmons BP. Guidelines for the prevention of intravascular infection. Atlanta, GA: Centers for Disease Control; 1981.

11. American Society of Hospital Pharmacists. ASHP technical assistance bulletin on handling cytotoxic and hazardous drugs. *Am J Hosp Pharm*. 1990; 47:1033–49.

12. Vaccari PL, Tonat K, DeChristoforo R, et al. Disposal of antineoplastic wastes at the National Institutes of Health. *Am J Hosp Pharm*. 1984; 41:87–93.

Chapter 15
Handling of Sterile Products Outside the Pharmacy

Douglas J. Scheckelhoff

While sterile products are within the pharmacy, storage and other handling conditions can be largely controlled (see Chapter 14). Since these products are then used in various patient settings, however, their handling outside the pharmacy also must be considered. Efforts must focus not only on the product's acceptability for patient use (stability, sterility, etc.) but also on the reduction of waste and preparation costs. How the product is transported from the pharmacy, how it is stored outside the pharmacy, and the methods used for return, recycling, and disposal are all important factors.[1-7]

DELIVERY METHODS

Institutional Setting

Within the institutional setting, sterile products are delivered not only by health care personnel but also by automated means (e.g., pneumatic tube system). With the advent of polyvinyl chloride (PVC) bags and other durable containers, delivery is now driven more by efficiency and timeliness than safety. Chemotherapy products, controlled substances, and some syringe dosage forms, however, are treated differently.

Because of the risk of exposure from a spill, chemotherapy dosage forms are not sent in pneumatic tube systems and are often placed within another protective bag or container.[1] Controlled substances usually require special handling—hand delivery with signature records of both parties—due to security needs. Syringes also may require special handling; if they are dropped or jarred in a pneumatic tube system, the syringe plunger may depress, causing leakage. (Foam padding specifically designed for use in pneumatic tubes can reduce this problem.)

Home Care Setting

Delivery of sterile products to the home care patient often creates unique challenges. Both the patient's distance from the pharmacy and the drug's stability affect how a product is delivered.[4]

Temperature control during transit of sterile products for home use is critical. To maintain temperatures near the midpoint of the product's specified acceptable range, the pharmacy must provide appropriate packaging. This packaging must ensure the product's effectiveness during transit and under expected environmental conditions.

The pharmacy should develop and follow written procedures for packaging. Additional precautions (e.g., double bagging) should protect the shipper, patient, and caregiver from leakage of hazardous substances. Furthermore, the shipper, patient, and caregiver should be trained to recognize and deal with accidental spills.

Some nonhazardous products also may need to be packaged for transport. If the container (e.g., preloaded syringe) is susceptible to jars or jolts, it should be packaged to protect its integrity. Therefore, it might be placed in a hard plastic or cardboard tube or within bubble packs or plastic pellets.

Transport procedures should be tested and documented to ensure that they are effective. Postdelivery temperature checks can ensure that packaging materials (ice packs, coolers, bubble packs, etc.) maintain adequate control. If packaging materials are changed, temperature checks should again be performed.

When commercial carriers are used, the pharmacy is responsible for their selection. Before using a carrier, the pharmacy should provide a written statement of shipping requirements—delivery schedules, transit time duration, handling, and external temperature control—and obtain the carrier's assurance for fulfilling them. Some carriers request special packaging and labeling before they will handle hazardous chemicals or biomedical waste.

Delivery personnel should know the shipping requirements for each package. Product labels generally provide temperature information; if products are boxed or labels are otherwise concealed, an exterior label (e.g., "Refrigerate") should be applied.

STORAGE METHODS

Institutional Setting

In the hospital setting, control of a product transfers from the pharmacy to other health care providers on a patient care unit. The importance of refrigeration and its impact on stability and recyclability should be understood by both nursing and pharmacy.[2,3]

As part of the pharmacy's inspection process, temperatures of patient care unit refrigerators should be recorded monthly. If solutions are frequently taken out of the refrigerator long before administration (e.g., at the beginning of a shift), the pharmacy must follow room temperature stability. This procedure greatly reduces recyclability and increases waste.

It is in the pharmacy's best interest to organize sterile products in the refrigerator in a manner that prevents nursing staff from collecting a day's supply at the patient's bedside hours before administration. The purchase of additional refrigerators for accessible locations also may be worthwhile. A few hundred dollars for a refrigerator can quickly be offset if it prevents only a few doses of an expensive antibiotic from being wasted.

Use of parenteral products that are stable at room temperature (e.g., ready-to-use or "RTU" products) or that can be "activated" (i.e., reconstituted) immediately prior to administration eliminates the need for refrigeration and the subsequent problems.

Home Care Setting

In the home environment, sterile products usually are stored in the patient's own refrigerator; a shelf, drawer, or other area segregated from food should be used to avoid contamination of the outside of the container. An additional plastic bag also can isolate sterile products from other items in the refrigerator. If the quantity and volume of solutions are great (e.g., parenteral nutrition solutions), however, a separate refrigerator can be supplied. Drugs or supplies that do not require refrigeration should be stored in a separate, restricted area (e.g., a lockable filing cabinet or cupboard).

Controls must be maintained in the home until the product is administered and all waste is appropriately disposed. Labels should state storage requirements and the expiration date. A thermometer should be provided and checked periodically by health care personnel to ensure that temperatures are acceptable. Patients should be trained to check products for expiration dating and to verify refrigerator temperatures regularly (e.g., daily). They also should be trained to contact the pharmacy if a refrigerator malfunctions or a drug is improperly stored.

Either pharmacy personnel or a home nurse should visit each home (at least weekly) and confirm that drug storage is adequate with regard to temperature control, cleanliness, separation of food and drug items, and avoidance of improper product use (e.g., a single-dose vial used as a multiple-dose container). Improperly stored, soiled, expired, or visibly defective products should be removed. Home visits should also assess compliance with waste disposal procedures.

RETURN METHODS

Parenteral products—discontinued or changed orders or missed doses—are often returned to the pharmacy via normal delivery methods.[3] In both the institutional and home settings, these items should be retrieved as quickly as possible to maximize their recycling potential. If these solutions are left unrefrigerated for pickup when the next pharmacy delivery is made, many hours may be lost. Based on the cost of these items, an active retrieval mechanism can reduce both effort and waste.

RECYCLING METHODS

Institutional Setting

Parenteral products returned to the pharmacy may be recycled if the pharmacist knows how they were stored and handled when outside the pharmacy.[4-6] Room temperature stability should be used if the pharmacist is uncertain that the product was refrigerated.

Recycling is typically based on expiration dates. Products usually are labeled with an actual expiration date (used with short stability drugs) or a standard expiration date (e.g., 24 hr). If the standard expiration date is used, the pharmacist must decide if the product should be recycled according to its actual expiration date (based on stability, infection control guidelines, storage conditions, etc.; see Chapter 12). Furthermore, products should only be used in time frames that are consistent with published data.[2,4,8]

If a product is recycled, this fact should be noted on the label. Therefore, if the IV is returned again, its true preparation time is still identifiable.

Home Care Setting

Products returned from the home environment usually are not recycled since their storage and handling cannot be controlled by the pharmacy. Most state boards of pharmacy prohibit reuse of repackaged or compounded items, including sterile products.

Reuse of intact items that have not been repackaged (e.g., intact vials or prefilled syringes) is acceptable, providing the packaging is tamper evident and the products are stable at room temperature.

WASTE DISPOSAL METHODS

Institutional Setting

Improper disposal of medical waste received great attention in the 1980s when used syringes were washed up on public beaches and found in playgrounds built over old landfills. Since then, disposal methods have been more regulated and the recycling of waste has received more consideration.

Disposal methods vary based on type of product and regulations governing the hospital. For example, since chemotherapy waste is considered hazardous, it usually must be incinerated. Moreover, the process must meet requirements specific for hazardous materials (relative to incineration temperature and duration).

Most drugs that are disposed of are not hazardous, however, and may or may not be regulated. Often, disposal methods are prescribed by the landfill where the waste is sent. Since landfill regulations and restrictions are often strict and increase disposal costs, many hospitals treat nonhazardous waste as hazardous material and send it for incineration.

Home Care Setting

Patients receiving hazardous drugs in the home should be instructed on proper waste disposal. Needles and other sharps should be placed in a hard plastic or cardboard container to prevent injury. A separate area in the home should be identified for storage of hazardous waste, and all family members should be instructed on the potential dangers.

A schedule for waste removal should be developed and agreed on by both the pharmacy and the patient. Patients should contact the home care pharmacy if waste is not removed according to this schedule.

SUMMARY

After sterile products have been prepared, their storage and handling in the patient care unit or home care setting are important considerations. The pharmacist must ensure that procedures are in place to guarantee proper delivery, storage, return, and recycling of these products as well as the destruction of any product waste or hazardous materials.

REFERENCES

1. American Society of Hospital Pharmacists. ASHP technical assistance bulletin on handling cytotoxic and hazardous drugs. *Am J Hosp Pharm.* 1990; 47:1033–49.
2. American Society of Hospital Pharmacists. ASHP technical assistance bulletin on quality assurance for pharmacy-prepared sterile products. *Am J Hosp Pharm.* 1993; 50:2386–98.
3. Birdwell SW, Meyer GE, Scheckelhoff DJ, et al. Survey of wastage from intravenous admixture in US hospitals. *Pharmacoeconomics.* 1993; 4:271–7.
4. Sterile drug products for home use. In: United States pharmacopeia, 23rd rev./national formulary, 18th ed. Rockville, MD: United States Pharmacopeial Convention; 1994:1963–75.
5. Billeter M, Nowak MM, Rapp RP, et al. Waste of IV admixtures in the ADD-vantage system and a traditional minibag system. *Am J Hosp Pharm.* 1990; 47:1598–1600.
6. Mitchell SR. Monitoring waste in an intravenous admixture program. *Am J Hosp Pharm.* 1987; 44: 106–11.

7. Salberg DJ, Newton RW, Leduc DT. Cost of wastage in a hospital intravenous admixture program. *Hosp Form.* 1984; 19:375–8.

8. Trissel LA. Handbook on injectable drugs, 8th ed. Bethesda, MD: American Society of Hospital Pharmacists; 1994.

Chapter 16
Process Validation

Philip J. Schneider

Because end-product sterility testing of parenteral products is often not practical (see Chapter 17), process validation has become a popular quality-control technique. This technique systematically demonstrates that a process will reproducibly meet its claim.[1]

Process validation—often referred to as media fills—involves manipulation of microbial growth media according to the aseptic process being validated. For example, to validate the process of preparing a TPN admixture, the same preparation process would be followed using a soybean casein digest medium.

An early study of process validation for IV admixture programs outlined two procedures:[2]

1. Aseptic transfer of sterile trypticase soy broth (TSB) from 30-ml vials to sterile empty 6-ml vials (to simulate aseptic transfer of a drug to an IV admixture).
2. Preparation of an IV admixture and filtration of it through a micropore filter followed by culture of the filter (to detect possible contamination).

The results of this study led to the recommendation for 40 test samples to validate operator technique.[2]

A later description of process validation[3] outlined four other processes:

❑ Preparation of a syringe dose from a TSB ampul using a 5-μm filter needle.
❑ Preparation of a syringe dose using lyophilized broth.
❑ Preparation of a 50-ml admixture from a TSB ampul.
❑ Preparation of a 50-ml admixture from a vial of lyophilized broth.

No sample sizes were recommended in this report.[3]

A method for initially validating and monitoring aseptic technique of IV admixture personnel also was reported.[4] A two-transfer process was used: one from an ampul and one from a reconstituted vial into a 50-ml IV admixture. To validate performance, the final recommendation was that 40 procedures be performed for every 800 admixtures.[4]

SCHEDULING OF PROCESS VALIDATION

Process validation should be scheduled under a "worst case" scenario—under conditions posing the greatest chance for product failure. Therefore, these tests are conducted independent of production runs, when the testing line is set up specifically for them.[5]

In the pharmacy, such process validation testing should take place immediately after a day's production is completed. According to the United States Pharmacopeial Convention (USP), process validation using media fills should be scheduled at times representative of peak fatigue, stress, and pacing demands.[5]

SAMPLING TECHNIQUES

Process validation of aseptic technique and aseptic processes is based on the concept that, when contaminated, a growth medium will support the organisms introduced by the operator. Therefore, the medium used (e.g., soybean casein digest media or TSB) must support the types of microbes typically found in operator-contaminated sterile products. Furthermore, the media must be manipulated according to the aseptic technique or process being validated. The media should be packaged and handled just like the ingredients of the actual sterile products. These tests can be done with commercially available kits or actual pharmacy supplies.

Commercial Kits

Several commercially available kits facilitate process validation using different sampling techniques. The Compounded Validation Test Media Kit (Baxter Healthcare) includes supplies for simulating the preparation of both simple and complex IV admixtures. The Attack Aseptic Technique Testing and Challenge Kit (Marsam Pharmaceutical) includes materials needed to simulate sterile product preparation using ampuls, vials, and powder fill vials.[6]

Compounded validation test media kit

The simple version of this test media kit validates processes such as the preparation of single, small volume parenteral doses (e.g., piggyback IVs). The operator must make only five separate 1-ml injections from a sterile water vial to a plastic IV bag containing the soybean casein digest broth.

The complex version of this kit is intended for TPN formulations, large volume parenterals, and batch-prepared, small volume parenterals. The operator must make five separate 1-ml injections from a sterile water vial to a plastic IV bag containing the growth media. Using the same syringe, the operator then makes five 1-ml injections from that bag to another plastic bag containing the media. The media from both bags are then combined through a Y-set into a third, empty, plastic IV bag. This final bag is then clamped, sealed, and disconnected, just like a real IV.

Both the simple and complex validation kits require that the final container be labeled and incubated for 7 days at 30–35° C followed by 7 days at 25° C. The containers are checked visually each day for turbulence, which indicates microbial growth and a positive test.

Attack aseptic technique testing and challenge kit

This kit, containing only vials and ampuls, is for a more basic test of an individual's aseptic technique. One dry-filled vial contains polyethylene glycol 8000 to simulate the constitution of a soluble drug. One ampul and two vials of sterile TSB are used to simulate transfer of drugs from these types of containers. The ampul and liquid vial challenges require an operator to draw the media from the containers and transfer it into sterile empty vials. The powder-filled vial challenge requires an operator to draw the media from a vial and reconstitute the powder-filled vial. The contents of the reconstituted vial are transferred into a sterile empty vial.

In all cases, the vials are then incubated for 14 days. If the contents become cloudy, the test is considered positive and a possible failure in aseptic technique. A positive test may also indicate that the procedures are faulty or that the environment is contaminated.

TPN Technique

The USP describes a process validation procedure that might simulate the preparation of a complex admixture such as a TPN formulation. The procedure requires two containers of media that can be pooled for each test. These two containers are paired in a work environment (e.g., laminar-airflow hood). One milliliter is drawn from the first container and transferred aseptically by syringe to the second; this process is repeated 10 times. Then the media from the second container is transferred by syringe to the first container for a total of 10 transfers. Thus, the process involves 10 syringe transfers for each media container. The containers are incubated at room temperature for 14 days with regular checks for media growth.[5]

SAMPLING SIZE

Initially, process validation was concerned with the manufacture of large quantities of products. Therefore, sample size recommendations based on statistical sampling techniques are not valid for IV admixture programs. The number of different procedures involved and the relatively small number of admixtures prepared renders statistical sampling inappropriate. The number of samples sufficient to detect one contamination at a 95% probability is 3000.

One appropriate method has been described for determining the number of test samples needed to monitor the sterility of IV admixture programs.[7] It uses cumulative sum control charts to determine sample size given acceptable and rejectable quality levels. Thus, with a maximum acceptable contamination rate of 3% and a rejectable quality level of 12%, a sampling of 5% of output is recommended to monitor the aseptic technique of a person preparing sterile products.[4] For example, if a technician prepares 800 admixtures per month, 40 validation samples need to be tested. Previous reports suggested that 40 tests are statistically appropriate for initial validation, based on the anticipated potential for contaminating an IV admixture drug preparation.[2,4] Furthermore, 10 samples per month per technician were recommended to detect a shift from the acceptable to the rejectable level of quality.[4]

Other recommendations indicate that sample size should be based on[1]

- ❏ The number of products normally filled during a given fill period.
- ❏ The number of products per unit of time based on production speed. (Sample size could be based on the number of IV admixtures prepared in 30 min, for example.)

FREQUENCY OF PROCESS VALIDATION

The USP also has recommended how often personnel should perform process validation procedures.[5] These recommendations are based on the complexity of the products.

Low-Risk Products

Typical IV admixtures that are prepared by aseptically processing sterile ingredients are low-risk products. Personnel should pass a validation initially, before being given the responsibility, by demonstrating that no contamination occurs in three consecutive media fills. Apparently, this small number of media-fill tests is based on the complexity of the test itself. The example cited involves the preparation of 20 units; 10 transfers from each unit are added to another unit for a total of 200 aseptic manipulations.[5] Validation procedures with fewer steps (e.g., commercially available kits) require more tests.

Followup monitoring of staff technique should take place quarterly thereafter unless a media fill is contaminated during quarterly validation, the procedures change significantly, or there is evidence that a person has contaminated a product. In this case, the person should be retrained and retested.

High-Risk Products

High-risk products involve (1) complex procedures, (2) products used beyond 1 day, and (3) products prepared using nonsterile ingredients.[5] To validate personnel, the testing should include media fills that simulate the specific product being prepared as well as aseptic technique. Therefore, the media fill should not only simulate the procedures used but also the number of units produced during the preparation process.

Product-specific validation should occur annually. Failure of a test may indicate a problem with either the person or the process. Before the person or process is used to prepare a product, three media fills should be successful.[5]

Program Validation

Although a specific number of validation tests cannot be recommended for a sterile products program, a facility should be evaluated when it first opens and be revalidated at least twice a year. Validation is necessary not only for the personnel preparing sterile products but also for the technique, procedures, and facility.

When the validation method is selected, the number of aseptic manipulations required for the test must be considered. In no case should this number be less than the number required to prepare the most complex product being produced. Pharmacists need to use good professional judgment when selecting the validation procedure, the number of procedures per time interval, and the frequency of testing.

SUMMARY

End-product sterility testing may be replaced by process validation as a quality-control measure for IV admixture programs, because process validation provides a better ongoing measure of an operator's technique. Commercially available media-fill containers and kits now make it easier to develop this procedure. Unfortunately, scientific methods are not practical for selecting a sample size or determining the frequency of testing. Pharmacists need to review the various published recommendations to determine a defendable sample size and frequency. Nevertheless, process validation should be part of every contemporary sterile products preparation program.

REFERENCES

1. Validation of aseptic filling for solution drug products. Technical Monograph 2. Philadelphia, PA: Parenteral Drug Association; 1980.

2. Morris BG, Avis KE, Bowles GC. Quality control plan for intravenous admixture programs. II: Validation of operator technique. *Am J Hosp Pharm.* 1980; 37:668–72.

3. Dirks I, Smith FM, Furtado D, et al. Method for teaching aseptic technique of intravenous admixture personnel. *Am J Hosp Pharm.* 1982; 39:457–9.

4. Brier KL. Evaluating aseptic technique of pharmacy personnel. *Am J Hosp Pharm.* 1983; 40:400–3.

5. Sterile drug products for home use. In: United States pharmacopeia, 23rd rev./national formulary, 18th ed. Rockville, MD: United States Pharmacopeial Convention; 1994:1963–75.

6. Turco S, Miele WH, Barnoski D. Evaluation of an aseptic technique testing and challenge kit (Attack®). *Hosp Pharm.* 1993; 28:11–3, 16–8.

7. Sanford RL. Cumulative sum control charts for admixture quality control. *Am J Hosp Pharm.* 1980; 37:655–9.

Chapter 17
End-Product Evaluation

Philip J. Schneider

The final testing of a sterile product is an important—although difficult—part of the preparation program. Public concern about the quality of pharmacist-prepared sterile products underscores the need for end-product evaluation.

In addition to microbial and pyrogen testing, end-product evaluation should include physical and analytical testing. Techniques now being practiced include weight, refractometry, pH, and laboratory analyses. This chapter reviews four types of end-product evaluation that pharmacists can use for prepared sterile products.

PHYSICAL TESTING

Physical testing is both inexpensive and quick. The prime concern is that the actual product contains the ingredients specified in the original prescription. If the drug, dose, and formulation are appropriate for the patient, the final product still should be evaluated for

- ❏ Container leaks and integrity.
- ❏ Particulates in solution.
- ❏ Solution color, volume, and odor.

Using both observation and calculation checks, a pharmacist should verify that the final product was prepared accurately with respect to

1. Ingredients (using vials, ampuls, and final solution container).
2. Quantities (using syringes drawn back to the volume used).
3. Containers (using the final solution container).

The components used should be placed on individual trays for pharmacist verification. The final physical test should be reflected by a pharmacist's signature on a dispensing document.[1]

ANALYTICAL TESTING

To evaluate the contents of a prepared sterile product, analytical techniques also may be needed. For example, traditional physical inspection techniques may not be reliable for products prepared using automated compounding devices.

Weight Verification

Weight verification is often used to evaluate products prepared from ingredients with different specific gravities such as TPN and cardioplegia solutions. Because concentrated dextrose solutions have a high specific gravity (1.17–1.24) compared to water (1), the weight of the final product can be estimated using this formula:

$$weight = specific\ gravity \times volume$$

With most automated compounding devices, the final solution can be weighed on the load cell. Sensitive electronic balances also can be used to compare actual to calculated weights.

Refractometry Verification

Refractometry also can be used to evaluate sterile products inexpensively. It is a qualitative test for the identity of an ingredient but is not a quantitative test of its actual concentration. This technique has applicability for controlled substances, particularly to monitor for diversion,[2-5] and parenteral nutrition solutions.[6] The refractive index differs for various solutions. For example, it is 1 Brix unit for lactated Ringer's injection but 5.5 Brix units for dextrose 5% and lactated Ringer's injection.[7]

Refractometry can only be used for solutions containing an organic compound (e.g., a drug or dextrose). It cannot be used for opaque products (e.g., total nutrient admixtures containing fat emulsion) or solutions of inorganic compounds (e.g., electrolytes).

pH Testing

The pH of the final solution can be measured using an electronic pH device or even simple pH paper. Then the measured pH can be compared to published values[8] as one indicator of proper product preparation.

Laboratory Analysis

Laboratory analysis can show the content of substances routinely measured in the clinical setting. Such measurement of the electrolyte content of TPN and cardioplegia solutions is particularly important because a significant error can be catastrophic.[9] Furthermore, measurement of drug concentrations (e.g., aminoglycosides, theophylline, and anticonvulsants) can resolve problems in patients being monitored by their serum concentrations (therapeutic drug monitoring).

MICROBIAL TESTING

For years, pharmacists have attempted to use end-product sterility testing (microbial testing) for quality control.

Nevertheless, this technique has a limited role in the ongoing evaluation of IV admixtures because

1. The sample size is not large enough for statistical evaluation. Typically, only a few dosage forms of identical content are prepared. For statistically valid sample sizes, all doses in a small batch would have to be tested. This requirement is obviously impractical in a practice setting.
2. Numerous processes are involved. Many different drugs, base solutions, and volumes are used in patient-specific IV admixtures. Sterility testing based on sample size requires that samples come from identical products.
3. The testing of a purportedly sterile product involves aseptic processing itself, creating the potential for contamination (adventitious contamination). Each time a sterile product is manipulated, it can be contaminated.

Despite these limitations, microbial testing has two roles in a sterile product preparation program:

❑ Testing of products suspected of contamination.
❑ Testing of batch-produced products that are quarantined before use.

There are two official methods of microbial testing: (1) direct transfer of a sample to sterile culture media and (2) membrane filtration. These methods are described in the *United States Pharmacopeia/National Formulary (USP/NF)*.[10]

Sterile Culture Media

Microbial growth in incubated testing media indicates that the parenteral product is contaminated. Identification of the contaminant often can indicate its source.

The most common method for sterile growth media testing is direct transfer. A sample aliquot of a prepared parenteral product is aseptically transferred into two sterile culture media. One medium, thyoglycollate, is incubated at 32° C for 14 days. The other medium, soybean casein digest, is incubated at 22° C for 14 days. Positive (intentionally contaminated samples with known organisms) and negative (no contamination) controls are incubated with the test samples. Any sample that becomes turbid during the incubation period is a positive test.

This technique can detect only *grossly* contaminated products. It might be used to test a quarantined batch prepared significantly in advance of use or a suspected product several days after preparation. Sterile culture media testing is of limited use for evaluating individual IV admixtures within a few hours of preparation.

Membrane Filtration

Parenteral products also can be tested using membrane filters. This technique is recommended if the product contains preservatives or a compound with intrinsic bacteriostatic activity (e.g., an antibiotic). It also is useful if product testing is needed within hours of preparation.

For this method, the *entire* product is filtered through a sterile, 0.45-μm filter. Then the membrane is washed with a sterile fluid to remove compounds having a bacteriostatic effect. The membrane is aseptically divided and placed into thyoglycollate medium and soybean casein digest and incubated at 32° and 22° C, respectively. Both positive and negative controls are used. Turbidity during a 7-day incubation is a positive test.[11]

Commercial kits are available to assist pharmacists in using the membrane filter technique for end-product sterility testing.

Total Nutrient Admixture Testing

Total nutrient admixture preparations pose a new challenge for sterility testing. Since they are not aqueous solutions, turbidity cannot be used as an endpoint for a positive test. However, a technique used for culturing blood has been applied; the system uses a culture bottle containing 70 ml of trypticase soy broth (TSB) and a plastic cylinder with an agar-coated slide unit. The total nutrient admixture sample is first cultured in TSB and then subcultured in the TSB after the broth is washed over the agar surface. Growth on the agar surface reflects a positive test.[12]

PYROGEN AND BACTERIAL ENDOTOXIN TESTING

Pyrogens and bacterial endotoxins are metabolic products of living microorganisms or the dead microorganisms themselves. When present in parenterals administered to patients, they can cause fever and chills. For the same reasons as microbial testing, both pyrogen and endotoxin testing have limited applicability for IV admixture programs. Nevertheless, they should be performed when contamination is suspected or large batches are prepared.

Two tests are used for pyrogens and bacterial endotoxins in parenteral products: the rabbit test and the limulus amebocyte lysate test. Detailed descriptions of these methods appear in the *USP/NF*.[13,14]

Rabbit Test

Since the rabbit is very sensitive to pyrogens, it is used in the official test for them. Samples of a parenteral product are injected into the ear veins of three rabbits, and their body temperatures are monitored. An increase indicates the presence of pyrogens.

Devices also can be tested for pyrogens. The device is washed with sterile water for injection, the washings are injected into the ear veins of the rabbits, and their body temperatures are monitored.

In pharmacy practice, commercial laboratories usually are used for this rabbit test.

Limulus Amebocyte Lysate Test

The limulus amebocyte lysate test was recognized recently by the USP as a test for bacterial endotoxins. Because it is less expensive and faster than the rabbit test, it has more applicability to pharmacy practice settings.

Amebocyte lysate is a lyophilized powder derived from red blood cells of horseshoe crabs. These cells contain a protein that clots in the presence of certain quantities of bacterial endotoxins. When a solution with bacterial endotoxins is added to the powder, the lysate causes the solution to gel within 1 hr.

SUMMARY

End-product evaluation in pharmacy practice often requires a quick physical check so that a dose is available for a patient when needed. For complex processes or when consequences of an error are critical, additional analytical testing, such as refractometry and weighing, should be considered. When large quantities of doses are prepared or when a specific product is in question, sophisticated end-product tests, including microbial and pyrogen testing, should be conducted. Virtually all of these tests can be performed by a pharmacist during everyday practice and should be part of any comprehensive compounding program.

REFERENCES

1. American Society of Hospital Pharmacists. ASHP technical assistance bulletin on quality assurance for pharmacy-prepared sterile products. *Am J Hosp Pharm.* 1993; 50:2386–98.

2. Gill DL Jr, Goodwin SR, Knudsen AK, et al. Refractometer screening of controlled substances in an operating room satellite pharmacy. *Am J Hosp Pharm.* 1990; 47:817–8.

3. Cheung JF, Chong S, Kitrenos JG, et al. Use of refractometers to detect controlled substance tampering. *Am J Hosp Pharm.* 1991; 48:1488–92.

4. Frankenfield DL, Johnson RE. Refractometry of controlled substances. *Am J Hosp Pharm.* 1991; 48:2120–30.

5. Donnelly AJ, Petryna HM, Newman LM, et al. A

simple, reliable, inexpensive method to aid in the detection of diversion of controlled substances by operating room personnel. *Anesthesiology*. 1990; 73:A1053. Abstract.

6. Meyer GE, Novelli KA, Smith JE. Use of refractive index measurement for quality assurance of pediatric parenteral nutrient solutions. *Am J Hosp Pharm*. 1987; 44:1617–20.

7. Donnelly AJ, Newman LM, Petryna HM, et al. Refractometric testing of alfentanil hydrochloride, fentanyl citrate, sufentanil citrate and midazolam hydrochloride. *Am J Hosp Pharm*. 1993; 50:298–300.

8. Trissel LA. Handbook on injectable drugs, 8th ed. Bethesda, MD: American Society of Hospital Pharmacists; 1994.

9. Bogdanich W. The great white lie. New York: Simon & Schuster; 1991.

10. Sterility tests. In: United States pharmacopeia, 23rd rev./national formulary, 18th ed. Rockville, MD: United States Pharmacopeial Convention; 1994: 1686–90.

11. Akers MJ, Wright GE, Carlson KA. Sterility testing of antimicrobial-containing injectable solutions prepared in the pharmacy. *Am J Hosp Pharm*. 1991; 48:2414–8.

12. Murray PR, Sandrock MJ. Sterility testing of a total nutrient admixture with a biphasic blood culture system. *Am J Hosp Pharm*. 1991; 48:2419–21.

13. Pyrogen test. In: United States pharmacopeia, 23rd rev./national formulary, 18th ed. Rockville, MD: United States Pharmacopeial Convention; 1994: 1718–9.

14. Bacterial endotoxins test. In: United States pharmacopeia, 23rd rev./national formulary, 18th ed. Rockville, MD: United States Pharmacopeial Convention; 1994:1696–7.

Chapter 18
Documentation of Sterile Product Preparation

Barbara T. McKinnon

It is often said that, "If it wasn't documented, it wasn't done." Documentation establishes a record of the activities performed.

Sterile product documents tell how a drug was processed and what quality attributes it possesses. This documentation helps to ensure that a system is in place to prepare products properly and also serves as a checklist for this preparation. Documentation must be performed precisely, unfailingly, consistently, quickly, and in sufficient detail to permit another individual to duplicate the process exactly.

USES OF DOCUMENTATION

Outside Organizations

Sterile product records may be inspected by numerous organizations including state boards of pharmacy, third-party payers, the Joint Commission on Accreditation of Healthcare Organizations, the Drug Enforcement Agency, and the Food and Drug Administration. These organizations use documentation records when determining payments, granting licensure, and, possibly, justifying continued accreditation of certain programs.

Legal Situations

If a patient pursues litigation related to a pharmacy-prepared sterile product, the attorney may subpoena the pharmacy's quality-assurance records and other relevant documents. Additionally, these records would be reviewed by the organization's attorney as well as its malpractice insurance carrier. In this situation, the quality of documentation may prevent a costly lawsuit or judgment.

Workload Justification

In addition to serving as a record of past actions, documentation of goods and services provided by the pharmacy can be used to determine workload statistics and productivity ratios. This information can subsequently support a formal request for adding staff, equipment, or workspace or for reallocating these same resources elsewhere.

Problem Identification

If problems are discovered with compounded sterile products, all documentation should be doublechecked as soon as possible. Whenever the quality of pharmacy-prepared sterile products is questioned, the following documents should be reviewed:

❑ Original prescription.
❑ Batch record.
❑ Results of quality-control tests.
❑ Calibration and setup procedures for involved equipment.
❑ Environmental quality-control results for the time of compounding.
❑ Validation and training records for involved personnel.

Results of the investigation then should be used in a continuous quality-improvement process to

1. Identify problems.
2. Take action to improve problem areas.
3. Evaluate the effectiveness of the action taken.

DOCUMENTED INFORMATION

Documentation can be brief as long as important facts are not omitted. Forms, worksheets, and computer software can prompt the user to document all essential data. Computerized labels, NCR forms, or addressographs may save time by avoiding duplicate data entries (e.g., patient names and locations). When possible, documentation should occur *when* and *where* the work is completed or while it is in progress.

Documentation errors must be handled carefully to avoid the appearance of a coverup. Correction fluid should never be used on pharmacy records; a single line should be drawn through the mistake, and the word "error" with the person's initials should be written by it.

Medication-Related Records

Maintenance of all medication-related records (including prescription documents and medication orders for hospital and home care patients) must follow the mandates established by federal and state laws. Prescription records must be readily retrievable for at least 2 years for inspection by state boards of pharmacy; however, records may need to be retained longer for other purposes (e.g., 5 years for Medicare). Often, NCR or faxed copies of physician's orders are sent to institutional pharmacies. These copies do not have to be kept for 2 years, however, if the original is in the patient's medical record and all other documents (e.g., patient medication profile and batch record) are filed.

Records for controlled substances and investigational drugs require special handling. Inventories and prescriptions for controlled substances may be kept separately or have the letter "C" stamped in the lower right corner for easy retrieval. Narcotic order forms must be stored for at least 2 years; state laws vary. Typically, a perpetual inventory is maintained for both controlled substances and investigational drugs. Additionally, a biennial controlled substance inventory is required.

The statute of limitations for litigation is 2 years for adults. For pediatric patients, however, litigation may be initiated until the child reaches the age of majority. Therefore, many hospitals and home care organizations utilize microfiche or compact disk files for long-term storage of their records.

The records that should be maintained for at least 2 years include[1]

❑ Patient profiles.
❑ Medication records.
❑ Purchase records.
❑ Biennial controlled substance inventories.
❑ Policies and procedures for cytotoxic waste.
❑ Lot numbers of components used in compounded sterile products.

Batch Preparation Records

As discussed in Chapter 11, batch preparation records must be maintained. For routinely compounded products, a set of master production records helps to ensure that all associated activities can be reproduced with a high degree of uniformity. During production, these records document that the product meets established specifications. Master production records contain the model requirements for the batch formula and compounding directions. Specifications for selection and handling of equipment are critical; substitution of a different item, such as a filter with a different pore size, can have serious consequences.

Batch production records show that each significant step prescribed for the compounding of a product was completed. Furthermore, signatures of the employees who performed and checked the procedures authenticate that the process was done correctly. Control records confirm that product specifications were met, based on analytical determinations of the process and the product. Environmental monitoring records show the conditions that existed during product preparation. Records of product quarantine and a copy of the product labeling also should be maintained.

Pharmacy Quality-Assurance Records

Records of the quality of pharmacy activities should be filed for an adequate time, consistent with organizational policies.[2] These documents include the

- Organization's policies and procedures.
- Logs of refrigerator and freezer temperatures.
- Certification of laminar-airflow hoods, biological safety cabinets, and cleanrooms.
- Results of environmental monitoring.

Personnel Training, Certification, and Recertification Records

Orientation and training of new pharmacists and technicians who may prepare sterile products must be documented. Some state boards now review such training during their routine annual pharmacy inspections.[3] It is not adequate simply to state that an employee passed an initial evaluation period. Specific training on aseptic techniques for a Class 100 environment, appropriate garb and personal hygiene, and storage and handling of drugs and supplies should be annotated.

Additionally, employees should be trained in the setup, calibration, and use of all compounding devices and equipment; this training should be recorded for each type of equipment used. Furthermore, the completion of an acceptable validation procedure should be documented before employees are certified to compound patient products under direct supervision. Personnel records also should include documentation of employee health procedures (e.g., annual physical and tuberculin skin test) and an offer to provide vaccination against hepatitis B.

At appropriate intervals, employees should be recertified to verify that they follow good technique and current institutional procedures. For example, an annual recertification could include

- Written test covering aseptic technique, use of a Class 100 environment, and environmental monitoring procedures.

- Demonstration of aseptic technique with media fills followed by immediate feedback.

Recertification records should be maintained in an employee's personnel file.

SUMMARY

Documentation is an important part of any sterile product preparation program. These records may be used to justify third-party payments, to prevent or provide a basis for legal action, to justify workload, and to discover errors in policies and procedures.

At a minimum, documentation should be collected for all activities related to medication supply and use, batch preparation processes, quality-assurance programs, and personnel training.

REFERENCES

1. Delapointe D, Williams DH, Anderson WA, et al. Model rules for sterile pharmaceuticals. The model state pharmacy act and model rules of the National Association of Boards of Pharmacy. Park Ridge, IL: National Association of Boards of Pharmacy; 1992.
2. American Society of Hospital Pharmacists. ASHP technical assistance bulletin on quality assurance for pharmacy-prepared sterile products. *Am J Hosp Pharm.* 1993; 50:2386–98.
3. Sterile product preparation in pharmacy practice. Tennessee Code Annotated, Sections 63-10-102(a) and (b), 63-10-101(e)(4)(6), and 63-10-206. *Tenn Pharmacist.* 1994; June:12–4.

Chapter 19

Policies and Procedures for Sterile Product Preparation

E. Clyde Buchanan

A good policy and procedure manual can promote the safe, efficient, and uniform performance of all departmental functions.[1] Each department involved in preparing sterile products should write its own policies and procedures based on specific circumstances.[2]

A policy—the general statement—provides a basis for decision-making. It addresses what must be done and, sometimes, why and when. A procedure—the "how to" document—provides the method for carrying out a policy. Procedures outline the complete cycle of a task, step by step, and assign responsibility to specific personnel.

Written policies and procedures can lead to numerous benefits:[1]

- ❒ Establishment of practice standards for both administrative and professional activities, in compliance with accrediting and certifying bodies.
- ❒ Coordination of resources (personnel, supplies, and equipment) for delivery of efficient and economic services.
- ❒ Reduction in waste (time and materials) resulting from errors, inexperience, and lack of supervision.
- ❒ Improvement in intradepartmental communications.
- ❒ Reduction in errors associated with oral transmission of information.
- ❒ Improvement in employees' security, job satisfaction, and productivity.
- ❒ Rapid detection of inefficient or inferior personnel performance.
- ❒ Establishment of means to evaluate the quality of services.
- ❒ Consistency in orienting and training new personnel.

The ASHP Technical Assistance Bulletin on Quality Assurance for Pharmacy-Prepared Sterile Products states that policies and procedures should be available to all involved personnel[3] (see Appendix 6). These policies and procedures should be updated at least annually, by the designated pharmacist and department head, to reflect current standards. Revisions then should be communicated to affected personnel. Before compounding sterile products, personnel should read the policies and procedures and verify (by signature) having done so.

This chapter notes the topics pertinent to preparation of sterile products that should be covered in a pharmacy's policy and procedure manual. These same topics are presented in detail throughout this book and the appendices.

PERSONNEL TRAINING AND EVALUATION

Job Description

Complete job descriptions for personnel preparing sterile products are essential to the hiring and orientation process. Job descriptions should include

- ❐ Basic qualifications (e.g., education level, certification, registration, and length and type of experience).
- ❐ Physical requirements (e.g., ability to lift moderately heavy weights, push carts, and perform rapid, repetitive, and accurate manipulations).
- ❐ Working conditions (e.g., shifts, environment, and garb).
- ❐ Responsibilities and competencies (e.g., ability to compound a pharmaceutical product that is free of microbial, particulate, and pyrogenic contaminants).

Job Orientation

Policies and procedures on orientating new employees to sterile compounding should include their roles and those of coworkers, garb, facilities, equipment, area-specific techniques, and reference books (see Chapter 2).

Training and Education

Personnel training and continuing education procedures should specify frequency, methods, requirements, and documentation. Educational topics should include (1) aseptic technique and quality control; (2) chemical, pharmaceutical, and clinical properties of drugs; (3) good manufacturing practices; (4) equipment operation; and (5) product handling (see Chapter 2).

Competency Evaluation

Policies and procedures for competency evaluation should specify the methods of observation and/or testing and the intervals between these evaluations. For example, personnel could be observed continually for aseptic technique, could demonstrate how to use new equipment, or could have periodic written tests of math skills. Perhaps the most important means of demonstrating continued competence is media-fill validation of aseptic technique (see Chapter 16).

ACQUISITION, STORAGE, AND HANDLING OF SUPPLIES

Acquisition

Policies and procedures for acquisition of sterile and nonsterile ingredients should include (see Chapter 11)

- ❐ Ingredient selection by *United States Pharmacopeia/National Formulary (USP/NF)* standards.
- ❐ Bulk drug substance dating procedures.
- ❐ Repackaging guidelines.
- ❐ Identification of ingredients by testing.
- ❐ System for purchase of equipment, containers, and closures.

Storage

Policies and procedures concerning storage should be based on USP or manufacturer-specified conditions. Written procedures are needed for temperature monitoring of refrigerators and freezers; light, ventilation, and humidity standards; stock rotation and inspection; and locations of quarantined products (both ingredients and end products) (see Chapters 14 and 15).

Handling

These policies and procedures should include the removal of outer packaging in the anteroom, handling of pouched supplies (e.g., syringes), decontamination of ampuls and vials, and disposal of used items, hazardous waste, and sharps. Inspection of sterile ingredients and containers just prior to compounding is part of aseptic technique.

Handling policies and procedures for expired drugs and supplies should encompass their removal and quarantine as well as their return or disposal. Product recall procedures should detail notification of recalls, removal from stock and nursing areas, and retrieval from patients (see Chapters 14 and 15).

FACILITIES

Policies and procedures should contain clear rules for cleanliness of work areas, including time periods between cleaning, selection of disinfectants, and cleaning methods. The traffic control policy for work areas should identify authorized personnel and equipment and supply access to the anteroom and cleanroom. If a sterile compounding area is less clean than Class 10,000, the products that can be prepared there must be specified. Safety features, such as emergency showers and eyewashes, also should be covered (see Chapter 4).

EQUIPMENT

These policies and procedures should encompass

❒ Location of equipment and supplies in relation to work areas (e.g., prohibition of particle-producing items, such as pencils and paper towels, in the cleanroom).

❒ Use and cleaning of fixtures and equipment (e.g., sinks, lockers, and carts).

❒ Cart entry past demarcation line in the anteroom.

❒ Methods for using all laminar-airflow hoods.

❒ Traffic near a hood.

❒ Starting, cleaning, stopping, and moving hoods.

Clear procedures are especially important for the use of automatic compounders and pumps since they have been implicated in serious errors nationwide. Such equipment must be calibrated for accuracy, monitored continually, and recertified periodically. Finally, sterilization methods for nonsterile equipment and vessels must be clearly written (see Chapter 5).

PERSONNEL CONDUCT AND GARB

Policies should prohibit staff from eating, drinking, smoking, and wearing makeup and jewelry in the cleanroom and under the hood. Hand-washing and drying rules should be spelled out, as well as regulations dealing with infectious conditions such as skin rashes, sunburn, and coughs. Policies also should prevent pregnant women from exposure to teratogenic products.

Garb policies and procedures should describe how to (1) remove street clothes; (2) don coats or gowns; (3) reuse coats and gowns on reentry to the cleanroom; (4) use masks, hair covers, and shoe covers; (5) use gloves for both hazardous and nonhazardous drugs; (6) rinse gloves between operations; and (7) use sticky mats to clean shoes (see Chapter 8).

PRODUCT PREPARATION

Product Integrity

Written policies and procedures should ensure stability, compatibility, purity, and physiologic norms for all products based on pharmaceutical standards and references. Procedures also should cover inspection of ingredients and containers for expiration dates and defects prior to compounding (see Chapter 3).

Aseptic Technique

These policies and procedures should outline the cleaning of containers prior to their introduction into the hood, touch avoidance of critical container areas, use of needles and syringes, manipulations relative to laminar airflow in a hood, and organization of work in the laminar-airflow

hood. Furthermore, requirements concerning the identification of cytotoxic and hazardous drugs and equipment and protective garb must be clearly stated. Particulate filtration methods also should be outlined (see Chapters 7 and 10).

Master Work Sheets

Policies and procedures should specify pharmacist verification of ingredients and their amounts, for both manual and automated additives (see Chapter 11). For each product, a master work sheet should delineate

❒ Ingredients and their quantities.

❒ Equipment and supplies to assemble prior to preparation.

❒ Compounding directions.

❒ Sterilization method.

❒ Sample label.

❒ Evaluation and testing requirements.

❒ Quarantine methods.

❒ Storage conditions.

❒ Expiration period.

Batch Preparation Records

For each batch, these records document the procedures, materials, and personnel involved. A batch preparation record identifies all solutions and ingredients with their corresponding amounts, concentrations, or volumes; manufacturer and lot numbers for each component; and signatures or initials of individuals measuring ingredients.

A unique lot or control number, an expiration date, and the preparation date are assigned to each batch. Personnel who prepare or approve the batch are indicated, as are the specific equipment used, end-product evaluation and testing specifications, storage requirements, and the actual yield compared to the anticipated yield (see Chapter 11).

STERILIZATION METHODS

Selection

Policies and procedures should state the sterilization method for each type of product. Although micropore filtration is used for heat-labile products, it cannot assure a pyrogen-free product. Autoclaving is preferred for batches of heat-stable products; if done properly, all units should be sterile and pyrogen free. Dry heat sterilization is usually reserved for highly heat-stable products that must remain in powder form (see Chapter 10).

Specific Requirements

Sterile filtration procedures should indicate both the filter material (e.g., hydrophilic or lipophilic) for different product types and methods for ensuring filter integrity. For autoclaving, the arrangement of units, the validation of cycles, and the maintenance of equipment must be described. For dry heat sterilization, procedures must clearly state how the oven heating process is validated and monitored, how the product is arranged in the oven, and how the oven is maintained.

Terminally sterilized products require quarantine and release procedures (e.g., duration, location, and documentation) (see Chapter 10).

ENVIRONMENTAL MONITORING

The designated pharmacist, along with infection control and microbiology personnel, should develop an environmental monitoring plan for cleanroom air, work surfaces, walls, floors, and ceilings. Monitoring devices should be specified. A continuous method for monitoring particulate matter in the air is mandatory to document "cleanroom" conditions.

Microbial sampling of the air and surfaces, done by growing viable colony-forming units of bacteria from samples, should be included. Procedures should specify upper limits of microbial counts, required actions when limits are exceeded, and the restarting of product preparation after an environment has failed (see Chapter 6).

PROCESS VALIDATION

These policies and procedures must specify when and how an operator's ability to compound sterile products is to be validated. New staff members must initially establish competence for each product type they are to handle (e.g., syringes, TPNs, and batch-reconstituted antibiotics) by use of media fills. Then staff members must be revalidated periodically (e.g., quarterly or annually) and whenever they learn to prepare a different product.

For ASHP's Risk Level 2 products, simulation of the process with media fills must verify that each product type can be prepared sterile. For ASHP's Risk Level 3, each distinct product's preparation method must be process validated and documented in the procedures.

Policies should set limits of acceptability for

❑ Individual operators.
❑ Each Risk Level 2 product type.
❑ Each individual Risk Level 3 product.

Procedures should specify required actions when these limits are exceeded (see Chapter 16).

EXPIRATION DATING

Expiration dating policies and procedures should cite the methods followed for setting expiration dates and the references used for determining product stability times, especially when strengths or storage times differ from manufacturer labeling. Expiration times include specific storage temperatures (e.g., 24 hr at room temperature and/or 7 days under refrigeration). The department should have a policy for handling products removed from and returned to refrigeration.

To determine an expiration date for products not covered by manufacturers' labeling or reliable literature, experimental stability testing is required. Sometimes the institution's laboratory personnel can help pharmacists test a product's shelf life (see Chapter 12).

LABELING

Policies and procedures for labeling should outline the required information for

❑ Products prepared in batches and stored prior to dispensing.
❑ Products dispensed for administration within the institution.
❑ Patient-use products.

Procedures should indicate where labels are obtained and stored in the pharmacy. They should also require sequestration of batch labels with their product batch (see Chapter 13).

END-PRODUCT EVALUATION

For Risk Level 1 products, end-product evaluation policies and procedures should include pharmacist inspection for leaks, container integrity, cloudiness, particulates, color, and volume. Also to be covered is pharmacist verification of ingredients, quantities, containers, reservoirs, and labels versus the drug order or prescription. Furthermore, a policy may specify that certain products require doublechecks (e.g., pediatric TPNs). Verification of automatic compounder settings also is extremely important, as is the disposal of defective products.

In addition to these policies, Risk Level 2 end-product evaluation should include a program of sterility testing, according to a formal sampling plan.

For Risk Level 3 products, methods for testing and documenting the sterility, nonpyrogenicity, and ingredient concentration should be described.

A quality-control program also must be explained, including the separation of responsibility for production and quality control; a sampling plan; methods of sterility, pyrogen, and ingredient potency testing; and in-use product sterility testing for suspected contamination (see Chapter 17).

MAINTAINING QUALITY OF COMPOUNDED PRODUCTS

Inside the Institution

Policies and procedures should document storage methods that ensure product identity, strength, and quality during transport and storage for both unrefrigerated and refrigerated products. These policies will differ from those developed for noncompounded products.

Special transport procedures for different product types also must be outlined. Furthermore, the selection of manual or automated delivery systems should be discussed (see Chapter 14).

Outside the Institution

These policies and procedures should cover packing for transport, in-transit temperatures, precautions for toxic product transport, commercial carrier expectations, evaluation of shipper performance, and in-home conditions. For the home, procedures should include (1) assurance of proper storage capability; (2) written instructions for storage, use, and unsuitability for use; and (3) home visitation and inspection.

Policies and procedures for patient or caregiver training must include the content of the training program and evaluation of patient or caregiver competence (see Chapter 15).

PATIENT MONITORING AND COMPLAINT SYSTEM

For outcome monitoring, policies and procedures should encompass reporting and handling of patient problems and trending of patient problems regarding sterile products.

HOUSEKEEPING PROCEDURES

These policies and procedures should cover cleaning and disinfecting of floors, work surfaces, and walls. Intervals between each type of cleaning should be specified, cleaning equipment and supplies should be listed, and the reuse of cleaning supplies should be outlined. When these procedures are developed, the institution's housekeeping department should be consulted.

Brands of disinfectants and changing intervals also should be specified. Infection control personnel can help to develop these policies.

QUALITY-ASSURANCE PROGRAM

The pharmacy should have written policies and procedures for monitoring, evaluating, correcting, and improving sterile preparation activities and processes. These policies and procedures should refer to those on training and education, competency evaluation, product preparation, sterilization methods, process validation, and end-product evaluation.

DOCUMENTATION RECORDS

Policies and procedures concerning documentation records should specify the location of stored records and the required storage time. The following records should be kept, but storage periods will vary according to laws, regulations, and professional standards (see Chapter 18):

- ❑ Training records and competence tests scores for each employee (e.g., aseptic technique observation and media fills).
- ❑ Refrigerator and freezer temperature logs or charts.
- ❑ Certification of laminar-airflow hoods and scales.
- ❑ Batch preparation records.
- ❑ Master work sheets.
- ❑ Environmental monitoring tests.
- ❑ Process validations.
- ❑ Drug recalls.
- ❑ Product problem reports to manufacturers and USP.
- ❑ Adverse drug reaction reports to manufacturers and the Food and Drug Administration.
- ❑ Patient complaints and problem handling and outcome.

SUMMARY

The establishment of policies and procedures is a critical step in any sterile product preparation program. A thorough policy and procedure manual must be available to all involved personnel. These employees also must show an understanding of each policy and procedure before being allowed to prepare sterile products. Moreover, their competency in performing these procedures and interpreting each policy should be assessed periodically.

REFERENCES

1. Hethcox JM. The policy and procedure manual. In: Brown TR, ed. Handbook of institutional pharmacy practice, 3rd ed. Bethesda, MD: American Society of Hospital Pharmacists; 1992:53–62.
2. Ginnow WK, King CM Jr. Revision and reorganization of a hospital pharmacy policies and proce-

dures manual. *Am J Hosp Pharm.* 1978; 35:698–704.

3. American Society of Hospital Pharmacists. ASHP technical assistance bulletin on quality assurance for pharmacy-prepared sterile products. *Am J Hosp Pharm.* 1993; 50:2386–98.

4. Sterile drug products for home use. In: United States pharmacopeia, 23rd rev./national formulary, 18th ed. Rockville, MD: United States Pharmacopeial Convention; 1994:1963–75.

5. American Society of Hospital Pharmacists. ASHP technical assistance bulletin on handling cytotoxic and hazardous drugs. *Am J Hosp Pharm.* 1990; 47:1033–49.

Appendix 1

CHAPTER 32—DRUGS GENERAL

SUBJECT: Hospital Pharmacies—Status as Drug Manufacturer

POLICY:

1. Compounding in hospitals—registration

We interpret Section 510 of the Federal Food, Drug, and Cosmetic Act as not requiring registration by the hospital pharmacy that compounds medication for inpatient dispensing, outpatient dispensing (sale or free), mailing to a patient within the State or out of the State, or for transferral to another unit of the same hospital (within the State or in another State) for dispensing by that unit of the hospital. However, if the hospital pharmacy compounds medication which it sells to another hospital or a drugstore, such sale is not at "retail" and registration is required.

2. Application of the "current good manufacturing practices" regulations to hospital pharmacies

Section 501(a)(2)(B) of the Act provides that a drug shall be deemed to be adulterated if the methods used in, or the facilities or controls used for its manufacture, processing, packing, or holding do not conform to current good manufacturing practice...." This section, through the operation of Section 301(k) is applicable to hospital pharmacies, as well as to manufacturers, whether or not the establishments are required to register with FDA under Section 510. However, the CGMP regulations set forth in 21 CFR 211 apply to those establishments which are both required to register under Section 510 and which prepare dosage forms. Therefore, if the hospital pharmacy is not required to register as described in paragraph one above, 21 CFR 211 does not apply. It is the policy of FDA not to routinely inspect such pharmacies for compliance with Section 501(a)(2)(B) if they operate within state or local laws governing the practice of pharmacy. However, when a hospital pharmacy is engaged in repacking or relabeling operations that are beyond the usual conduct of dispensing or selling drugs at retail, the exemptions in the Act cease to apply; the establishment is required to register and is subject to regular inspections under Section 704 of the Act.

3. Labeling of "prepackaged drugs"

We believe that drugs packaged for use as ward stock should be labeled with the information required by regulation 201.100(b).

DATE: 10/01/80
ISSUING OFFICE: EDRO, Division of Field Regulatory Guidance
AUTHORITY: Associate Commissioner for Regulatory Affairs

139

4. <u>Investigational drugs</u>

We do not believe that preparation of investigational drugs by a hospital pharmacy for use by an investigator in the hospital or in another hospital, requires registration under Section 510 of that Act. However, if the new drug has been or is to be shipped in interstate commerce for clinical trials, the "sponsor" of the investigation should file a "Notice of Claimed Investigational Exemption for a New Drug" before the shipment is made or the trials started. This "Notice" would necessarily include the name and address of the pharmacy and provide information regarding manufacture of the new drug by the pharmacy.

Submission of Forms FD-1571, 1572, and 1573 is only required when the finished new drug or the "new drug substance" used in its manufacture, is in interstate commerce.

When interstate commerce is involved and the various forms must be submitted, the hospital or some other responsible person may act as the "sponsor" and file the Form FD-1571. Such "sponsor" should obtain completed Form FD-1572 or 1573 as appropriate from the actual investigators.

The physician-investigator may delegate to a hospital pharmacist responsible to him, or any other person responsible to him, the maintenance of the required records concerning the use of the investigational drug.

5. <u>New drug applications</u>

We recognize that a physician may prescribe an unusual preparation that requires compounding by the pharmacy from drugs readily available for other uses and which is not generally regarded as safe and effective for the intended use. If the pharmacy merely acts to fill each individual prescription as received, it is our opinion that clearance under the "new drug" provisions of the Act is not required.

If the hospital prepares a bulk quantity of an unusual drug in anticipation of prescriptions from the physician who developed the formula, or from other physicians who have been induced to use the unusual medication, we believe the situation would then differ from the one described in the preceding paragraph. If such drug is shipped interstate or a major ingredient used in manufacturing the drug is received from an out-of-state supplier, we would regard the article as a "new drug" in interstate commerce and therefore subject to the investigational new drug regulations.

6. <u>Prepacking</u>

We do not believe that "prepackaging" by the hospital pharmacy for dispensing within the hospital, or for outpatient dispensing, or for transferral to another unit of the hospital, would require registration under Section 510 of the Act. However, repacking of a drug which is sold to another hospital, whether or not such other hospital is under the control of the same corporation, would require registration under Section 510.

7. Antibiotic certification

Hospital pharmacies are not exempt from the antibiotic certification regulations. Antibiotic preparations compounded by the hospital pharmacy are subject to the applicable regulations, regardless of whether the item that is compounded by the hospital pharmacy is available in the usual commercial channels. However, we point out that the pharmacist may, without further certification, compound an antibiotic preparation on the basis of a prescription issued by a licensed practitioner, if the antibiotic ingredient used for compounding the prescription is taken from a certified container packaged for dispensing. The compounded prescription is exempt from certification "for a reasonable time to permit the delivery of the drug compounded on such prescription."

CHAPTER 32—DRUGS GENERAL

SUBJECT: Manufacture, Distribution, and Promotion of Adulterated, Misbranded, or Unapproved New Drugs for Human Use by State-Licensed
Pharmacies

BACKGROUND

This compliance policy guide (CPG) reflects longstanding FDA policy that
has been articulated in related CPGs, warning letters, and federal court
decisions.

FDA recognizes that pharmacists traditionally have extemporaneously compounded and manipulated reasonable quantities of drugs upon receipt of a
valid prescription for an individually identified patient from a licensed
practitioner. This traditional activity is not the subject of this CPG.

With respect to such activities, it is important to note that 21 U.S.C.
360(g)(1) exempts retail pharmacies from the registration requirements
that include, among other things, a mandatory biennial FDA inspection. The
exemption applies to "pharmacies" that operate in accordance with state
law and dispense drugs "upon prescriptions of practitioners licensed to
administer such drugs to patients <u>under the care of such practitioners in
the course of their professional practice, and which do not manufacture</u>,
prepare, propagate, <u>compound</u>, or process drugs or devices for sale <u>other
than in the regular course of their business of dispensing</u> or selling
drugs or devices <u>at retail</u>" (emphasis added). See also 21 U.S.C. Sections
374(a)(2) (exempting pharmacies that meet the foregoing criteria from
certain inspection provisions) and 353(b)(2) (exempting drugs dispensed by
filling a valid prescription from certain misbranding provisions).

It should be noted, however, that while retail pharmacies that meet the
statutory criteria are exempted from certain requirements of the Federal
Food, Drug, and Cosmetic Act (Act), they are not the subject of any general exemption from the new drug, adulteration, or misbranding provisions
of the Act.

FDA believes that an increasing number of establishments with retail pharmacy licenses are engaged in manufacturing, distributing, and promoting
unapproved new drugs for human use in a manner that is clearly outside the
bounds of traditional pharmacy practice and that constitute violations of
the Act. Some "pharmacies" that have sought to find shelter under and
expand the scope of the exemptions identified above, have claimed that

ISSUING OFFICE: Office of Enforcement, Division of Compliance Policy
AUTHORITY: Associate Commisioner for Regulatory Affairs
DATE: 03/16/92
FORM FDA 2678a(9/88)

their manufacturing, distribution, and marketing practices are only retail dispensing; however, the practices of these entities are far more consistent with those of drug manufacturers and wholesalers than with retail pharmacies. The activities of the self-styled pharmacies are consistent with the activities of manufacturers in that they direct promotional activities at licensed practitioners and patients. The promotional activities include employing detail persons and hiring marketing consultants to promote the company's specialization of compounding specific products or therapeutic classes of drugs. The firms also receive and use in large quantity bulk drug substances to manufacture unapproved drug products and to manufacture drug products in large quantity, in advance of receiving a valid prescription for the products. Moreover, the firms serve physicians and patients with whom they have no established individual or professional relationship.

When less significant violations of the Act related to a pharmacy have occurred, FDA has worked cooperatively with state regulatory agencies; generally, FDA will continue to defer such actions to state authorities. However, FDA regards the more extreme examples of the foregoing conduct as significant violations that constitute deliberate efforts to circumvent the new drug, adulteration or misbranding provisions of the Act.

There is a very real potential for causing harm to the public health when drug products are manufactured and distributed in commercial amounts without FDA's prior approval and without adequate record keeping (to retrace and recall harmful products), without labeling, or without adequate manufacturing controls to assure the safety, purity, potency, quality, and identity of the drug product. In one recent instance, an outbreak of eye infections in regional hospitals, and the loss of an eye by each of two patients, was attributed to a drug product compounded by a pharmacy.

FDA has issued warning letters to several firms that were clearly manufacturing drugs for human use under the guise of traditional pharmacy practice. For example, one establishment manufactured over 300,000 dosage units of albuterol sulfate and other inhalation therapy drugs per month for 6,000 patients, most of whom live out of state. Another firm manufactured a large quantity of a drug product at dosage levels that have not been determined by adequate and well controlled studies to be effective for the indicated use. A recent inspection of another company operating with a pharmacy license revealed that the firm had hundreds of bulk drug ingredients on hand to manufacture about 165 different products. A review of the manufacturing dates of the "compounded" drugs on hand during the inspection of this firm revealed that 37 products had been produced over a year prior to the inspection, six products had been made between six and eleven months prior to the inspection, and 111 products had no recorded manufacturing date.

The agency has initiated enforcement action when pharmacy practice extends beyond the reasonable and traditional practice of a retail pharmacy. The courts have upheld FDA's interpretation in those cases. See United States v. Sene X Eleemosynary Corp., 479 F. Supp. 970 (S.D. Fla. 1979), aff'd, [1982-1983 Transfer Binder] Food Drug Cosm. L. Rep. (CCH) para. 38,207 at 39,117 (11th Cir. 1983); Cedars N. Towers Pharmacy, Inc., v. United States, [1978-79 Transfer Binder] Food Drug Cosm. L. Rep. (CCH) para. 38,200 at 38,826 (S.D. Fla. Aug. 28, 1978). See also United States v. Algon Chemical, Inc., 879 F.2d 1154 (3d Cir. 1989), United States v. 9/1 Kg. Containers, 854 F.2d 173 (7th Cir. 1988), cert. denied, 489 U.S. 1010 (1989), and United States v. Rutherford, 442 U.S. 544 (1979), regarding limitations on sale of unapproved and otherwise unlawful products to licensed practitioners.

POLICY

FDA recognizes that a licensed pharmacist may compound drugs extemporaneously after receipt of a valid prescription for an individual patient (i.e.,, an oral or written order of a practitioner licensed by state law to administer or order the administration of the drug to an individual patient identified and treated by the practitioner in the course of his or her professional practice).

Pharmacies that do not otherwise engage in practices that extend beyond the limits set forth in this CPG may prepare drugs in very limited quantities before receiving a valid prescription, provided they can document a history of receiving valid prescriptions that have been generated solely within an established professional practitioner-patient-pharmacy relationship, and provided further that they maintain the prescription on file for all such products dispensed at the pharmacy as required by state law.

If a pharmacy compounds finished drugs from bulk active ingredient materials considered to be unapproved new drug substances, as defined in 21 CFR 310.3(g), such activity must be covered by an FDA-sanctioned investigational new drug application (IND) that is in effect in accordance with 21 U.S.C. Section 355(i) and 21 CFR 312.

In certain circumstances, it may be appropriate for a pharmacist to compound a small quantity of a drug that is only slightly different than an FDA-approved drug that is commercially available. In these circumstances, patient-by-patient consultation between physician and pharmacist must result in documentation that substantiates the medical need for the particular variation of the compound.

Pharmacies may not, without losing their status as retail entities, com-

GUIDE | 7132.16

pound, provide, and dispense drugs to third parties for resale to individual patients.

FDA will generally continue to defer to state and local officials regulation of the day-to-day practice of retail pharmacy and related activities. FDA anticipates that cooperative efforts between the states and the agency will result in coordinated investigations, referrals, and follow-up actions by the states.

FDA may, in the exercise of its enforcement discretion, initiate federal enforcement actions against entities and responsible persons when the scope and nature of a pharmacy's activity raises the kinds of concerns normally associated with a manufacturer and that results in significant violations of the new drug, adulteration, or misbranding provisions of the Act. In determining whether to initiate such an action, the agency will consider whether the pharmacy engages in any of the following acts:

1. Soliciting business (e.g., promoting, advertising, or using sales persons) to compound specific drug products, product classes, or therapeutic classes of drug products.

2. Compounding, regularly, or in inordinate amounts, drug products that are commercially available in the marketplace and that are essentially generic copies of commercially available, FDA-approved drug products.

3. Receiving, storing, or using drug substances without first obtaining written assurance from the supplier that each lot of the drug substance has been made in an FDA-approved facility.

4. Receiving, storing, or using drug components not guaranteed or otherwise determined to meet official compendia requirements.

5. Using commercial scale manufacturing or testing equipment for compounding drug products.

6. Compounding inordinate amounts of drugs in anticipation of receiving prescriptions in relation to the amounts of drugs compounded after receiving valid prescriptions.

7. Offering compounded drug products at wholesale to other state licensed persons or commercial entities for resale.

8. Distributing inordinate amounts of compounded products out of state.

9.   Failing to operate in conformance with applicable state law regu-
      lating the practice of pharmacy.

The foregoing list of factors is not intended to be exhaustive and other
factors may be appropriate for consideration in a particular case.

FDA guidelines and other CPGs interpret or clarify agency positions concerning nuclear pharmacy, hospital pharmacy, shared service operations,
mail order pharmacy, and the manipulation of approved drug products.

REGULATORY ACTION GUIDANCE

Pharmacies engaged in promotion and other activities analogous to manufacturing and distributing drugs for human use are subject to the same provisions of the Act as manufacturers. District offices are encouraged to
consult with state regulatory authorities to assure coherent application
of this CPG to establishments which are operating outside of the traditional practice of pharmacy.

FDA-initiated regulatory action may include issuing a warning letter,
seizure, injunction, and/or prosecution. Charges may include, but need not
be limited to, violations of 21 U.S.C Sections 351(a)(2)(B), 352(a),
352(f)(1), 352(o), and 355(a) of the Act.

ISSUED: 03/16/92

Appendix 3

CHAPTER 32c—DRUGS—NDA/IND

SUBJECT: Regulatory Action Regarding Approved New Drugs and Antibiotic Drug Products Subjected to Additional Processing or other Manipulations

BACKGROUND

FDA is issuing this policy guide to describe the circumstances in which the agency may initiate regulatory action regarding the marketing of approved new drugs and antibiotics that have been subjected to further processing or other manipulation, such as repacking, that is not covered by an approval under sections 505 or 507. (See U.S. v. Baxter Healthcare Corp., et al., CCH 38,166 Docket Nos. 89-2087/8 (7th Cir. May, 1990)).

Section 505 of the Federal Food, Drug, and Cosmetic Act (the Act) requires FDA approval of any new drug prior to marketing. Under the terms of that section, approval must be based on, among other things, the processes, facilities and controls used in the manufacture of the product. This is because various aspects of the manufacturing process, such as sterilization, mixing, filling, and packaging, can have a significant effect on safety and efficacy of a drug product.

Under section 507 of the Act, FDA requires an approved application, similar to an NDA under section 505, for any antibiotic to be exempted from the statutory requirement of batch certification. Thus, the agency conducts the same review, including an inspection of the manufacturer's facility, for approval of an antibiotic under section 507 as for approval of a new drug under section 505.

Under these provisions, each step in the manufacture and processing of a new drug or antibiotic, from handling of raw ingredients to final packaging, must be approved by FDA, whether carried out by the original manufacturer or by some subsequent handler or repacker of the product. Pharmacists are not exempt from these statutory requirements; however, the agency regards mixing, packaging, and other manipulations of approved drug by licensed pharmacists, consistent with the approved labeling of the product, as an approved use of the product if conducted within the practice of pharmacy, i.e., filling prescriptions for identified patients. Processing and repacking (including repackaging) of approved drugs by pharmacists for resale to hospitals, other pharmacies, etc., are beyond the practice of pharmacy and are thus subject to the requirements of premarket approval.

ISSUING OFFICE: Office of Enforcement, Division of Compliance Policy
AUTHORITY: Associate Commisioner for Regulatory Affairs
DATE: 01/18/91
FORM FDA 2678a(9/88)

GUIDE 7132c.06

The only repacking outside the practice of pharmacy that has been sanctioned in the absence of FDA approval is that of solid oral dosage forms of products already approved under section 505. See U.S. v. Kaybel, Inc., et al., 430 F.2d 1346 (3d Cir. 1970) (repacking of approved Enovid (estrogen) tablets from large bottles into small bottles allowed without an additional approval under section 505).

The repacking of approved new drugs and antibiotics by entities outside the terms of the respective approvals has become much more common due to the increased demand for varied product package sizes, including products for "unit-dose" dispensing by doctors, pharmacists, and institutions. Agency policy concerning unit-dose labeling for oral and liquid oral dosage forms is stated in CPG 7132b.10. The expiration dating and stability requirements for unit-dose repackaged drugs are covered in CPG 7132b.11. Custom repackers have responded to this increased demand by performing manipulations that are well beyond the intended uses approved in the labeling for pharmacists and physicians. Such manipulations result in new products whose safety and effectiveness have not been established. During the drug approval process, specifications are set for active ingredients, identity and limits for degradation products, sterility assurance, and closure integrity. Repacking by a new manufacturer may result in an unanticipated interaction between the pharmaceutical entity and the new packaging, such as absorption and degradation, which may affect the quality and purity of the product.

STERILE DRUG PRODUCTS

The FDA has an even greater concern about the manipulation of approved sterile drug products, especially when the sterile container is opened or otherwise entered to conduct manipulations such as dissolving, diluting or aliquoting, refilling, resterilizing, or repackaging in new containers. The moment a sterile container is opened and manipulated, a quality standard (sterility) is destroyed and previous studies supporting the standard(s) are compromised and are no longer valid. These quality standards that include product stability and sterility must be restored.

Non-invasive manipulations may also raise questions of sterility, as when intact containers are repacked into a tray with other drugs, needles, gauze, etc., and the resulting package is sterilized and marketed as a unit for clinical use. Sterilization is an operation that must be documented and rigorously reviewed, and the FDA has consistently maintained that sterility is an absolute concept that must be ensured not only by sterility testing of the finished product, but also by validation of the sterilization process. Requirements for sterilization are covered in CPG 7132a.06.

GUIDE   7132c.06

POLICY

To protect the public health and to carry out its responsibility under sections 505 and 507, FDA will seek to ensure that all significant phases of the manufacture and processing of new drugs and antibiotics are approved. The agency may initiate regulatory action regarding the marketing of any new drug or antibiotic that has been subjected, for example, to any of the following manipulations, unless the manipulation is covered by an approval under sections 505 or 507: (1) mixing, (2) granulating, (3) milling, (4) molding, (5) lyophilizing, (6) tableting, (7) encapsulating, (8) coating, (9) sterilization, (10) repacking (including repackaging). The details of each manipulation, including the site(s) at which they will occur, must be the subject of an approved application or supplement filed pursuant to sections 505 or 507.

EXCEPTIONS

Consistent with its enforcement policy subsequent to the Kaybel decision, the agency does not intend to initiate regulatory action with regard to the repacking of already-approved, solid oral dosage form drug products if (1) the repacking operation does not include any of the steps identified above, (2) the drug to be repacked is approved under sections 505 and 507, and (3) the labeling used for the repacked product is identical to that of the approved drug except for labeling changes necessary for compliance with section 502(b) of the Act.

In addition, the agency continues to regard manipulations that are performed within the practice of pharmacy, consistent with the approved labeling of the product, as approved uses of the product.

REGULATORY ACTION GUIDANCE

Recommendation for regulatory action should be discussed with the Office of Compliance (HFD-310) prior to referral of the case.

ISSUED: 01/18/91

Appendix 4
Good Compounding Practices Applicable to State Licensed Pharmacies

The following Good Compounding Practices (GCPs) are meant to apply only to the compounding of drugs by State-licensed pharmacies.

Subpart A—General Provisions

The recommendations contained herein are considered to be the minimum current good compounding practices for the preparation of drug products by State-licensed pharmacies for dispensing and/or administration to humans or animals.

The following definitions from the NABP *Model State Pharmacy Act* apply to these Good Compounding Practices. States may wish to insert their own definitions to comply with State Pharmacy Practice Acts.

> ***"Compounding"***—*the preparation, mixing, assembling, packaging, or Labeling of a drug or device (i) as the result of a Practitioner's Prescription Drug Order or initiative based on the Practitioner/patient/ pharmacist relationship in the course of professional practice, or (ii) for the purpose of, or as an incident to, research, teaching, or chemical analysis and not for sale or Dispensing. Compounding also includes the preparation of Drugs or Devices in anticipation of Prescription Drug Orders based on routine, regularly observed prescribing patterns.*

> ***"Manufacturing"***—*the production, preparation, propagation, conversion, or processing of a Drug or Device, either directly or indirectly, by extraction from substances of natural origin or independently by means of chemical or biological synthesis, and includes any packaging or repackaging of the substance(s) or Labeling or relabeling of its container, and the promotion and marketing of such Drugs or Devices. Manufacturing also includes the preparation and promotion of commercially available products from bulk compounds for resale by pharmacies, Practitioners, or other Persons.*

> ***"Component"***—*any ingredient intended for use in the compounding of a drug product, including those that may not appear in such product.*

Based on the existence of a pharmacist/patient/prescriber relationship and the presentation of a valid prescription, pharmacists may compound, in reasonable quantities, drug products that are commercially available in the marketplace.

Pharmacists shall receive, store, or use drug substances for compounding that have been made in an FDA-approved facility. Pharmacists shall also receive, store, or use drug components in compounding prescriptions that meet official compendia requirements. If neither of these requirements can be met, pharmacists shall use their professional judgment to procure alternatives.

Pharmacists may compound drugs in very limited quantities prior to receiving a valid prescription based on a history of receiving valid prescriptions that have been generated solely within an established pharmacist/patient/prescriber relationship, and provided that they maintain the prescriptions on file for all such products dispensed at the pharmacy (as required by State law). The compounding of inordinate amounts of drugs in anticipation of receiving prescriptions without any historical basis is considered manufacturing.

Pharmacists shall not offer compounded drug products to other State-licensed persons or commercial entities for subsequent resale, except in the course of professional practice for a prescriber to administer to an individual patient. Compounding pharmacies/pharmacists may advertise or otherwise promote the fact that they provide prescription compounding services; however, they shall not solicit business (e.g., promote, advertise, or use salespersons) to compound specific drug products.

The distribution of inordinate amounts of compounded products pursuant to a legitimate prescription out of state without a prescriber/patient/pharmacist relationship is considered manufacturing. Pharmacists engaged in the compounding of drugs shall operate in conformance with applicable State law regulating the practice of pharmacy.

Subpart B—Organization and Personnel

As in the dispensing of all prescriptions, the pharmacist has the responsibility and authority to inspect and approve or reject all components, drug product containers, closures, in-process materials, labeling, and the authority to prepare and review all compounding records to assure that no errors have occurred in the compounding process. The pharmacist is also responsible for the proper maintenance, cleanliness, and use of all equipment used in prescription compounding practice.

All pharmacists who engage in compounding of drugs shall be proficient in the art of compounding and shall maintain that proficiency through current awareness and training. Also, every pharmacist who engages in drug compounding must be aware of and familiar with all details of the Good Compounding Practices.

Personnel engaged in the compounding of drugs shall wear clean clothing appropriate to the operation being performed. Protective apparel, such as a coat/jacket, apron, or hand or arm coverings, shall be worn as necessary to protect drug products from contamination.

Only personnel authorized by the responsible pharmacist shall be in the immediate vicinity of the drug compounding operation. Any person shown at any time (either by medical examination or pharmacist determination) to have an apparent illness or open lesion(s) that may adversely affect the safety or quality of a drug product being compounded shall be excluded from direct contact with components, drug product containers, closures, in-process materials, and drug products until the condition is corrected or determined by competent medical personnel not to jeopardize the safety or quality of the product(s) being compounded. All personnel who normally assist the pharmacist in compounding procedures shall be instructed to report to the pharmacist any health conditions that may have an adverse effect on drug products.

Subpart C—Drug Compounding Facilities

Pharmacies engaging in compounding shall have a specifically designated and adequate area (space) for the orderly placement of equipment and materials to be used to compound medications. The drug compounding area for sterile products shall be separate and distinct from the area used for the compounding or dispensing of non-sterile drug products. The area(s) used for the compounding of drugs shall be maintained in a good state of repair.

Bulk drugs and other materials used in the compounding of drugs must be stored in adequately labeled containers in a clean, dry area or, if required, under proper refrigeration.

Adequate lighting and ventilation shall be provided in all drug compounding areas. Potable water shall be supplied under continuous positive pressure in a plumbing system free of defects that could contribute contamination to any compounded drug product. Adequate washing facilities, easily accessible to the compounding area(s) of the pharmacy, shall be provided. These facilities shall include, but not be limited to, hot and cold water, soap or detergent, and air-driers or single-source towels.

The area(s) used for the compounding of drugs shall be maintained in a clean and sanitary condition. It shall be free of infestation by insects, rodents, and other vermin. Trash shall be held and disposed of in a timely and sanitary manner. Sewage, trash, and other refuse in and from the pharmacy and immediate drug compounding area(s) shall be disposed of in a safe and sanitary manner.

Sterile Products

If sterile (aseptic) products are being compounded, conditions set forth in the *NABP Model Rules for Sterile Pharmaceuticals* must be followed.

If radiopharmaceuticals are being compounded, conditions set forth in the NABP *Model Rules for Nuclear/Radiologic Pharmacy* must be followed.

Special Precaution Products

If drug products with special precautions for contamination, such as penicillin, are involved in a compounding operation, appropriate measures, including either the dedication of equipment for such operations or the meticulous cleaning of contaminated equipment prior to its return to inventory, must be utilized in order to prevent cross-contamination.

Subpart D—Equipment

Equipment used in the compounding of drug products shall be of appropriate design, adequate size, and suitably located to facilitate operations for its intended use and for its cleaning and maintenance. Equipment used in the compounding of drug products shall be of suitable composition so that surfaces that contact components, in-process materials, or drug products shall not be reactive, additive, or absorptive so as to alter the safety, identity, strength, quality, or purity of the drug product beyond that desired.

Equipment and utensils used for compounding shall be cleaned and sanitized immediately prior to use to prevent contamination that would alter the safety, identity, strength, quality, or purity of the drug product beyond that desired. In the case of equipment, utensils, and containers/closures used in the compounding of sterile drug products, cleaning, sterilization, and maintenance procedures as set forth in the NABP *Model Rules for Sterile Pharmaceuticals* must be followed.

Previously cleaned equipment and utensils used for compounding drugs must be protected from contamination prior to use. Immediately prior to the initiation of compounding operations, they must be inspected by the pharmacist and determined to be suitable for use.

Automatic, mechanical, or electronic equipment, or other types of equipment or related systems that will perform a function satisfactorily may be used in the compounding of drug products. If such equipment is used, it shall be routinely inspected, calibrated (if necessary), or checked to assure proper performance.

Subpart E—Control of Components and Drug Product Containers and Closures

Components, drug product containers, and closures used in the compounding of drugs shall be handled and stored in a manner to prevent contamination. Bagged or boxed components of drug product containers and closures used in the compounding of drugs shall be stored off the floor in such a manner as to permit cleaning and inspection.

Drug product containers and closures shall not be reactive, additive, or absorptive so as to alter the safety, identity, strength, quality, or purity of the compounded drug beyond the desired result. Components, drug product containers, and closures for use in the compounding of drug products shall be rotated so that the oldest approval stock is used first. Container closure systems shall provide adequate protection against foreseeable external factors in storage and use that can cause deterioration or contamination of the compounded drug product. Drug product containers and closures shall be clean and, where indicated by the intended use of the drug, sterilized and processed to remove pyrogenic properties to assure that they are suitable for their intended use.

Drug product containers and closures intended for the compounding of sterile products must be handled, sterilized, stored, etc. in keeping with the NABP *Model Rules for Sterile Pharmaceuticals*. Methods of cleaning, sterilizing, and processing to remove pyrogenic properties shall be written and followed for drug product containers and closures used in the preparation of sterile pharmaceuticals, if these processes are performed by the pharmacist, or under the pharmacist's supervision, following the NABP *Model Rules for Sterile Pharmaceuticals*.

Subpart F—Drug Compounding Controls

There shall be written procedures for the compounding of drug products to assure that the finished products have the identity, strength, quality, and purity they purport or are represented to process. Such procedures shall include a listing of the components (ingredients), their amounts (in weight or volume), the order of component addition, and a description of the compounding process. All equipment and utensils and the container/closure system, relevant to the sterility and stability of the intended use of the drug, shall be listed. These written procedures shall be followed in the execution of the drug compounding procedure.

Components for drug product compounding shall be accurately weighed, measured, or subdivided as appropriate. These operations should be checked and rechecked by the compounding pharmacist at each stage of the process to ensure that each weight or measure is correct as stated in the written compounding procedures. If a component is removed from the original container to another (e.g., a powder is taken from the original container, weighed, placed in a container, and stored in another container) the new container shall be identified with the:

(a) component name, and
(b) weight or measure.

To assure the reasonable uniformity and integrity of compounded drug products, written procedures shall be established and followed that describe the tests or examinations to be conducted on the product being compounded (e.g., compounding of capsules). Such control procedures shall be established to monitor the output and to validate the performance of those compounding processes that may be responsible for causing variability in the final drug product. Such control procedures shall include, but are not limited to, the following (where appropriate):

(a) capsule weight variation;
(b) adequacy of mixing to assure uniformity and homogeneity;
(c) clarity, completeness, or pH of solutions.

Appropriate written procedures designed to prevent microbiological contamination of compounded drug products purporting to be sterile shall be established and followed. Such procedures shall include validation of any sterilization process.

Subpart G—Labeling Control of Excess Products

In the case where a quantity of a compounded drug product in excess of that to be initially dispensed in accordance with Subpart A is prepared, the excess product shall be labeled or documentation referenced with the complete list of ingredients (components), the preparation date, and the assigned expiration date based upon professional judgment, appropriate testing, or published data. It shall also be stored and accounted for under conditions dictated by its composition and stability characteristics (e.g., in a clean, dry place on a shelf or in the refrigerator) to ensure its strength, quality, and purity.

At the completion of the drug finishing operation, the product shall be examined for correct labeling.

Subpart H—Records and Reports

Any procedures or other records required to be maintained in compliance with these Good Compounding Practices shall be retained for the same period of time as each State requires for the retention of prescription files.

All records required to be retained under these Good Compounding Practices, or copies of such records, shall be readily available for authorized inspection during the retention period at the establishment where the activities described in such records occurred. These records or copies thereof shall be subject to photocopying or other means of reproduction as part of such inspection.

Records required under these Good Compounding Practices may be retained either as the original records or as true copies, such as photocopies, microfilm, microfiche, or other accurate reproductions of the original records.

Reprinted, with permission, from *Natl Pharm Compliance News.* 1993; May:2–3 and Oct:2–3.

Appendix 5
National Association of Boards of Pharmacy
Model Rules for Sterile Pharmaceuticals

Section 1. Scope and Purpose

The purpose of this section is to provide standards for the preparation, labeling, and distribution of sterile products by pharmacies, pursuant to or in anticipation of a Prescription Drug Order. The primary focus of these Rules is the assurance of product quality and characteristics, such as sterility and potency, that would be associated with environmental quality, preparation activities, and checks and tests carried out in the Pharmacy. These standards are intended to apply to all sterile products, notwithstanding the location of the patient (e.g., home, hospital, nursing home, hospice, doctor's office).

Section 2. Definitions

(a) "Biological Safety Cabinet" means a containment unit suitable for the preparation of low to moderate risk agents where there is a need for protection of the product, personnel, and environment according to National Sanitation Foundation (NSF) Standard 49.

(b) "Class 100 Environment" means an atmospheric environment which contains less than 100 particles 0.5 microns in diameter per cubic foot of air according to Federal Standard 209D.

(c) "Cytotoxic" means a pharmaceutical that has the capability of killing living cells.

(d) "Enteral" means within or by way of the intestine.

(e) "Parenteral" means a sterile preparation of Drugs for injection through one or more layers of the skin.

(f) "Sterile Pharmaceutical" means a dosage form free from living micro-organisms (aseptic).

Section 3. Policy and Procedure Manual

A policy and procedure manual shall be prepared and maintained for the Compounding, Dispensing, and Delivery of Sterile Pharmaceutical Prescription Drug Orders.

(a) The policy and procedure manual shall include a quality assurance program for the purpose of monitoring personnel qualifications, training and performance, product integrity, equipment, facilities, and guidelines regarding patient education.

(b) The policy and procedure manual shall be current and available for inspection by a Board of Pharmacy-designated agent.

Section 4. Physical Requirements

(a) The Pharmacy shall have a designated area with entry restricted to designated personnel for preparing Parenteral products. This area shall be structurally isolated from other areas with restricted entry or access, and must be designed to avoid unnecessary traffic and airflow disturbances from activity within the controlled facility. It shall be used only for the preparation of these specialty products. It shall be of sufficient size to accommodate a laminar airflow hood and to provide for the proper storage of Drugs and supplies under appropriate conditions of temperature, light, moisture, sanitation, ventilation, and security.

(b) The Pharmacy preparing Parenteral products shall have:

(1) Appropriate environmental control devices capable of maintaining at least Class 100 conditions in the workplace where critical objects are exposed and critical activities are performed; furthermore, these devices are capable of maintaining Class 100 conditions during normal activity. Examples of appropriate devices include laminar airflow hoods and zonal laminar flow of High Efficiency Particulate Air (HEPA) filtered air;

(2) Appropriate disposal containers for used needles, syringes, etc., and if applicable, for Cytotoxic waste from the preparation of chemotherapy agents and infectious wastes from patients' homes;

(3) When Cytotoxic Drug products are prepared, appropriate environmental control also includes appropriate biohazard cabinetry;

(4) Temperature-controlled Delivery container;

(5) Infusion Devices, if appropriate.

(c) The Pharmacy shall maintain supplies adequate to maintain an environment suitable for the aseptic preparation of sterile products.

(d) The Pharmacy shall have sufficient current reference materials related to sterile products to meet the needs of Pharmacy staff.

Section 5. Records and Reports

In addition to standard record and reporting requirements, the following additional records and reports must be maintained for sterile pharmaceuticals:

(a) A policy and procedure manual, including policies and procedures for Cytotoxic and/or infectious waste, if applicable, and;

(b) Lot numbers of the components used in Compounding sterile prescriptions.

Section 6. Delivery Service

The Pharmacist-in-Charge shall assure the environmental control of all products shipped. Therefore, any Compounded, sterile pharmaceutical must be shipped or Delivered to a patient in appropriate temperature-controlled (as defined by USP Standards) Delivery containers and stored appropriately in the patient's home.

Section 7. Disposal of Cytotoxic and/or Hazardous Wastes

The Pharmacist-in-Charge is responsible for assuring that there is a system for the disposal of Cytotoxic and/or infectious waste in a manner so as not to endanger the public health.

Section 8. Emergency Kit

When sterile pharmaceuticals are provided to home care patients, the Dispensing Pharmacy may supply the nurse with emergency Drugs, if the physician has authorized the use of these Drugs by a protocol, in an emergency situation (e.g., anaphylactic shock).

Section 9. Cytotoxic Drugs

In addition to the minimum requirements for a Pharmacy established by rules of the Board, the following additional requirements are necessary for those pharmacies that prepare Cytotoxic Drugs to insure the protection of the personnel involved.

(a) All Cytotoxic Drugs should be Compounded in a vertical flow, Class II, Biological Safety Cabinet. Other products should not be Compounded in this cabinet.

(b) Protective apparel shall be worn by personnel Compounding Cytotoxic Drugs. This shall include disposable masks, gloves, and gowns with tight cuffs.

(c) Appropriate safety and containment techniques for Compounding Cytotoxic Drugs shall be used in conjunction with the aseptic techniques required for preparing sterile products.

(d) Disposal of Cytotoxic waste shall comply with all applicable local, State, and Federal requirements.

(e) Written procedures for handling both major and minor spills of Cytotoxic agents must be developed and must be included in the policy and procedure manual.

(f) Prepared doses of Cytotoxic Drugs must be Dispensed, labeled with proper precautions inside and outside, and shipped in a manner to minimize the risk of accidental rupture of the primary container.

Section 10. Patient Training

If appropriate, the Pharmacist must demonstrate or document the patient's training and competency in managing this type of therapy provided by the Pharmacist to the patient in the home environment. A Pharmacist must be involved in the patient training process in any area that relates to Drug Compounding, Labeling, storage, stability, or incompatibility. The Pharmacist must be responsible for seeing that the patient's competency in the above areas is reassessed on an ongoing basis.

Section 11. Quality Assurance

There shall be a documented, ongoing quality assurance control program that monitors personnel performance, equipment, and facilities. Appropriate samples of finished products shall be examined to assure that the Pharmacy is capable of consistently preparing sterile products meeting specifications.

(a) All clean rooms and laminar flow hoods shall be certified by an independent contractor according to Federal Standard 209D, or National Sanitation Foundation Standard 49 for operational efficiency at least every six months. Appropriate records shall be maintained.

(b) There shall be written procedures developed requiring sampling if microbial contamination is suspected.

(c) If bulk Compounding of Parenteral solutions is performed using non-sterile chemicals, extensive end-product testing must be documented prior to the release of the product from quarantine. This process must include appropriate tests for particulate matter and testing for pyrogens.

(d) There shall be written justification of the chosen beyond-use dates for Compounded products.

(e) There shall be documentation of quality assurance audits at regular, planned intervals, including infection control and sterile technique audits.

Reprinted, with permission, from Model rules for sterile pharmaceuticals. Chicago, IL: National Association of Boards of Pharmacy; 1993:12.1–3.

Appendix 6
ASHP Technical Assistance Bulletin on Quality Assurance for Pharmacy-Prepared Sterile Products

Pharmacists are responsible for the correct preparation of sterile products.[a] Patient morbidity and mortality have resulted from incorrectly prepared or contaminated pharmacy-prepared products.[1–5] These ASHP recommendations are intended to help pharmacists ensure that pharmacy-prepared sterile products are of high quality.

The National Coordinating Committee on Large Volume Parenterals (NCCLVP), which ceased to exist in the 1980s, published a series of recommendations in the 1970s and early 1980s,[6–12] including an article on quality assurance (QA) for centralized intravenous admixture services in hospitals.[7] The NCCLVP recommendations, however, are somewhat dated and do not cover the variety of settings in which pharmacists practice today nor the many types of sterile preparations pharmacists compound in current practice settings.

The Joint Commission on Accreditation of Healthcare Organizations (JCAHO) publishes only general standards relating to space, equipment and supplies, and record keeping for the preparation of sterile products in hospitals.[13] The 1993 JCAHO home care standards provide somewhat more detailed, nationally recognized pharmaceutical standards for home care organizations.[14] These standards, however, also lack sufficient detail to provide pharmacists with adequate information on quality assurance activities.

The Food and Drug Administration (FDA) publishes regulations on Current Good Manufacturing Practices[15,16] that apply to sterile products made by pharmaceutical manufacturers for shipment in interstate commerce. The FDA has also published a draft guideline on the manufacture of sterile drug products by aseptic processing.[17] Both of these documents apply to the manufacture of sterile products by licensed pharmaceutical manufacturers. The Centers for Disease Control and Prevention (CDC) has published guidelines for hand washing, prevention of intravascular infections,[18] and hospital environmental control.[19] The United States Pharmacopeial Convention, Inc., (USPC) establishes drug standards for packaging and storage, labeling, identification, pH, particulate matter, heavy metals, assay, and other requirements[16]; as of this writing, there is an effort under way at USPC to develop an informational chapter on compounding sterile products intended for home use.[20]

Although the aforementioned guidelines provide assistance to pharmacists, each has certain limitations (e.g., outdated, limited scope). None of these guidelines addresses sterile product storage and administration with newer types of equipment (e.g., portable infusion devices,[21,22] indwelling medication reservoirs) or the use of automated sterile-product compounding devices.[23]

This document was developed to help pharmacists establish quality assurance procedures for the preparation of sterile products. The recommendations in this Technical Assistance Bulletin are applicable to pharmacy services in various practice settings including but not limited to hospitals, community pharmacies, nursing homes, and home health care organizations. ASHP has published a practice standard on handling cytotoxic and hazardous drugs[24]; when preparing sterile preparations involving cytotoxic or hazardous drugs, pharmacists should consider the advice in that document.

The ASHP Technical Assistance Bulletin on Quality Assurance for Pharmacy-Prepared Sterile Products *does not* apply to the *manufacture* of sterile pharmaceuticals, as defined in state and federal laws and regulations, *nor* does it apply to the preparation of medications by pharmacists, nurses, or physicians in emergency situations for *immediate* administration to patients. Not all recommendations may be applicable to the preparation of pharmaceuticals.

These recommendations are referenced with supporting scientific data when such data exist. In the absence of published supporting data, recommendations are based on expert opinion or generally accepted pharmacy procedures. Pharmacists are urged to use professional judgment in interpreting these recommendations and applying them in practice. It is recognized that, in certain emergency situations, a pharmacist may be requested to compound products under conditions that do not meet the recommendations. In such situations, it is incumbent upon the pharmacist to employ professional judgment in weighing the potential patient risks and benefits associated with the compounding procedure in question.

Objectives. The objectives of these recommendations are to provide

1. Information to pharmacists on quality assurance and quality control activities that may be applied to the preparation of

Approved by the ASHP Board of Directors, September 24, 1993. Developed by the ASHP Council on Professional Affairs.

The assistance of the following individuals is acknowledged: E. Clyde Buchanan, M.S.; Philip J. Schneider, M.S., FASHP; Howard Switzky; Lawrence A. Trissel, FASHP; and Larry Pelham, M.S.

Reprinted from *Am J Hosp Pharm.* 1993; 50:2386–90.

sterile products in pharmacies; and

2. A scheme to match quality assurance and quality control activities with the potential risks to patients posed by various types of products.

Multidisciplinary input. Pharmacists are urged to participate in the quality improvement, risk management, and infection control programs of their organizations. In so doing, pharmacists should report findings about quality assurance in sterile preparations to the appropriate staff members or committees (e.g., risk management, infection control practitioners) when procedures that may lead to patient harm are known or suspected to be in use. Pharmacists should also cooperate with managers of quality improvement, risk management, and infection control to develop optimal sterile product procedures.

Definitions. Definitions of selected terms, as used for the purposes of this document, are located in the appendix. For brevity in this document, the term *quality assurance* will be used to refer to both quality assurance and quality control (as defined in the appendix), as befits the circumstances.

Risk level classification

In this document, sterile products are grouped into three levels of risk to the patient, increasing from least (level 1) to greatest (level 3) potential risk and having different associated quality assurance recommendations for product integrity and patient safety. This classification system should assist pharmacists in selecting which sterile product preparation procedures to use. Compounded sterile products in risk levels 2 and 3 should meet or exceed all of the quality assurance recommendations for risk level 1. When circumstances make risk level assignment unclear, recommendations for the higher risk level should prevail. Pharmacists must exercise their own professional judgment in deciding which risk level applies to a specific compounded sterile product or situation. Consideration should be given to factors that increase potential risk to the patient, such as multiple system breaks, compounding complexities, high-risk administration sites, immunocompromised status of the patient, use of nonsterile components, microbial growth potential of the finished sterile drug product, storage conditions, and circumstances such as time between compounding and initiation of administration. The following risk assignments, based on the expertise of knowledgeable practitioners, represent one logical arrangement in which pharmacists may evaluate risk. Pharmacists may construct alternative arrangements that could be supported on the basis of scientific information and professional judgment.

Risk level 1. Risk level 1 applies to compounded sterile products that exhibit characteristics 1, 2, *and* 3 stated below. All risk level 1 products should be prepared with sterile equipment (e.g., syringes, vials), sterile ingredients and solutions, and sterile contact surfaces for the final product. Of the three risk levels, risk level 1 necessitates the least amount of quality assurance. Risk level 1 includes the following:

1. Products
   A. Stored at room temperature (see the appendix for temperature definitions) and completely administered within 28 hours from preparation; or
   B. Stored under refrigeration for 7 days or less before complete administration to a patient over a period not to

exceed 24 hours (Table 1); or
   C. Frozen for 30 days or less before complete administration to a patient over a period not to exceed 24 hours.
2. Unpreserved sterile products prepared for administration to one patient, or batch-prepared products containing suitable preservatives prepared for administration to more than one patient.
3. Products prepared by closed-system aseptic transfer of sterile, nonpyrogenic, finished pharmaceuticals obtained from licensed manufacturers into sterile final containers (e.g., syringe, minibag, portable infusion-device cassette) obtained from licensed manufacturers.

Risk level 2. Risk level 2 sterile products exhibit characteristic 1, 2, *or* 3 stated below. All risk level 2 products should be prepared with sterile equipment, sterile ingredients and solutions, and sterile contact surfaces for the final product and by using closed-system transfer methods. Risk level 2 includes the following:

1. Products stored beyond 7 days under refrigeration, or stored beyond 30 days frozen, or administered beyond 28 hours after preparation and storage at room temperature (Table 1).
2. Batch-prepared products without preservatives that are intended for use by more than one patient. (Note: Batch-prepared products without preservatives that will be administered to multiple patients carry a greater risk to the patients than products prepared for a single patient because of the potential effect of product contamination on the health and well-being of a larger patient group.)
3. Products compounded by combining multiple sterile ingredients, obtained from licensed manufacturers, in a sterile reservoir, obtained from a licensed manufacturer, by using closed-system aseptic transfer before subdivision into multiple units to be dispensed to patients.

Risk level 3. Risk level 3 products exhibit either characteristic 1 *or* 2:

1. Products compounded from nonsterile ingredients or compounded with nonsterile components, containers, or equipment.
2. Products prepared by combining multiple ingredients—sterile or nonsterile—by using an open-system transfer or open reservoir before terminal sterilization or subdivision into multiple units to be dispensed.

Quality assurance for risk level 1

RL 1.1: Policies and procedures. Up-to-date policies and procedures for compounding sterile products should be written and available to all personnel involved in these activities. Policies and procedures should be reviewed at least annually by the designated pharmacist and department head and updated, as necessary, to reflect current standards of practice and quality. Additions, revisions, and deletions should be communicated to all personnel involved in sterile compounding and related activities. These policies and procedures should address personnel education and training requirements, competency evaluation, product acquisition, storage and handling of products and supplies, storage and delivery of final products, use and maintenance of facilities and equipment, appropriate garb and conduct for personnel working in the controlled area, process validation, preparation technique, labeling, documentation, and quality control.[9] Further, written policies and procedures should address

Table 1.

Assignment of Products to Risk Level 1 or 2 According to Time and Temperature Before Completion of Administration

Risk Level	Room Temperature (15 to 30 °C)	Days of Storage	
		Refrigerator (2 to 8 °C)	Freezer (−20 to −10 °C)
1	Completely administered within 28 hr	≤7	≤30
2	Storage and administration exceeds 28 hr	>7	>30

personnel access and movement of materials into and near the controlled area. Policies and procedures for monitoring environmental conditions in the controlled area should take into consideration the amount of exposure of the product to the environment during compounding. Before compounding sterile products, all personnel involved should read the policies and procedures and sign to verify their understanding.

RL 1.2: Personnel education, training, and evaluation. Pharmacy personnel preparing or dispensing sterile products should receive suitable didactic and experiential training and competency evaluation through demonstration, testing (written or practical), or both. Some aspects that should be included in training programs include aseptic technique; critical-area contamination factors; environmental monitoring; facilities, equipment, and supplies; sterile product calculations and terminology; sterile product compounding documentation; quality assurance procedures; aseptic preparation procedures; proper gowning and gloving technique; and general conduct in the controlled area. In addition to knowledge of chemical, pharmaceutical, and clinical properties of drugs, pharmacists should also be knowledgeable about the principles of Current Good Manufacturing Practices.[15,16] Videotapes[25] and additional information on the essential components of a training, orientation, and evaluation program are described elsewhere.[7,12,26,27] All pharmacy personnel involved in cleaning and maintenance of the controlled area should be knowledgeable about cleanroom design (if applicable), the basic concepts of aseptic compounding, and critical-area contamination factors. Nonpharmacy personnel (e.g., housekeeping staff) involved in the cleaning or maintenance of the controlled area should receive adequate training on applicable procedures.

The aseptic technique of each person preparing sterile products should be observed and evaluated as satisfactory during orientation and training and at least on an annual basis thereafter. In addition to observation, methods of evaluating the knowledge of personnel include written or practical tests and process validation.

RL 1.3: Storage and handling. Solutions, drugs, supplies, and equipment used to prepare or administer sterile products should be stored in accordance with manufacturer or USP requirements. Temperatures in refrigerators and freezers used to store ingredients and finished sterile preparations should be monitored and documented daily to ensure that compendial

storage requirements are met. Warehouse and other pharmacy storage areas where ingredients are stored should be monitored to ensure that temperature, light, moisture, and ventilation remain within manufacturer and compendial requirements. To permit adequate floor cleaning, drugs and supplies should be stored on shelving areas above the floor. Products that have exceeded their expiration dates should be removed from active storage areas. Before use, each drug, ingredient, and container should be visually inspected for damage, defects, and expiration date.

Unnecessary personnel traffic in the controlled area should be minimized. Particle-generating activities, such as removal of intravenous solutions, drugs, and supplies from cardboard boxes, should not be performed in the controlled area. Products and supplies used in preparing sterile products should be removed from shipping containers outside the controlled area before aseptic processing is begun. Packaging materials and items generating unacceptable amounts of particles (e.g., cardboard boxes, paper towels, reference books) should not be permitted in the controlled area or critical area. The removal of immediate packaging designed to retain the sterility or stability of a product (e.g., syringe packaging, light-resistant pouches) is an exception; obviously, this type of packaging should not be removed outside the controlled area. Disposal of packaging materials, used syringes, containers, and needles should be performed at least daily, and more often if needed, to enhance sanitation and avoid accumulation in the controlled area.

In the event of a product recall, there should be a mechanism for tracking and retrieving affected products from specific patients to whom the products were dispensed.

RL 1.4: Facilities and equipment. The controlled area should be a limited-access area sufficiently separated from other pharmacy operations to minimize the potential for contamination that could result from the unnecessary flow of materials and personnel into and out of the area. Computer entry, order processing, label generation, and record keeping should be performed outside the critical area. The controlled area should be clean, well lighted, and of sufficient size to support sterile compounding activities. For hand washing, a sink with hot and cold running water should be in close proximity. Refrigeration, freezing, ventilation, and room temperature control capabilities appropriate for storage of ingredients, supplies, and pharmacy-prepared sterile products in accordance with manufacturer, USP, and state or federal requirements should exist. The controlled area should be cleaned and disinfected at regular intervals with appropriate agents, according to written policies and procedures. Disinfectants should be alternated periodically to prevent the development of resistant microorganisms. The floors of the controlled area should be nonporous and washable to enable regular disinfection. Active work surfaces in the controlled area (e.g., carts, compounding devices, counter surfaces) should be disinfected, in accordance with written procedures. Refrigerators, freezers, shelves, and other areas where pharmacy-prepared sterile products are stored should be kept clean.

Sterile products should be prepared in a Class 100 environment.[28] Such an environment exists inside a certified horizontal- or vertical-laminar-airflow hood. Facilities that meet the recommendations for risk level 3 preparation would be suitable for risk level 1 and 2 compounding. Cytotoxic and other hazardous products should be prepared in a Class II biological-safety cabinet.[24] Laminar-airflow hoods are designed to be operated continuously. If a laminar-airflow hood is turned off between aseptic processing, it should be operated long enough to allow complete purging of room air from the critical area (e.g., 15–30 minutes), then disinfected before use. The critical-area work surface and all accessible interior surfaces of the hood should be disinfected with an appropriate agent before work begins and periodically thereafter, in accordance with written policies and procedures. The exterior surfaces of the laminar-airflow hood should be cleaned periodically with a mild detergent or suitable disinfectant; 70% isopropyl alcohol may damage the hood's clear plastic surfaces. The laminar-airflow hood should be certified by a qualified contractor at least every six months or when it is relocated to ensure operational efficiency and integrity.[29] Prefilters in the laminar-airflow hood should be changed periodically, in accordance with written policies and procedures.

A method should be established to calibrate and verify the accuracy of automated compounding devices used in aseptic processing.

RL 1.5: Garb. Procedures should generally require that personnel wear clean clothing covers that generate low amounts of particles in the controlled area. Clean gowns or closed coats with sleeves that have elastic binding at the cuff are recommended. Hand, finger, and wrist jewelry should be minimized or eliminated. Head and facial hair should be covered. Masks are recommended during aseptic preparation procedures.

Personnel preparing sterile products should scrub their hands and arms (to the elbow) with an appropriate antimicrobial skin cleanser.

RL 1.6: Aseptic technique and product preparation. Sterile products should be prepared with aseptic technique in a Class 100 environment. Personnel should scrub their hands and forearms for an appropriate length of time with a suitable antimicrobial skin cleanser at the beginning of each aseptic compounding process and when re-entering the controlled area. Personnel should wear appropriate attire (see RL 1.5: Garb). Eating, drinking, and smoking should be prohibited in the controlled area. Talking should be minimized in the critical area during aseptic preparation.

Ingredients used to compound sterile products should be determined to be stable, compatible, and appropriate for the product to be prepared, according to manufacturer or USP guidelines or appropriate scientific references. The ingredients of the preparation should be predetermined to be suitable to result in a final product that meets physiological norms for solution osmolality and pH, as appropriate for the intended route of administration. Each ingredient and container should be inspected for defects, expiration date, and product integrity before use. Expired, inappropriately stored, or defective products should not be used in preparing sterile products. Defective products should be promptly reported to the FDA.[30]

Only materials essential for preparing the sterile product should be placed in the laminar-airflow hood. The surfaces of ampuls, vials, and container closures (e.g., vial stoppers) should be disinfected by swabbing or spraying with an appropriate disinfectant solution (e.g., 70% isopropyl alcohol) before placement in the hood. Materials used in aseptic preparation should be arranged in the critical area of the hood in a manner that prevents interruption of the unidirectional airflow between the high-efficiency particulate air (HEPA) filter and critical sites of needles, vials, ampuls, containers, and transfer sets. All aseptic procedures should be performed at least 6 inches inside the front edge of the laminar-airflow hood, in a clear path of unidirectional airflow between the HEPA filter and work materials (e.g., needles, stoppers). The number of personnel preparing sterile products in the hood at one time should be minimized. Overcrowding of the critical work area may interfere with unidirectional airflow and increase the potential for compounding errors. Likewise, the number of units being prepared in the hood at one time should be consistent with the amount of work space in the critical area. Automated compounding devices and other equipment placed in or adjacent to the critical area should be cleaned, disinfected, and placed to avoid contamination or disruption of the unidirectional airflow between the HEPA filter and sterile surfaces.

Aseptic technique should be used to avoid touch contamination of sterile needles, syringe parts (e.g., plunger, syringe tip), and other critical sites. Solutions from ampuls should be properly filtered to remove particles. Solutions of reconstituted powders should be mixed carefully, ensuring complete dissolution of the drug with the appropriate diluent. Needle entry into vials with rubber stoppers should be done cautiously to avoid the creation of rubber core particles. Before, during, and after the preparation of sterile products, the pharmacist should carefully check the identity and verify the amounts of the ingredients in sterile preparations against the original prescription, medication order, or other appropriate documentation (e.g., computerized patient profile, label generated from a pharmacist-verified order) before the product is released or dispensed. Additional information on aseptic technique is available elsewhere.[6,25,31]

For preparation involving automated compounding devices, data entered into the compounding device should be verified by a pharmacist before compounding begins and end-product checks should be performed to verify accuracy of ingredient delivery. These checks may include weighing and visually verifying the final product. For example, the expected weight (in grams) of the final product, based on the specific gravities of the ingredients and their respective volumes, can be documented on the compounding formula sheet, dated, and initialed by the responsible pharmacist. Once compounding is completed, each final product can be weighed and its weight compared with the expected weight. The product's actual weight should fall within a pre-established threshold for variance.[32] Visual verification may be aided by marking the beginning level of each bulk container before starting the automated mixing process and checking each container after completing the mixing process to determine whether the final levels appear reasonable in comparison with expected volumes. The operator should also periodically observe the device during the mixing process to ensure that the device is operating properly (e.g., check to see that all stations are operating).[33] If there are doubts whether a product or component has been properly prepared or stored, then the product should not be used. Refractive index measurements may also be used to verify the addition of certain ingredients.[34]

RL 1.7: Process validation. Validation of aseptic processing procedures provides a mechanism for ensuring that processes consistently result in sterile products of acceptable quality. For most aseptic preparation procedures, process validation is actually a method of assessing the adequacy of a person's aseptic technique. It is recommended that each individual involved in the preparation of sterile products successfully complete a validation process on technique before being allowed to prepare sterile products. The validation process should follow a written procedure that includes evaluation of technique through process simulation.[35–37]

Process simulation testing is valuable for assessing the compounding process, especially aseptic fill operations.[17] It allows for the evaluation of opportunities for microbial contamination during all steps of sterile product preparation. The sterility of the final product is a cumulative function of all processes involved in its preparation and is ultimately determined by the processing step providing the lowest probability of sterility.[38] Process simulation testing is carried out in the same manner as normal production except that an appropriate microbiological growth medium is used in place of the actual products used during sterile preparation. The growth medium is processed as if it were a product being compounded for patient use; the same personnel, procedures, equipment, and materials are involved. The medium samples are then incubated and evaluated. If no microbial growth is detected, this provides evidence that adequate aseptic technique was used. If growth is detected, the entire sterile preparation process must be evaluated, corrective action taken, and the process simulation test performed again.[17,38] No products intended for patient use should be prepared by an individual until the process simulation test indicates that the individual can competently perform aseptic procedures. It is recommended that personnel competency be revalidated at least annually, whenever the quality assurance program yields an unacceptable result, and whenever unacceptable techniques are observed; this revalidation should be documented.

RL 1.8: Expiration dating. All pharmacy-prepared sterile products should bear an appropriate expiration date. The expiration date assigned should be based on currently available drug stability information and sterility considerations. Sources of drug stability information include references (e.g., *Remington's Pharmaceutical Sciences, Handbook on Injectable Drugs*), manufacturer recommendations, and reliable, published research. When interpreting published drug stability information, the pharmacist should consider all aspects of the final sterile product being prepared (e.g., drug reservoir, drug concentration, storage conditions).[15,16] Methods used for establishing expiration dates should be documented. Appropriate inhouse (or contract service) stability testing may be used to determine expiration dates.

RL 1.9: Labeling. Sterile products should be labeled with at least the following information:

1. For patient-specific products: the patient's name and any other appropriate patient identification (e.g., location, identification number); for batch-prepared products: control or lot number;

2. All solution and ingredient names, amounts, strengths, and concentrations (when applicable);
3. Expiration date (and time, when applicable);
4. Prescribed administration regimen, when appropriate (including rate and route of administration);
5. Appropriate auxiliary labeling (including precautions);
6. Storage requirements;
7. Identification (e.g., initials) of the responsible pharmacist;
8. Device-specific instructions (when appropriate); and
9. Any additional information, in accordance with state or federal requirements.

It may also be useful to include a reference number for the prescription or medication order in the labeling; this information is usually required for products dispensed to outpatients. The label should be legible and affixed to the final container in a manner enabling it to be read while the sterile product is being administered (when possible).

RL 1.10: End-product evaluation. The final product should be inspected and evaluated for container leaks, container integrity, solution cloudiness, particulates in the solution, appropriate solution color, and solution volume when preparation is completed and again when the product is dispensed. The responsible pharmacist should verify that the product was compounded accurately with respect to the use of correct ingredients, quantities, containers, and reservoirs; different methods may be used for end-product verification (e.g., observation, calculation checks, documented records).

RL 1.11: Documentation. The following should be documented and maintained on file for an adequate period of time, according to organizational policies and procedures and state regulatory requirements: (1) the training and competency evaluation of employees in sterile product procedures, (2) refrigerator and freezer temperatures, and (3) certification of laminar-airflow hoods. Pharmacists should also maintain appropriate dispensing records for sterile products, in accordance with state regulatory requirements.

Quality assurance for risk level 2

Because the risks associated with contamination of a sterile product are increased with long-term storage and administration, more stringent requirements are appropriate for risk level 2 preparation.

RL 2.1: Policies and procedures. In addition to all recommendations for risk level 1, the written quality assurance program should define and identify necessary environmental monitoring devices and techniques to be used to ensure an adequate environment for risk level 2 sterile product preparation. Examples include the use of airborne particle counters, air velocity and temperature meters, viable particle samplers (e.g., slit samplers), agar plates, and swab sampling of surfaces and potential contamination sites. All aspects of risk level 2 sterile product preparation, storage, and distribution, including details such as the choice of cleaning materials and disinfectants and the monitoring of equipment accuracy, should be addressed in written policies and procedures. Limits of acceptability (threshold or action levels) for environmental monitoring and process simulation and actions to be implemented when thresholds are exceeded should be defined in written policies. For sterile batch compounding, written policies and procedures should be established for the use of master formulas and work sheets and for appropriate documentation. Policies and procedures should also address personnel attire in the controlled area, lot number determination and documentation, and any other quality assurance procedures unique to compounding risk level 2 sterile products.

RL 2.2: Personnel education, training, and evaluation. All recommendations for risk level 1 should be met. In addition to recommendations for risk level 1, assessment of the competency of personnel preparing risk level 2 sterile products should include an appropriate process simulation procedure (as described in RL 1.7: Process validation). However, process simulation procedures for assessing the preparation of risk level 2 sterile products should be representative of all types of manipulations, products, and batch sizes personnel preparing risk level 2 products are likely to encounter.

RL 2.3: Storage and handling. All storage and handling recommendations for risk level 1 should be met.

RL 2.4: Facilities and equipment. In addition to all recommendations for risk level 1, the following are recommended for risk level 2 sterile product preparation:

1. Risk level 2 products should be prepared in a Class 100 horizontal- or vertical-laminar-airflow hood that is properly situated in a controlled area that meets Class 100,000 conditions (or better) for acceptable airborne particle levels. Class 100,000 conditions mean that no more than 100,000 particles 0.5 μm and larger may exist per cubic foot of air.[28] A positive pressure relative to adjacent pharmacy areas is recommended.

2. Cleaning materials (e.g., mops, sponges, germicidal disinfectants) for use in the controlled area or cleanroom should be carefully selected. They should be made of materials that generate a low amount of particles. If reused, cleaning materials should be cleaned and disinfected between uses.

3. The critical-area work surfaces (e.g., interior of the laminar-airflow hood) should be disinfected frequently and before and after each batch preparation process with an appropriate agent, according to written policies and procedures. Floors should be disinfected at least daily. Carpet or porous floors, porous walls, and porous ceiling tiles are not desirable in the controlled area because these surfaces cannot be properly disinfected. Exterior hood surfaces and other hard surfaces in the controlled area, such as shelves, carts, tables, and stools, should be disinfected weekly and after any unanticipated event that could increase the risk of contamination. Walls should be cleaned at least monthly.

4. To ensure that an appropriate environment is maintained for risk level 2 sterile product preparation, an effective written environmental monitoring program is recommended.[26] Sampling of air and surfaces according to a written plan and schedule is recommended.[17,26] The plan and frequency should be adequate to document that the controlled area is suitable and that the laminar-airflow hood(s) or biological-safety cabinet(s) meet the Class 100 requirements. Limits of acceptability (thresholds or action levels) and appropriate actions to be taken in the event thresholds are exceeded should be specified.

5. To help reduce the number of particles in the controlled area, an adjacent support area (e.g., anteroom) of high cleanliness, separated from the controlled area by a barrier (e.g., plastic curtain, partition, wall), is desirable. Appropri-

ate activities for the support area include, but are not limited to, hand washing, gowning and gloving, removal of packaging and cardboard items, and cleaning and disinfecting hard-surface containers and supplies before placing these items in the controlled area.

RL 2.5: Garb. All recommendations for risk level 1 should be met. Gloves, gowns, and masks are recommended for the preparation of all risk level 2 sterile products. It must be emphasized that, even if sterile gloves are used, gloves do not remain sterile during aseptic compounding; however, they do assist in containing bacteria, skin, and other particles that may be shed, even from scrubbed hands. Clean gowns, coveralls, or closed jackets with sleeves having elastic binding at the cuff are recommended; these garments should be made of low-shedding materials. Shoe covers may be helpful in maintaining the cleanliness of the controlled area. During sterile product preparation, gloves should be rinsed frequently with a suitable agent (e.g., 70% isopropyl alcohol) and changed when their integrity is compromised (i.e., when they are punctured or torn).

RL 2.6: Aseptic technique and product preparation. All recommendations for risk level 1 sterile production preparation should be met.

A master work sheet should be developed for each batch of sterile products to be prepared. Once approved by the designated pharmacist, a verified duplicate (e.g., photocopy) of the master work sheet should be used as the preparation work sheet from which each batch is prepared and on which all documentation for that batch occurs. A separate preparation work sheet should be used for each batch prepared. The master work sheet should consist of the formula, components, compounding directions or procedures, a sample label, and evaluation and testing requirements.[39] The preparation work sheet should be used to document the following:

1. Identity of all solutions and ingredients and their corresponding amounts, concentrations, or volumes;
2. Manufacturer lot number for each component;
3. Component manufacturer or suitable identifying number;
4. Container specifications (e.g., syringe, pump cassette);
5. Lot or control number assigned to batch;
6. Expiration date of batch-prepared products;
7. Date of preparation;
8. Identity (e.g., initials, codes, signatures) of personnel involved in preparation;
9. End-product evaluation and testing specifications;
10. Storage requirements;
11. Specific equipment used during aseptic preparation (e.g., a specific automated compounding device); and
12. Comparison of actual yield to anticipated yield, when appropriate.

A policy and procedure could be developed that allows separate documentation of batch formulas, compounding instructions, and records. However documentation is done, a procedure should exist for easy retrieval of all records pertaining to a particular batch. Each group of sterile batch-prepared products should bear a unique lot number. Under no circumstances should identical lot numbers be assigned to different products or different batches of the same product. Lot numbers may be alphabetic, numeric, or alphanumeric.

The process of combining multiple sterile ingredients into a single, sterile reservoir for subdivision into multiple units for dispensing may necessitate additional quality control procedures. It is recommended that calculations associated with this process be verified by a second pharmacist, when possible; this verification should be documented. Because this process often involves making multiple entries into the intermediate sterile reservoir, the likelihood of contamination may be greater than that associated with the preparation of other risk level 2 sterile products.

RL 2.7: Process validation. Each individual involved in the preparation of risk level 2 sterile products should successfully complete a validation process, as recommended for risk level 1. Process simulation procedures for compounding risk level 2 sterile products should be representative of all types of manipulations, products, and batch sizes that personnel preparing risk level 2 sterile products are likely to encounter.

RL 2.8: Expiration dating. All recommendations for risk level 1 should be met.

RL 2.9: Labeling. All recommendations for risk level 1 should be met.

RL 2.10: End-product evaluation. All recommendations for risk level 1 should be met. Moreover, the growth media fill procedure should be supplemented with a program of end-product sterility testing, according to a formal sampling plan.[40-42] Written policies and procedures should specify measurements and methods of testing. Policies and procedures should include a statistically valid sampling plan and acceptance criteria for the sampling and testing. The criteria should be statistically adequate to reasonably ensure that the entire batch meets all specifications. Products not meeting all specifications should be rejected and discarded. There should be a mechanism for recalling all products of a specific batch if end-product testing procedures yield unacceptable results. On completion of final testing, products should be stored in a manner that ensures their identity, strength, quality, and purity. Detailed information on end-product sterility testing is published elsewhere.[7,16]

RL 2.11: Documentation. All recommendations for risk level 1 should be met. Additionally, documentation of end-product sampling and batch-preparation records should be maintained for an adequate period of time, according to organizational policies and procedures and state regulatory requirements. Documentation for sterile batch-prepared products should include the

1. Master work sheet;
2. Preparation work sheet; and
3. End-product evaluation and testing results.

Quality assurance for risk level 3

General comment on risk level 3. Risk level 3 addresses the preparation of products that pose the greatest potential risk to patients. The quality assurance activities described in this section are clearly more demanding—in terms of processes, facilities, and final product assessment—than for risk levels 1 and 2. Ideally, the activities described for risk level 3 would be used for all high-risk products. The activities may be viewed as most important in circumstances in which the medical need for such high-risk products is *routine*. In circumstances where the medical need for such a product is immediate (and there is not a suitable alternative) or when the preparation of such a product is rare,

professional judgment must be applied as to the extent to which some activities (e.g., strict facility design, quarantine and final product testing before product dispensing) should be applied.

RL 3.1: Policies and procedures. There should be written policies and procedures related to every aspect of preparation of risk level 3 sterile products. These policies and procedures should be detailed enough to ensure that all products have the identity, strength, quality, and purity purported for the product.[13,16] All policies and procedures should be reviewed and approved by the designated pharmacist. There should be a mechanism designed to ensure that policies and procedures are communicated, understood, and adhered to by personnel cleaning or working in the controlled area or support area. Policies and procedures should be reviewed at least annually by the designated pharmacist and department head. Written policies and procedures should define and identify the environmental monitoring activities necessary to ensure an adequate environment for risk level 3 sterile product preparation.

In addition to the policies and procedures required for risk levels 1 and 2, there should be written policies and procedures for the following:

1. Component handling and storage;
2. Any additional personnel qualifications commensurate with the preparation of risk level 3 sterile products;
3. Personnel responsibilities in the controlled area (e.g., cleaning, maintenance, access to controlled area);
4. Equipment use, maintenance, calibration, and testing;
5. Sterilization;
6. Master formula and master work sheet development and use;
7. End-product evaluation and testing;
8. Appropriate documentation for preparation of risk level 3 sterile products;
9. Use, control, and monitoring of environmentally controlled areas and calibration of monitoring equipment;
10. Validation of processes for preparing risk level 3 sterile products;
11. Quarantine of products and release from quarantine, if applicable;
12. A mechanism for recall of products from patients in the event that end-product testing procedures yield unacceptable results; and
13. Any other quality control procedures unique to the preparation of risk level 3 sterile products.

RL 3.2: Personnel education, training, and evaluation. Persons preparing sterile products at risk level 3 must have specific education, training, and experience to perform all functions required for the preparation of risk level 3 sterile products. However, final responsibility should lie with the pharmacist, who should be knowledgeable in the principles of good manufacturing practices and proficient in quality assurance requirements, equipment used in the preparation of risk level 3 sterile products, and other aspects of sterile product preparation. The pharmacist should have sufficient education, training, experience, and demonstrated competency to ensure that all sterile products prepared from sterile or nonsterile components have the identity, strength, quality, and purity purported for the products.[7,13] In addition to the body of knowledge required for risk levels 1 and 2, the pharmacist should possess sufficient knowledge in the following areas:

1. Aseptic processing[17,38,43];
2. Quality control and quality assurance as related to environmental, component, and end-product testing;
3. Sterilization techniques[16]; and
4. Container, equipment, and closure system selection.

All pharmacy personnel involved in the cleaning and maintenance of the controlled area should be specially trained and thoroughly knowledgeable in the special requirements of Class 100 critical-area technology and design. There should be documented, ongoing training for all employees to enable retention of expertise.

RL 3.3: Storage and handling. In addition to recommendations for risk levels 1 and 2, risk level 3 policies and procedures for storage and handling should include the procurement, identification, storage, handling, testing, and recall of components and finished products.

Components and finished products ready to undergo end-product testing should be stored in a manner that prevents their use before release by a pharmacist, minimizes the risk of contamination, and enables identification. There should be identifiable storage areas that can be used to quarantine products, if necessary, before they are released.[15]

RL 3.4: Facilities and equipment. Preparation of risk level 3 sterile products should occur in a Class 100 horizontal- or vertical-laminar-airflow hood that is properly situated in a controlled area that meets Class 10,000 conditions for acceptable airborne particle levels *or* in a properly maintained and monitored Class 100 cleanroom (without the hood).[28] The controlled area should have a positive pressure differential relative to adjacent, less clean areas of at least 0.05 inch of water.[17] Solutions that are to be terminally sterilized may be prepared in a Class 100 laminar-airflow hood located inside a controlled area that meets Class 100,000 conditions.

To allow proper cleaning and disinfection, walls, floors, and ceilings in the controlled area should be nonporous. To help reduce the number of particles in the controlled area, an adjacent support area (e.g., anteroom) should be provided.

During the preparation of risk level 3 sterile products, access to the controlled area or cleanroom should be limited to those individuals who are required to be in the area and are properly attired. The environment of the main access areas directly adjacent to the controlled area (e.g., anteroom) should meet at least Federal Standard 209E Class 100,000 requirements.[28] To help maintain a Class 100 critical-area environment during compounding, the adjacent support area (e.g., anteroom) should be separated from the controlled area by a barrier (e.g., plastic curtain, partition, wall). Written policies and procedures for monitoring the environment of the controlled area and adjacent areas should be developed.[17,26]

No sterile products should be prepared in the controlled area if it fails to meet established criteria specified in the policies and procedures. A calibrated particle counter capable of measuring air particles 0.5 μm and larger should be used to monitor airborne particulate matter. Before product preparation begins, the positive-pressure air status should meet or exceed the requirements. Air samples should be taken at several places in the controlled area with the appropriate environmental monitoring

devices (e.g., nutrient agar plates). Surfaces on which work actually occurs, including laminar-airflow hood surfaces and tabletops, should be monitored using surface contact plates, the swab–rinse technique, or other appropriate methods.[37,42]

Test results should be reviewed and criteria should be preestablished to determine the point at which the preparation of risk level 3 sterile products will be disallowed until corrective measures are taken. When the environment does not meet the criteria specified in the policies and procedures, sterile product processing should immediately cease and corrective action should be taken. In the event that this occurs, written policies and procedures should delineate alternative methods of sterile product preparation to enable timely fulfillment of prescription orders.

Equipment should be adequate to prevent microbiological contamination. Methods should be established for the cleaning, preparation, sterilization, calibration, and documented use of all equipment.

Critical-area work surfaces should be disinfected with an appropriate agent before the preparation of each product. Floors in the controlled area should be disinfected at least daily. Exterior hood surfaces and other hard surfaces in the controlled area, such as shelves, tables, and stools, should be disinfected weekly and after any unanticipated event that could increase the risk of contamination. Walls and ceilings in the controlled area or cleanroom should be disinfected at least weekly.

Large pieces of equipment, such as tanks, carts, and tables, used in the controlled area or cleanroom should be made of a material that can be easily cleaned and disinfected; stainless steel is recommended. Equipment that does not come in direct contact with the finished product should be properly cleaned, rinsed, and disinfected before being placed in the controlled area. All nonsterile equipment that will come in contact with the sterilized final product should be properly sterilized before introduction into the controlled area; this precaution includes such items as tubing, filters, containers, and other processing equipment. The sterilization process should be monitored and documented.[17]

RL 3.5: Garb. All recommendations for risk levels 1 and 2 should be met. Additionally, cleanroom garb should be worn inside the controlled area at all times during the preparation of risk level 3 sterile products. Attire should consist of a low-shedding coverall, head cover, face mask, and shoe covers. These garments may be either disposable or reusable. Head and facial hair should be covered. Before donning these garments over street clothes, personnel should thoroughly wash their hands and arms up to the elbows with a suitable antimicrobial skin cleanser.[19] Sterile disposable gloves should be worn and rinsed frequently with an appropriate agent (e.g., 70% isopropyl alcohol) during processing. The gloves should be changed if the integrity is compromised. If persons leave the controlled area *or support area* during processing, they should regown with clean garments before re-entering.

RL 3.6: Aseptic technique and product preparation. All recommendations for risk levels 1 and 2 should be met. Methods should ensure that components and containers remain free from contamination and are easily identified as to the product, lot number, and expiration date. If components are not finished sterile pharmaceuticals obtained from licensed manufacturers, pharmacists should ensure that these components meet USP standards. Products prepared from nonsterile ingredients should be tested to ensure that they do not exceed specified endotoxin limits.[16] As each new lot of components and containers is received, the components should be quarantined until properly identified, tested, or verified by a pharmacist.

The methods for preparing sterile products and using process controls should be designed to ensure that finished products have the identity, strength, quality, and purity they are intended to have. Any deviations from established methods should be documented and appropriately justified.

A master work sheet should be developed for the preparation of each risk level 3 sterile product. Once approved by the pharmacist, a verified duplicate of the master work sheet should be used as the controlling document from which each sterile end product or batch of prepared products is compounded and on which all documentation for that product or batch occurs. The master work sheet should document all the requirements for risk level 2 plus the following:

1. Comparison of actual with anticipated yield;
2. Sterilization method(s); and
3. Quarantine specifications.

The preparation work sheet should serve as the batch record for each time a risk level 3 sterile product is prepared. Each batch of pharmacy-prepared sterile products should bear a unique lot number, as described in risk level 2.

There should be documentation on the preparation work sheet of all additions of individual components plus the signatures or initials of those individuals involved with the measuring or weighing and addition of these components.

The selection of the final packaging system (including container and closure) for the sterile product is crucial to maintaining product integrity. To the extent possible, presterilized containers obtained from licensed manufacturers should be used. If an aseptic filling operation is used, the container should be sterile at the time of the filling operation. If nonsterile containers are used, methods for sterilizing these containers should be established. Final containers selected should be capable of maintaining product integrity (i.e., identity, strength, quality, and purity) throughout the shelf life of the product.[44]

For products requiring sterilization, selection of an appropriate method of sterilization is of prime importance. Methods of product sterilization include sterile filtration, autoclaving, dry heat sterilization, chemical sterilization, and irradiation.[16,45] Selection of the sterilization technique should be based on the properties of the product being processed. The pharmacist must ensure that the sterilization method used is appropriate for the product components and does not alter the pharmaceutical properties of the final product. A method of sterilization often used by pharmacists is sterile filtration.[46] In sterile filtration, the product should be filtered into presterilized containers under aseptic conditions. Sterilizing filters of 0.22 μm or smaller porosity should be used in this process. Colloidal or viscous products may require use of a 0.45-μm filter; however, extreme caution

should be exercised in these circumstances, and more stringent end-product sterility testing is essential.[26,47,48]

To ensure that a bacteria-retentive filter did not rupture during filtration of a product, an integrity test should be performed on all filters immediately after filtration. This test may be accomplished by performing a bubble point test, in which pressurized gas is applied to the upstream side of the filter with the downstream outlet immersed in water and the pressure at which a steady stream of bubbles begins to appear is noted.[46,48] The observed pressure is then compared with the manufacturer's specification for the filter. To compare the used filter with the manufacturer's specifications, which would be based on the filtration of water through the filter, it is necessary to first rinse the filter with sterile water for injection. An observed value lower than the manufacturer's specification indicates that the filter was defective or ruptured during the sterilization process. Methods should be established for handling, testing, and resterilizing any product processed with a filter that fails the integrity test.

RL 3.7: Process validation. In addition to risk level 1 and 2 recommendations, written policies and procedures should be established to validate all processes involved in the preparation of risk level 3 sterile products (including all procedures, equipment, and techniques) from sterile or nonsterile components. In addition to evaluating personnel technique, process validation provides a mechanism for determining whether a particular process will, when performed by qualified personnel, consistently produce the intended results.

RL 3.8: Expiration dating. In addition to risk level 2 recommendations, there should be reliable methods for establishing all expiration dates including laboratory testing of products for sterility, pyrogenicity, and chemical content, when necessary. These tests should be conducted in a manner based on appropriate statistical criteria, and the results documented.

RL 3.9: Labeling. All recommendations for risk levels 1 and 2 should be met.

RL 3.10: End-product evaluation. For each preparation of a sterile product or a batch of sterile products, there should be appropriate laboratory determination of conformity with established written specifications and policies. Any reprocessed material should undergo complete final product testing. It is advisable to quarantine sterile products compounded from nonsterile components, pending the results of end-product testing. If products prepared from nonsterile components must be dispensed before satisfactory completion of end-product testing, there must be a procedure to allow for immediate recall of the products from patients to whom they were dispensed.

RL 3.11: Documentation. In addition to the recommendations for risk levels 1 and 2, documentation for risk level 3 sterile products should include

1. Preparation work sheet;
2. Sterilization records of final products (if applicable);
3. Quarantine records (if applicable); and
4. End-product evaluation and testing results.

[a]Unless otherwise stated in this document, the term "sterile products" refers to sterile drug or nutritional substances that are prepared (e.g., compounded or repackaged) by pharmacy personnel.

Appendix A—Glossary

Aseptic preparation: The technique involving procedures designed to preclude contamination (of drugs, packaging, equipment, or supplies) by microorganisms during processing.

Batch preparation: Compounding of multiple sterile-product units, in a single discrete process, by the same individual(s), carried out during one limited time period.

Cleanroom: A room in which the concentration of airborne particles is controlled and there are one or more clean zones. (A clean zone is a defined space in which the concentration of airborne particles is controlled to meet a specified airborne-particulate cleanliness class.) Cleanrooms are classified based on the maximum number of allowable particles 0.5 μm and larger per cubic foot of air. For example, the air particle count in a Class 100 cleanroom may not exceed a total of 100 particles of 0.5 μm and larger per cubic foot of air.[28]

Closed-system transfer: The movement of sterile products from one container to another in which the container-closure system and transfer devices remain intact throughout the entire transfer process, compromised only by the penetration of a sterile, pyrogen-free needle or cannula through a designated stopper or port to effect transfer, withdrawal, or delivery. Withdrawal of a sterile solution from an ampul in a Class 100 environment would generally be considered acceptable; however, the use of a rubber-stoppered vial, when available, would be preferable.

Compounding: For purposes of this document, compounding simply means the mixing of substances to prepare a medication for patient use. This activity would include dilution, admixture, repackaging, reconstitution, and other manipulations of sterile products.

Controlled area: For purposes of this document, a controlled area is the area designated for preparing sterile products.

Critical areas: Any area in the controlled area where products or containers are exposed to the environment.[37]

Critical site: An opening providing a direct pathway between a sterile product and the environment or any surface coming in contact with the product or environment.

Critical surface: Any surface that comes into contact with previously sterilized products or containers.[37]

Expiration date: The date (and time, when applicable) beyond which a product should not be used (i.e., the product should be discarded beyond this date and time). NOTE: Circumstances may occur in which the expiration date and time arrive while an infusion is in progress. When this occurs, judgment should be applied in determining whether it is appropriate to discontinue that infusion and replace the product. Organizational policies on this should be clear.

HEPA filter: A high-efficiency particulate air (HEPA) filter composed of pleats of filter medium separated by rigid sheets of corrugated paper or aluminum foil that direct the flow of air forced through the filter in a uniform parallel flow. HEPA filters remove 99.97% of all air particles 0.3 μm or larger. When HEPA filters are used as a component of a horizontal- or vertical-laminar-airflow hood, an environment can be created consistent with standards for a Class 100 cleanroom.[49]

Quality assurance: For purposes of this document, quality assurance is the set of activities used to ensure that the processes used in the preparation of sterile drug products lead to products that meet predetermined standards of quality.

Quality control: For purposes of this document, quality control is the set of testing activities used to determine that the ingredients, components (e.g., containers), and final sterile products prepared meet predetermined requirements with respect to identity, purity, nonpyrogenicity, and sterility.

Repackaging: The subdivision or transfer from a container or device to a different container or device, such as a syringe or ophthalmic container.

Sterilizing filter: A filter that, when challenged with a solution containing the microorganism *Pseudomonas diminuta*, at a minimum concentration of 10^7 organisms per square centimeter of filter surface, will produce a sterile effluent.[16,17]

Temperatures (USP): Frozen means temperatures between –20 and –10 °C (–4 and 14 °F). Refrigerated means temperatures between 2 and 8 °C (36 and 46 °F). Room temperature means temperatures between 15 and 30 °C (59 and 86 °F).[16]

Validation: Documented evidence providing a high degree of assurance that a specific process will consistently produce a product meeting its predetermined specifications and quality attributes.[17]

References

1. Hughes CF, Grant AF, Leckie BD et al. Cardioplegic solution: a contamination crisis. *J Thorac Cardiovasc Surg.* 1986; 91:296–302.
2. Associated Press. Pittsburgh woman loses eye to tainted drugs; 12 hurt. *Baltimore Sun.* 1990; Nov 9:3A.
3. Anon. ASHP gears up multistep action plan regarding sterile drug products. *Am J Hosp Pharm.* 1991; 48:386,389–90. News.
4. Dugleaux G, Coutour XL, Hecquard C et al. Septicemia caused by contaminated parenteral nutrition pouches: the refrigerator as an unusual cause. *J Parenter Enter Nutr.* 1991; 15:474–5.
5. Solomon SL, Khabbaz RF, Parker RH et al. An outbreak of *Candida parapsilosis* bloodstream infections in patients receiving parenteral nutrition. *J Infect Dis.* 1984; 149:98–102.
6. National Coordinating Committee on Large Volume Parenterals. Recommended methods for compounding intravenous admixtures in hospitals. *Am J Hosp Pharm.* 1975; 32:261–70.
7. National Coordinating Committee on Large Volume Parenterals. Recommended guidelines for quality assurance in hospital centralized intravenous admixture services. *Am J Hosp Pharm.* 1980; 37:645–55.
8. National Coordinating Committee on Large Volume Parenterals. Recommendations for the labeling of large volume parenterals. *Am J Hosp Pharm.* 1978; 35:49–51.
9. National Coordinating Committee on Large Volume Parenterals. Recommended standard of practice, policies, and procedures for intravenous therapy. *Am J Hosp Pharm.* 1980; 37:660–3.
10. National Coordinating Committee on Large Volume Parenterals. Recommended procedures for in-use testing of large volume parenterals suspected of contamination or of producing a reaction in a patient. *Am J Hosp Pharm.* 1978; 35:678–82.
11. National Coordinating Committee on Large Volume Parenterals. Recommended system for surveillance and reporting of problems with large volume parenterals in hospitals. *Am J Hosp Pharm.* 1975; 34:1251–3.
12. Barker KN, ed. Recommendations of the NCCLVP for the compounding and administration of intravenous solutions. Bethesda, MD: American Society of Hospital Pharmacists; 1981.
13. Joint Commission on Accreditation of Healthcare Organizations. 1993 Accreditation manual for hospitals. Oakbrook Terrace, IL: Joint Commission on Accreditation of Healthcare Organizations; 1992.
14. Joint Commission on Accreditation of Healthcare Organizations. 1993 Accreditation manual for home care. Vol. 1. Standards. Oakbrook Terrace, IL: Joint Commission on Accreditation of Healthcare Organizations; 1993.
15. Food and Drug Administration. Title 21 Code of Federal Regulations. Part 21—current good manufacturing practice for finished pharmaceuticals, United States.
16. The United States pharmacopeia, 22nd rev., and The national formulary, 17th ed. Rockville, MD: The United States Pharmacopeial Convention; 1989.
17. Division of Manufacturing and Product Quality, Office of Compliance, Food and Drug Administration. Guideline on sterile drug prod-

ucts produced by aseptic processing. Rockville, MD: Food and Drug Administration; 1987.

18. Centers for Disease Control. Guideline for prevention of intravascular infections. *Am J Infect Control.* 1983; 11(5):183–93.

19. Centers for Disease Control. Guideline for handwashing and hospital environmental control. *Am J Infect Control.* 1986; 4(8):110–29.

20. Anon. Sterile drug products for home use. *Pharmacopeial Forum.* 1993; 19:5380–409.

21. Stiles ML, Tu Y-H, Allen LV Jr. Stability of morphine sulfate in portable pump reservoirs during storage and simulated administration. *Am J Hosp Pharm.* 1989; 46:1404–7.

22. Duafala ME, Kleinberg ML, Nacov C ct al. Stability of morphine sulfate in infusion devices and containers for intravenous administration. *Am J Hosp Pharm.* 1990; 47:143–6.

23. Seidel AM. Quality control for parenteral nutrition compounding. Paper presented at 48th ASHP Annual Meeting; San Diego, CA: 1991 Jun 6.

24. American Society of Hospital Pharmacists. ASHP technical assistance bulletin on handling cytotoxic and hazardous drugs. *Am J Hosp Pharm.* 1990; 47:1033–49.

25. American Society of Hospital Pharmacists. Aseptic preparation of parenteral products. (Videotape and study guide.) Bethesda, MD: American Society of Hospital Pharmacists; 1985.

26. Avis KE, Lachman L, Lieberman HA, eds. Pharmaceutical dosage forms: parenteral medications. Vol 2. New York: Marcel Dekker; 1992.

27. American Society of Hospital Pharmacists. ASHP technical assistance bulletin on outcome competencies and training guidelines for institutional pharmacy technician training programs. *Am J Hosp Pharm.* 1982; 39:317–20.

28. Federal Standard No. 209E. Airborne particulate cleanliness classes in cleanrooms and clean zones. Washington, DC: General Services Administration; 1992.

29. Bryan D, Marback RC. Laminar-airflow equipment certification: what the pharmacist needs to know. *Am J Hosp Pharm.* 1984; 41:1343–9.

30. Kessler DA. MedWatch: the new FDA medical products reporting program. *Am J Hosp Pharm.* 1993; 50:1921–36.

31. Hunt ML. Training manual for intravenous admixture personnel, 4th ed. Chicago: Baxter Healthcare Corporation and Pluribus Press, Inc.; 1989.

32. Murphy C. Ensuring accuracy in the use of automatic compounders. *Am J Hosp Pharm.* 1993; 50:60. Letter.

33. Brushwood DB. Hospital liable for defect in cardioplegia solution. *Am J Hosp Pharm.* 1992; 49:1174–6.

34. Meyer GE, Novielli KA, Smith JE. Use of refractive index measurement for quality assurance of pediatric parenteral nutrition solutions. *Am J Hosp Pharm.* 1987; 44:1617–20.

35. Morris BG, Avis KN, Bowles GC. Quality-control plan for intravenous admixture programs. II: validation of operator technique. *Am J Hosp Pharm.* 1980; 37:668–72.

36. Dirks I, Smith FM, Furtado D et al. Method for testing aseptic technique of intravenous admixture personnel. *Am J Hosp Pharm.* 1982; 39:457 9.

37. Brier KL. Evaluating aseptic technique of pharmacy personnel. *Am J Hosp Pharm.* 1983; 40:400–3.

38. Validation of aseptic filling for solution drug products. Technical monograph no. 2. Philadelphia: Parenteral Drug Association, Inc.; 1980.

39. Boylan JC. Essential elements of quality control. *Am J Hosp Pharm.* 1983; 40:1936–9.

40. Choy FN, Lamy PP, Burkhart VD et al. Sterility-testing program for antibiotics and other intravenous admixtures. *Am J Hosp Pharm.* 1982; 39:452–6.

41. Doss HL, James JD, Killough DM et al. Microbiologic quality assurance for intravenous admixtures in a small hospital. *Am J Hosp Pharm.* 1982; 39:832–5.

42. Posey LM, Nutt RE, Thompson PD. Comparison of two methods for detecting microbial contamination in intravenous fluids. *Am J Hosp Pharm.* 1982; 28:659–62.

43. Frieben WR. Control of aseptic processing environment. *Am J Hosp Pharm.* 1983; 40:1928–35.

44. Neidich RL. Selection of containers and closure systems for injectable products. *Am J Hosp Pharm.* 1983; 40:1924–7.

45. Phillips GB, O'Neill M. Sterilization. In: Gennaro AR, ed. Remington's pharmaceutical sciences. 18th ed. Easton, PA: Mack Publishing; 1990:1470–80.

46. McKinnon BT, Avis KE. Membrane filtration of pharmaceutical solutions. *Am J Hosp Pharm.* 1993; 50:1921–36.

47. Olson W. Sterilization of small-volume parenteral and therapeutic proteins by filtration. In: Olson W, Groves MJ, eds. Aseptic pharmaceutical manufacturing: technology for the 1990s. Prairie View, IL: Interpharm; 1987:101–49.

48. Eudailey WA. Membrane filters and membrane filtration processes for health care. *Am J Hosp Pharm.* 1983; 40:1921–3.

49. Turco S, King RE. Extemporaneous preparation. In: Turco S, King RE, eds. Sterile dosage forms. Philadelphia: Lea & Febiger; 1987:55–61.

⟨1206⟩ Sterile Drug Products for Home Use

A home-use sterile drug product (HSD) is a drug product requiring sterility, such as injectables and ophthalmics, that is prepared in and dispensed from a licensed pharmacy for intended administration by the patient or by a family member or other caregiver in a setting other than an organized, professionally staffed health care facility. The residence or other location to which an HSD is delivered typically is not equipped to ensure injectable drug quality as described in this chapter and is not under the *direct supervision* of the dispensing pharmacist.

This chapter explains in detail various procedures necessary to prepare and dispense sterile drug products intended for home use: the validation of sterilization and aseptic processes, the quality and control of environmental conditions for aseptic operations, personnel training, aseptic techniques, finished product release testing, storage and expiration dating, the control of product quality beyond the pharmacy, patient or caregiver training, patient monitoring and complaints, and finally, a quality assurance program. This information is not prescriptive, nor does it exclude alternate practices. However, alternatives when used should be shown on the basis of valid evidence to be at least as suitable, effective, and reliable as the practices provided herein.

RESPONSIBILITY OF THE DISPENSING PHARMACIST

A pharmacist dispensing any HSD is responsible for ensuring that the product has been prepared, labeled, controlled, stored, dispensed, and distributed properly. This includes the responsibility for ensuring that the HSD is kept under appropriate controlled conditions at the location of use and that it is administered properly through adequate labeling and verbal or written instructions. The dispensing pharmacist is also responsible for ensuring that the HSD retains its quality attributes within acceptable limits through a written quality assurance program. This program should ensure that for the entire labeled life of the product, or until manipulated by the patient or caregiver, the potency, pH, sterility, freedom from pyrogens, particulate limits, container integrity, appearance, and other qualities or characteristics that the HSD is expected to have do exist. The quality assurance program should encompass every HSD under the pharmacy's control and includes all phases of its preparation, distribution, storage, administration, and use. The dispensing pharmacy should employ proper analytical testing, where appropriate, to ensure the microbiological, chemical, and physical quality of all HSDs. These responsibilities apply equally to commercially available injectable drug products that are dispensed to patients without compounding or other manipulation and to HSDs that have been repackaged, reconstituted, diluted, admixed, blended, or otherwise manipulated (collectively referred to as "Compounded") in any way prior to dispensing. Emphasis in this chapter is placed upon the quality and the control of the processes utilized, personnel performance, and the environmental conditions under which the processes are performed. Other factors, such as testing and stability, are addressed to the extent necessary for the limited quantities of products with relatively short expiration dating periods normally associated with home care pharmacy practice. This chapter is not intended to address issues concerning the manufacture of sterile drug products.

RISK LEVELS

With reference to the microbiological quality (i.e., sterility) of the finished drug product, an HSD, in general, is compounded under either relatively *low-risk* or *high-risk* conditions, as determined by the potential for the introduction of microbial contamination. This contamination may result from the use of nonsterile components; novel, complex, or prolonged aseptic processes; or open exposure of the drug product or product containment devices to the atmosphere. In addition, long storage time between compounding and initiation of administration may affect the microbiological quality of the finished drug product.

The characteristics itemized below to distinguish between the high-risk and low-risk levels are intended to provide conceptual guidance and are not intended to be prescriptive. The pharmacist is expected to exercise professional judgment on a case-by-case basis when determining the risk level that would be appropriate for a particular process.

Low-Risk

An HSD is considered to be aseptically processed under low-risk conditions when all of the following conditions prevail:
(1) The finished product is compounded with commercially available, sterile drug products.
(2) Compounding involves only basic, and relatively few, aseptic manipulations that are promptly executed.
(3) "Closed system" transfers are used: the container-closure system remains essentially intact throughout the aseptic process, compromised only by the penetration of a sterile, pyrogen-free needle or cannula through the designated stopper or port to affect transfer, withdrawal, or delivery in accordance with the labeled instructions for the pertinent, commercially available devices.

Examples of low-risk processes include the following:
(1) Transferring sterile drug products from vials or ampuls into sterile final containers using a sterile needle and syringe.
(2) Transferring sterile drug products into sterile elastomeric infusion containers with the aid of a mechanical pump and an appropriate sterile transfer tubing device, with or without the subsequent addition of sterile drug products to the infusion container with a sterile needle and syringe.
(3) Compounding sterile nutritional solutions by combining *Dextrose Injection* and *Amino Acids Injection* via gravity transfer into sterile empty containers, with or without the subsequent addition of sterile drug products to the final container with a sterile needle and syringe.

High-Risk

Category I—A high-risk HSD may fall into either of two subclassifications. High-risk HSDs in *Category I* are those prepared from commercially available, sterile components where one or more of the following conditions prevail:
(1) Compounding involves the intermediate closed system pooling of sterile drug products.
(2) Compounding includes complex and/or numerous aseptic manipulations executed over a prolonged period.
(3) An individual finished product is administered as a multiday infusion via a portable pump or reservoir.

Examples of high-risk category I processes include the following:
(1) Compounding sterile nutritional solutions using an automated compounding device involving repeated attachment of fluid containers to proximal openings of the compounder tubing set and empty final containers to the distal opening. The process concludes with the transfer of additives into the filled final container from individual

drug product containers or from a pooled additive solution.

    (2) Preparing ambulatory pump reservoirs by adding more than one drug product with the evacuation of air from the reservoir prior to dispensing.

    (3) Preparing ambulatory pump reservoirs for multi-day (i.e., ambient temperature) administration.

Category II—High-risk HSDs in *Category II* are those involving either of the following:

    (1) A nonsterile drug substance or an injectable drug product prepared in-house from a nonsterile substance is used to compound the HSD.

    (2) "Open systems" are used, for example, when combining ingredients in a nonsealed reservoir before filling or when fluid passes through the atmosphere during a fill-seal operation.

Examples of high-risk category II processes include the following:

    (1) Compounding injectable morphine solutions from nonsterile morphine substance and suitable vehicles.

    (2) Compounding sterile nutritional solutions from nonsterile ingredients with initial mixing in a nonsealed or nonsterile reservoir.

Key factors for *building quality into products* include at least the following general principles:

    (1) Personnel are capable and qualified to perform their assigned duties.

    (2) Ingredients used in compounding have their expected identity, quality, and purity.

    (3) Critical processes are validated to ensure that procedures, when used, will consistently result in the expected qualities in the finished product.

    (4) The production environment is suitable for its intended purpose (addressing such matters as environmental cleanliness, control, monitoring, and the setting of action limits, as appropriate).

    (5) Appropriate release checks or testing procedures are performed to ensure that finished products have their expected potency, purity, quality, and characteristics at the time of release.

    (6) Appropriate stability evaluation is performed for establishing reliable expiration dating to ensure that finished products have their expected potency, purity, quality, and characteristics at least until the labeled expiration date.

    (7) There is assurance that processes are always carried out as intended or specified and are under control.

    (8) Preparation conditions and procedures are adequate for preventing mixups.

    (9) There are adequate procedures and records for investigating and correcting failures or problems in preparation, testing, or in the product itself.

    (10) There is adequate separation of quality control functions and decisions from those of production.

VALIDATION

The sterilization or aseptic processing of an HSD should be in accordance with properly designed and validated written procedures. The act of validation of a sterilization or aseptic process involves planned testing designed to demonstrate that microorganisms will be effectively destroyed, removed, or prevented from inadvertently being introduced by personnel or by process-related activities.

Sterilization Processes

A high-risk HSD prepared from nonsterile ingredients or components should be sterilized using an appropriate sterilization process, such as filtration or heat sterilization. In general, each sterilization process should be validated to demonstrate suitability for its intended purpose and specific manner of intended uses.

STERILIZATION BY FILTRATION

A sterilization filtration process should be capable of removing microorganisms from the liquid HSD. Commercially available pre-

sterilized filtration devices should be certified to be appropriate for human use in sterile pharmaceutical applications, have a pore size of 0.2 µm or smaller (generally recognized as a sterilizing filter), and have been lot tested for retention of *Pseudomonas diminuta* at a minimum concentration of 10^7 organisms per cm^2 under specified operating parameters. The individual devices should be tested for membrane and housing integrity, nonpyrogenicity, and extractables by the manufacturer. Such devices should be capable of sterilizing an HSD (see *Sterilization and Sterility Assurance of Compendial Articles* ⟨1211⟩). Before using such devices, the pharmacist should thoroughly evaluate their suitability for the intended HSD and conditions of use.

The size and configuration of filtration devices should accommodate the volume being filtered to permit complete filtration within a reasonable period of time and without clogging to the point where mid-process filter changes would be required.

Filters and associated devices and apparatus (housing, gaskets, etc.) should be physically and chemically compatible with the product to be filtered and should be capable of withstanding the temperatures, pressures, and hydrostatic stresses imposed on the system. These capabilities are to be established through appropriate product-specific testing. To establish compatibility, the pharmacy may rely on vendor certification or on definitive evidence, specific to product and filter, obtained from a critical review of the literature or from reliable unpublished research.

Validation should be established experimentally for all filtration apparatus involving assembly in the pharmacy of the membrane (filtration medium) into its housing or holder. The pharmacy may rely on vendor certification of validation for commercially available presterilized ready-to-use filter devices or for pharmacy-assembled apparatus. (The sterilization process used for pharmacy-assembled apparatus must be properly validated.) When relying on vendor certification of filtration validation, the pharmacy should request data from the vendor sufficient to ensure that an adequate challenge was used (minimum concentration of 10^7 organisms *Pseudomonas diminuta* per cm^2 of filter surface); and to ensure that the filtration apparatus and configuration, duration of filtration, filtration operating conditions (filtration rate and temperature), and the critical product formulation parameters (pH, viscosity, ionic strength, and osmolarity) used to generate the supplied data are representative of the pharmacy's product, apparatus, specified operating parameters, etc., in regard to the factors that might physically or chemically alter filter integrity, affect microbial capture mechanisms, or shrink the microorganism during filtration.

Each filter device used for product sterilization should be checked for integrity at the time of use. Integrity testing of commercially available, sterile, self-contained filter devices requiring no preuse assembly may be performed at the conclusion of the filtration process. Filter integrity test kits suitable for pharmacy use (for example, those consisting of a small gauge and a three-way stopcock assembly) are commercially available for testing the bubble point of small disk-type filters. For pharmacy-assembled apparatus, as defined above, prefiltration integrity testing is recommended in addition to postfiltration testing. Quantitative integrity testing, such as the bubble-point or forward flow tests (see *Sterilization and Sterility Assurance of Compendial Articles* ⟨1211⟩) should be used, as appropriate for larger filtration devices or when Category II high-risk HSDs are sterilized.

Filtration should be performed in accordance with written procedures that list those filters determined to be acceptable for the various HSDs to be filtered in the pharmacy or in accordance with master batch formulas that include definitive filter specifications. Filtration procedures and master batch formulas should also describe acceptable techniques for using and for checking the integrity of all listed filters. Fluid-filter compatibility must be established prior to the filtration of any HSD not included in the procedure.

HEAT STERILIZATION

Terminal sterilization should be used when sterilizing *Category II* high-risk HSDs. Sterilization may be accomplished in the final sealed container as a validated, controlled moist heat process (see

Table 1. Validation of Aseptic Processing.

Validation Purpose	Validation Requirements	
	Low Risk	High Risk*
General	Personnel validation	Process validation
Initial	3 consecutive media-fill runs without contamination	3 consecutive media-fill runs without contamination
Revalidation	1 media-fill run quarterly without contamination	annual media-fill run without contamination
Failure revalidation	3 consecutive media-fill runs without contamination	3 consecutive media-fill runs without contamination

*NOTE—Personnel should have first passed low-risk validation.

Sterilization and Sterility Assurance of Compendial Articles ⟨1211⟩). In the absence of heat sterilization capabilities, or where heat labile drug products or container-closure systems preclude heat sterilization, an HSD may be sterilized by filtration and aseptically processed and controlled in accordance with the standards set forth in this chapter.

Heat sterilization processes should be validated to ensure that the likelihood of survival of the most resistant microorganisms likely to constitute product bioburden is no greater than 10^{-6} under the specified operating conditions and parameters, such as sterilization time and temperature, size and nature of load, and chamber loading configuration. The validation and monitoring of heat sterilization processes should be in writing with all critical parameters specified, should be followed each time of use, and should be supervised by a pharmacist knowledgeable of the technology involved in the sterilization of drug products. Monitoring data should be recorded properly to ensure, retrospectively, that the processes were carried out as specified and that all critical parameters were within specified limits during processing.[1]

Aseptic Processing

All aseptic processing operations and configurations should be adequately established by media-fill validation.[2] Media fills should simulate as closely as possible actual aseptic operations. All manipulations, handling, environmental conditions, and other factors likely to influence the risk of process-associated contamination should be represented by the media-fill simulations. The intensity of such challenges should represent the greatest risk that would be expected during normal production. Media-fill validations should be repeated with sufficient frequency to ensure the ongoing capability of performing properly each aseptic processing operation used in the pharmacy. The frequency and results of media-fill runs should be documented.

The culture medium selected should be capable of supporting the growth of a broad spectrum of microorganisms likely to be production-associated contaminants in the pharmacy. Commercially available media can be obtained that, when reconstituted as directed by the manufacturer, are certified to have growth-promoting properties. Soybean-Casein Digest Medium is acceptable (see *Sterility* ⟨71⟩). Incubation of medium-filled units should take at least 14 days and may be at room temperature for 14 days or may be at room temperature for the first 7 days, with the final 1 to 7

[1]PDA Technical Monograph No. 1, Validation of Steam Sterilization Cycles, 1978.

[2]FDA Guideline on Sterile Drug Products Produced by Aseptic Processing, June 1987, pp. 20–27; PDA Technical Monograph No. 2, Validation of Aseptic Filling for Solution Drug Products, 1980.

days at 30° to 35°. Alternate suitable incubation schedules may be used as determined by the pharmacy to ensure enough growth of any potential contaminating microorganisms to be visually detectable. Microorganisms in all medium-filled units showing visible evidence of microbial growth should be promptly identified, and if this growth exceeds the action limits, an immediate investigation should be made with prompt correction of any identifiable causes of the failure. Review of environmental monitoring data obtained during the media fill should be included in the investigation, as well as a review of the cleaning, sanitizing, disinfection, production procedures, aseptic technique, personnel practices, and other factors as appropriate. Revalidation should occur after all media-fill failures (see Table 1).

Low-Risk Operations

The primary objective of the validation of aseptic processing involving low-risk operations is to ensure that personnel are capable of using effective aseptic technique to compound an HSD successfully under the most rigorous conditions encountered during normal work assignments. In carrying out validation of the process, personnel should perform media fills consisting of a planned repetitive sequence of compounded or repackaged units. The number of manipulations of each unit and the number of units in each media fill should reflect the most complex and prolonged aseptic manipulations likely to be encountered by an operator as a normal workload requirement. The number of units per media-fill run should be enough to ensure that the operator is capable of replicating acceptable aseptic procedures. Media transfers could be used to represent procedures such as syringe transfers, use of automated compounding devices, multiple additive procedures, and various aseptic assemblies and connections (see *Example of a Validation Procedure for Low-risk Operations*).

EXAMPLE OF A VALIDATION PROCEDURE FOR LOW-RISK OPERATIONS

Scenario—A pharmacy prepares antibiotics, hydration solutions, and parenteral nutrition solutions for home use. The most complex and prolonged aseptic manipulations are required for the parenteral nutrition solutions. The parenteral nutrition solution is made by combining the amino acid and dextrose by gravity transfer into 2-liter empty flexible bags, and then adding a maximum of 10 additives to a bag via syringe transfer. Typically, the pharmacy prepares no more than a 2- or 3-week supply of the solutions at one time.

Example of a validation procedure—One hundred mL of sterile Soybean Casein Digest Medium is transferred via gravity into plastic bags. Twenty units are completed in this manner, to approximate the number of units typically compounded at one time. After all twenty units have been filled, the media containers are lined up in pairs. One mL of media is drawn from one container and transferred aseptically by syringe transfer to another media unit and repeated for a total of ten transfers. Then media from the other units is syringe transferred to the first unit for a total of ten syringe transfers. This process is continued until all twenty units have undergone ten syringe transfers. The media fill units are incubated at room temperature for a total of fourteen days, with frequent checks for growth.

Media fills should be representative of peak periods of fatigue, stress, and pacing demands. For example, media fills could be scheduled immediately after normal production activity has ended. Media fills should not be performed during normal production.

Operators should pass an initial validation, performing three media fills with no contamination, before they are allowed to make HSDs for patients. Subsequently, each operator should perform at least one media fill involving low-risk operations quarterly. If one contaminated unit results from a media fill, the operator should be retrained and then perform three consecutive media fills with no contaminated unit before again being allowed to compound HSDs for patients. Operators should also be revalidated if the nature of their aseptic compounding assignments changes to the extent that their previous media fills are not representative of their revised assignments.

High-Risk Operations

In the case of high-risk operations, the focus of validation is on the process as well as personnel capability. Thus, the primary objective of the validation of aseptic processing for high-risk operations is to ensure that the aseptic process is capable of being carried out consistently under control by any qualified operator, before the process is utilized for production of units intended for administration to patients. Accordingly, each type of high-risk operation should be validated independently, rather than having operators perform representative sets of aseptic activities, as is the case with low-risk aseptic operations.

Personnel assigned to high-risk aseptic operations should be validated for low-risk operations as described above. In addition, these personnel should participate at least annually in the validation of each high-risk aseptic operation to which assigned.

For example, for high-risk operations involving nonsterile components, the media-fill run should simulate as closely as possible the most intensive conditions likely to be encountered during the normal production activities. The number of units in a media-fill run should be no less than the largest number of units encountered during production involving the process being validated. However, the fill volume of media-fill units need not equal the fill volume of finished product units.

A media-fill run should be performed at least annually for each unique high-risk batch processing procedure and configuration. A media-fill failure for most home care operations (less than 1000 units) is one or more contaminated units after incubation. For batches equal to or greater than 1000 units, a media-fill failure is greater than one contaminated unit. When a media-fill failure occurs, three consecutive successful media fills should occur before the process failing the media fill may be used for the compounding of an HSD for patients.

ENVIRONMENTAL QUALITY AND CONTROL

Achieving and maintaining sterility and overall freedom from contamination of a pharmaceutical product is dependent upon the quality status of the components incorporated, the process utilized, personnel performance, and the environmental conditions under which the process is performed. The standards required for the environmental conditions depend upon the amount of exposure of the HSD to the immediate environment anticipated during processing. The quality and control of environmental conditions for low-risk and high-risk operations is explained in this section. In addition, operations using nonsterile components require the use of a method of preparation designed to produce a sterile product.

Critical Site Exposure

The degree of exposure of the product during processing will be affected by the length of time of exposure, the size of the critical site exposed, and the nature of the critical site.

A critical site is any opening providing a direct pathway between a sterile product and the environment or any surface coming in direct contact with the product and the environment. The risk of such a site picking up contamination from the environment increases with time of exposure. Therefore, the processing plan and the intent of the operator should give due consideration to organization, efficiency, and speed in order to keep such exposure time to a minimum. For example, an ampul should not be opened unnecessarily in advance of use.

The size of the critical site affects the risk of contamination entering the product: the greater the exposed area, the greater the risk. An open vial or bottle exposes to contamination a critical site of much larger area than the tip of a 26-gauge needle. Therefore, the risk of contamination when entering an open vial or bottle is much greater than during the momentary exposure of a needle tip.

The nature of a critical site also affects the risk of contamination. The relatively rough, permeable surface of a rubber closure retains microorganisms and other contaminants, after wiping with an alcohol pad, more readily than does the smooth glass surface of the neck of an ampul. Therefore, the surface disinfection can be expected to be more effective for an ampul.

The prevention or elimination of airborne particles must be given high priority. Mobile or airborne contaminants are much more likely to reach critical sites than contaminants that are adhering to the floor or other surfaces below the work level. Further, particles that are relatively large or of high density settle from the airspace more quickly and thus can be removed from the vicinity of critical sites.

Environmentally Controlled Workspaces

LAFW AND BUFFER ROOM

An environmentally controlled workspace suitable for the aseptic processing of an HSD consists of a suitably constructed, properly functioning, and regularly certified device, which sweeps the workspace or an entire room with HEPA-filtered air at a velocity of 90 feet per minute ± 20%, such as a laminar airflow workbench (LAFW). Such a workspace is required for both low-risk and high-risk operations. The air blower for the workspace should be operated without interruption in order to sweep the workspace continually. Since the airflow velocity is relatively gentle, an LAFW must be located in an environmentally controlled room or a space otherwise separated from less controlled work areas, such as the main pharmacy, by partitions, plastic curtains, or preferably, a solid wall. Hereinafter, this area surrounding an LAFW shall be called the "Buffer Room." (Figure 1 shows an example of a floor plan for an environmentally controlled workspace and adjacent areas, as a basis for illustrating the following discussion.) Clean and sanitized supplies may be accumulated and stored for a limited period of time in the Buffer Room in order to be conveniently available for use in preparing products in the LAFW.

Since an LAFW is normally a self-contained unit, the air circulated is drawn from the Buffer Room and does not contribute fresh air. Therefore, such a unit does not create positive air pressure in the Buffer Room. However, units can be installed to draw in fresh outside air through a HEPA filter and provide positive air pressure, but they cannot be movable.

The direction of flow may be horizontal or vertical. (A suitable biological safety cabinet with vertical airflow should be used for processing cytotoxic and other hazardous agents to protect the operator as well as the product.) The air quality within the LAFW adjacent to critical sites should meet a Class 100 (MCB-1) clean room specification during normal work activity. (See Table 2 for the definition of clean room classes. Also, see *Microbiological Evaluation and Classification of Clean Rooms and Clean Zones* ⟨1116⟩.)

The environmental quality within the Buffer Room should be demonstrably better than that of adjacent areas, such as the main pharmacy, to reduce the risk of contaminants being blown, dragged, or otherwise introduced into the LAFW. For example, strong air currents from briefly opened doors, personnel walking past the LAFW, or the airstream from the heating, ventilating, and air-conditioning (HVAC) system can easily exceed the velocity of clean air from the LAFW. Also, operators introducing supplies into the LAFW or reaching in with their arms can drag contaminants along with those movements.

The level of cleanliness of the air in the Buffer Room, in conjunction with the expertise of the operator, is critical to maintaining the Class 100 (MCB-1) conditions within the LAFW. The air entering the Buffer Room should be fresh, HEPA-filtered, conditioned air. The air in the Buffer Room should meet the requirements for at least a Class 100,000 (see Table 2) clean room for low-risk operations and a Class 10,000 (MCB-2) for high-risk operations. In addition to cleaning the inflowing air and providing at least 10 air changes per hour, cooling is essential because of the continual buildup of heat from the circulation of air through the blower and HEPA filter of the LAFW. It should be noted that the

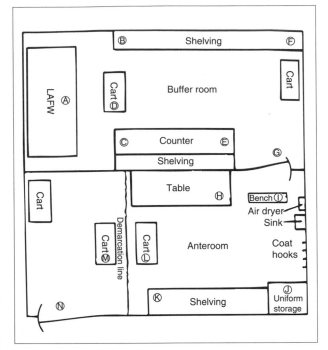

Fig. 1. Example of a floor plan.
(Encircled letters are suggested environmental sampling sites.)

dirt can accumulate. If ceilings consist of inlaid panels, the panels should be impregnated with a polymer to render them impervious and hydrophobic, and they should be caulked around each perimeter to seal them to the support frame. Walls may be of panels locked together and sealed or of epoxy-coated gypsum board. Preferably, floors are overlaid with wide sheet vinyl flooring with heat-welded seams and coving to the sidewall. Dust-collecting overhangs, such as ceiling utility pipes, or ledges, such as window sills, should be avoided. The exterior lens surface of ceiling lighting fixtures should be smooth, mounted flush, and sealed. Any other penetrations through the ceiling or walls should be sealed.

The Buffer Room should contain no sinks or floor drains. Work surfaces should be constructed of smooth, impervious materials, such as stainless steel or molded plastic, so that they are readily cleanable and sanitizable. Carts should be of stainless steel wire or sheet metal construction with good quality, cleanable casters to promote mobility. Storage shelving, counters, and cabinets should be smooth, impervious, free from cracks and crevices, nonshedding, cleanable, and sanitizable. Their number, design, and manner of installation should promote effective cleaning and sanitizing.

ACCESS CONTROL TO THE BUFFER ROOM (ANTEROOM)

Access to the Buffer Room should be planned and strictly controlled because of the need to protect the aseptic operations performed in an LAFW from contaminating substances, while permitting supplies and personnel to enter the area from relatively uncontrolled storerooms, from the main pharmacy, or from administrative areas. Access should be strictly limited to only designated, qualified personnel. The number of personnel in the Buffer Room at any one time should not exceed those essential to perform the required tasks.

An Anteroom or other separated area should be available for the decontamination of supplies, equipment, and personnel before they enter the Buffer Room. (This decontamination area is hereafter referred to as the Anteroom, as shown in Figure 1.) The size of the room should be sufficient to accommodate this activity with the heaviest work load anticipated. Minimally this would require space for two or more carts and space for personnel to clean, sanitize, and transfer supplies from the stockroom cart to the clean room cart. A floor demarcation should identify the maximum distance into the room that stockroom carts can penetrate.

The Anteroom should also be designed for uncartoning and disinfecting large-volume parenteral (LVP) bottles, pouches of hypodermic syringes, ampuls, vials, pouches of LVP bags, transfer set packages, and other required supplies. Here, also, carts for use in the Buffer Room should be cleaned and disinfected.

One or more sinks and a forced air hand dryer or disposable nonshedding towels should be available near the entrance door to the Buffer Room so that personnel can scrub their hands and arms before donning hair covers, shoe covers, clean gowns, and face masks. After donning hair and shoe covers, foamed alcohol may

circulation of air from the Buffer Room through the HEPA filter of the LAFW enhances the cleanliness of the air, particularly during nonuse periods.

Tasks carried out within the Buffer Room should be limited to those for which a controlled environment is necessary. Only the furniture, equipment, supplies, and other goods required for the tasks to be performed may be brought into this room, and they should be nonpermeable, nonshedding, and resistant to disinfectants. Whenever such items are brought into the room, they should first be cleaned and sanitized. Whenever possible, equipment and other items used in the Buffer Room should not be taken from the room except for calibration, servicing, or other activity associated with the proper maintenance of the item.

The surfaces of ceilings, walls, floors, fixtures, shelving, counters, and cabinets in the Buffer Room should be smooth, impervious, free from cracks and crevices, and nonshedding, thereby promoting cleanability and minimizing spaces in which microorganisms and other contaminants may accumulate. The surfaces should be resistant to damage by sanitizing agents. Junctures of ceilings to walls should be coved or caulked to avoid cracks and crevices where

Table 2. Class Limits in Particles per Cubic Foot.
(Size equal to or greater than particle sizes shown.)*

Class	Measured Particle Size (micrometers)				
	0.1	0.2	0.3	0.5	5.0
1	35	7.5	3	1	—
10	350	75	30	10	—
100	—	750	300	100	—
1,000	—	—	—	1,000	7
10,000	—	—	—	10,000	70
100,000	—	—	—	100,000	700

*The Class limit particle concentrations shown in Table 2 are defined for class purposes only and do not necessarily represent the size distribution to be found in any particular situation. Federal Standard No. 209E, General Services Administration, Washington, DC 20407, September 11, 1992.

be used to resanitize the hands. Faucet handles should be designed so that they can be shut off with the elbows or feet. An alternate procedure being used increasingly is to disinfect the hands and arms with a foamed alcohol, or other effective sanitizer, instead of scrubbing with detergent and water. The hot air hand dryer is then not needed. A means of demarcation should be provided between the Buffer Room side and the general entry side of the Anteroom to enhance the gowning procedure. One option, a movable bench (preferably of stainless steel), shown in Figure 1, provides a barrier and place for personnel to sit down to don shoe covers just before entering the Buffer Room. A storage area for clean gowning supplies should be conveniently located nearby. The door into the Buffer Room should remain automatically, positively closed and capable of being opened with elbow hooks or other means without using clean hands. The Anteroom should be designed to reduce to as low as possible the risk of recontamination of cleaned and sanitized supplies and personnel prior to entry into the Buffer Room.

An Anteroom as just described is necessary for high-risk operations. For low-risk operations, a carefully controlled area adjacent to the Buffer Room but without rigid walls may be acceptable. However, essentially the same attention for organization and cleanliness of the anteroom area is to be given in conjunction with both high- and low-risk operations.

Cleaning and Sanitizing the Workspaces

The cleaning, sanitizing, and organizing of the LAFW should be the responsibility of trained operators (pharmacists and technicians) following written procedures and should be performed at the beginning of each shift. All items should be removed from the LAFW and all surfaces wiped clean with a freshly prepared mild detergent followed by an approved sanitizing agent,[3] allowing sufficient time for the agent to exert its antimicrobial effect. The chosen sanitizing agent should be rotated with one of a different action at least quarterly. Recleaning should be performed if spillage or other events indicate the need.

Work surfaces near the LAFW in the Buffer Room should be cleaned in a similar manner, including counter tops and supply carts. Storage shelving should be emptied of all supplies and then cleaned and sanitized at least weekly, using approved agents.

Floors in the Buffer Room should be cleaned by mopping once daily when no aseptic operations are in progress. Mopping may be performed by trained and supervised custodial personnel, using approved agents described in the written procedures. Only approved cleaning and sanitizing agents should be utilized, with careful consideration of compatibilities, effectiveness, and inappropriate or toxic residues. Their schedules of use and methods of application should be in accord with written procedures. All cleaning tools, such as wipers, sponges, and mops, should be nonshedding and dedicated to use in the Buffer Room. Floor mops may be used in both the Buffer Room and the Anteroom, but only in that order. Most wipers should be discarded after one use. If cleaning tools are reused, their cleanliness should be maintained by thorough rinsing and sanitization after use and by storing in a clean environment between uses. Trash should be collected in suitable plastic bags and removed with minimal agitation.

In the Anteroom supplies and equipment removed from shipping cartons should be wiped with a sanitizing agent, such as sterile 70% isopropyl alcohol (IPA[4]), which is checked periodically for contamination. Alternatively, if supplies are planned to be received in sealed pouches, the pouches can be removed as the supplies are introduced into the Buffer Room without the need to sanitize the individual supply items. No shipping or other external cartons may be taken into the Buffer Room. Cleaning and sanitizing of the Anteroom should be performed at least weekly by trained and supervised custodial personnel, in accordance with written

procedures. However, floors are cleaned and sanitized daily, always proceeding from the Buffer Room to the Anteroom. Storage shelving should be emptied of all supplies and cleaned and sanitized at planned intervals, preferably monthly.

These cleaning and sanitizing procedures apply to both low-risk and high-risk operations.

Personnel and Gowning

Personnel are critical keys to the maintenance of asepsis when carrying out their assigned responsibilities. They must be thoroughly trained in aseptic techniques and be highly motivated to maintain these standards each time they prepare a sterile product.

Prior to entering the Buffer Room, operators should remove outer lab jackets or the like, makeup, and jewelry and should thoroughly scrub hands and arms to the elbow. After drying hands and arms they should properly don clean, nonshedding uniform components, including hair covers, shoe covers, knee-length coats or coveralls, and sterile latex gloves, in that order. The coats should fit snugly at the wrists and be zipped or snapped closed in the front. Shoe covers should be donned so that feet then touch the floor only on the clean side of the bench or other demarcation. Face masks should be donned just prior to beginning work at the horizontal LAFW, as talking, sneezing, or coughing normally generates an air velocity that exceeds the velocity of air from the LAFW. When working at a vertical LAFW, the wearing of a mask is optional where a solid transparent shield establishes a physical barrier between the face of the operator and the workspace. However, any facial hair should be completely covered in all instances.

Sterile latex gloves should be put on, aseptically—being sure to protect the outer surfaces from contamination—as the last uniform component. Latex gloves are effective in containing bacteria, skin scales, and other particles shed by the most scrupulously scrubbed hands. However, the outer sterile surfaces do not remain sterile since they will contact the room air, sanitized supply items, work counters, and other surfaces that, while clean, are not sterile. Therefore, operators must perform aseptic manipulations in a manner designed to prevent touching critical sites with the gloved fingers or hands. Further, operators should attempt to maintain gloved hand surfaces as free from contamination as possible by repeated rinsing with a sterile sanitizing agent, such as IPA, during use.

Sterile latex gloves must be worn when operator protection as well as product protection is essential, such as during operations involving cytotoxic or otherwise hazardous sterile products.

Proper scrubbing and gowning immediately prior to entry into the Buffer Room is required of all personnel, without exception. Should the operator find it necessary to leave the room, the coat may be carefully removed at the entrance and hung inside out for redonning upon re-entry, but only during the same shift. However, hair covers, masks, shoe covers, and gloves should be discarded and new ones donned prior to re-entry.

For high-risk operations, it is especially critical to minimize the risk of contamination on lab coats, coveralls, and other garb to be worn in the Buffer Room. Preferably, fresh clean garb should be donned upon each entry into the Buffer Room to avoid liberating contaminants from previously worn garb. Alternatively, garb that has been worn may be removed with the intention of regarbing for re-entry into the Buffer Room and stored during the interim under proper control and protection in the Anteroom. Garb worn or taken outside the confines of the Anteroom should not be worn in the Buffer Room.

Dispersion of particles from body surfaces, such as from skin rashes, sunburn, or cosmetics, increases the risk of contamination of critical sites and should be appropriately controlled or minimized. If severe, the operator should be excluded from the Buffer Room until the condition is remedied, especially for high-risk operations.

Suggested Standard Operating Procedures (SOPs)

The pharmacy should have written, properly approved SOPs designed to ensure the quality of the environment in which an HSD is prepared. The following procedures are recommended:

---

[3]Approved by the pharmacist in charge.

[4]NOTE—70% isopropyl alcohol (IPA) may harbor resistant microbial spores. Therefore, IPA used in aseptic areas should always be filtered through a 0.2-μm hydrophobic filter to render it sterile.

(1) Access to the Buffer Room should be restricted to qualified personnel with specific responsibilities or assigned tasks in the area.

(2) All cartoned supplies should be decontaminated in the Anteroom by removing them from shipping cartons and wiping with a disinfecting agent, such as sterile IPA, while being transferred to a clean, sanitized cart or other conveyance for introduction into the Buffer Room. Individual pouched supplies need not be wiped because the pouches can be removed as these supplies are introduced into the Buffer Room.

(3) Supplies required frequently or otherwise needed close at hand but not necessarily needed for the scheduled operations of the shift should be decontaminated and stored on the shelving in the Anteroom.

(4) Carts used to bring supplies from the storeroom should not be rolled beyond the demarcation line in the Anteroom, and carts used in the Buffer Room should not be rolled outward beyond the demarcation line unless cleaned and sanitized before returning.

(5) Generally, supplies required for the scheduled operations of the shift should be prepared and brought into the Buffer Room, preferably on one or more movable carts. Supplies that are required for back-up or general support of operations may be stored on the designated shelving in the Buffer Room, but excessive accumulation of supplies should be avoided.

(6) Objects that shed particles should not be brought into the Buffer Room, including pencils, cardboard cartons, paper towels, and cotton items.

(7) Traffic flow into and out of the Buffer Room should be minimized.

(8) All personnel preparing to enter the Buffer Room should remove all jewelry from hands and arms.

(9) All personnel entering the Buffer Room should first scrub hands and arms with soap, including using a scrub brush on the fingers and nails. An air dryer or disposable non-shedding towels should be used to dry hands and arms after washing.

(10) All personnel entering the Buffer Room, after scrubbing, should don attire as described under *Personnel and Gowning*.

(11) No chewing gum, candy, or food items may be brought into the Buffer Room.

(12) At the beginning of each shift and when spillage occurs, the LAFW surface should be wiped with a clean, non-linting wiper or sponge dampened with distilled water. The entire inside of the LAFW should then be wiped with another clean wiper wet with an approved disinfectant, such as IPA.

(13) The blower of the LAFW should be operated continuously. However, in the event of a long period of nonuse, the blower may be turned off and the opening covered with a plastic curtain or other shield. Before reuse, all internal surfaces should be sanitized and the blower operated for a minimum of 30 minutes.

(14) Traffic in the area of the LAFW should be minimized and controlled. The LAFW should be shielded from all less clean air currents that are of higher velocity than the clean laminar airflow.

(15) Supplies to be utilized in the LAFW for the planned procedures should be accumulated and then decontaminated by wiping the outer surface with IPA or removing the outer wrap at the edge of the LAFW as the item is introduced into the aseptic work area.

(16) After proper introduction into the LAFW of supply items required for and limited to the assigned operations, they should be so arranged that a clear, uninterrupted path of HEPA-filtered air will bathe all critical sites at all times during the planned procedures. That is, no objects may be placed behind an exposed critical site in a horizontal position or above in the vertical laminar flow workbench.

(17) All supply items should be arranged in the LAFW to re-

duce clutter and to provide maximum efficiency and order for the flow of work.

(18) All procedures should be performed in a manner designed to minimize the risk of touch contamination. Gloves should be sanitized with adequate frequency.

(19) All rubber stoppers of vials and bottles and the neck of ampuls should be sanitized with IPA prior to the introduction of a needle or spike for the removal of product.

(20) After the preparation of every admixture, the contents of the container should be thoroughly mixed and then inspected for the presence of particulate matter, evidence of incompatibility, or other defects.

(21) After procedures are completed, used syringes, bottles, vials, and other supplies should be removed, but with a minimum of exit and re-entry into the LAFW to minimize the risk of dragging contamination into the aseptic workspace.

Environmental Control and Monitoring Program

Because achieving or maintaining sterility is essential in the preparation of sterile products, the assessment of the level of control of the environment in which those products are prepared is recommended. The level of environmental control achieved may be evaluated by measuring the viable and the total (viable and nonviable) number of particles in the environment. Viable particle counting is recommended for environmental assessment in conjunction with the preparation of an HSD. Total particle counting is recommended for facility classification.

Viable particle counts are indicative of the portion of the total particle counts that represent microorganisms, normally reported as Colony Forming Units (cfu's), since typical viable particle counting results do not distinguish between single microorganisms and clusters. The difficulties in obtaining consistent and quantitative growth of microorganisms and the time lag between sampling and obtaining results because of growth time are important environmental monitoring limitations.

Total particle counts are usually performed by means of electronic instruments that give results instantly, based upon the measurement of particles in a prescribed volume of air. Clean room classifications (see Table 2) are based upon such measurements. A number of different types of instruments are available. Measurements can be made one at a time, or, with most instruments, automatically obtained on a planned, ongoing schedule. Instantaneous results permit assessment of environmental particulates at any given time and permit rapid changes in the control program should the results indicate a problem. However, these results do not distinguish between viable and nonviable particulates.

This section focuses on the measurement and monitoring of programs for viable particles.[5]

TESTING PROGRAM

A testing program is based upon the use of various methods for collecting an environmental sample nutrient, usually solid, culture medium, incubating at a temperature and for a time period conducive to the multiplication of any collected microorganisms, and then counting the discrete colonies that have developed on the surface of the medium. The count, reported as cfu's, is a measure of microbial contamination of the environment at the time and under the conditions of sampling. For more details, see *Microbiological Evaluation and Classification of Clean Rooms and Clean Zones* ⟨1116⟩.

In general, test methods for airborne environmental microbial contaminants either determine the number of cfu's collected in a measured volume of air ("quantitative" or "volumetric") or during a specified period of time. Any test method sensitive enough to show trends in environmental quality under specified conditions of the sampling used is acceptable. In general, quantitative methods are preferred over nonquantitative methods. When using either approach, the sample size should be sufficient to give a result

---

[5]The PDA Technical Report No. 13, 1990, may be consulted for details and monitoring methods not covered in this section.

of statistical significance. The testing program should also include surface sampling.

Dynamic monitoring, that is, testing under operating conditions during work activity, should be used routinely in order to give a cfu count during the processing of an HSD that demonstrates the critical effects of the presence and movement of operators. The latter is possible when comparing results from dynamic monitoring with results from static monitoring when no processing is being performed. Static monitoring generally evaluates the status of the facilities, operating equipment, and housekeeping.

The greatest value of ongoing microbial monitoring is achieved when microbial recoveries show trends. For a given environmental area, a baseline count is determined under the best environmental control believed to be possible for the area. Sampling should be done in selected locations and in a manner intended to reflect best the environmental conditions in the area. The encircled letters on Figure 1 illustrate possible sampling locations. To establish the baseline count, a large number of samples should be taken in multiple locations over a period of time to reflect time of day and week, workload conditions, and, preferably, seasonal variations. Analysis of these results would give counts normally expected to be achievable and the identification of a reduced number of selected sites expected to reflect the environmental conditions in the area with subsequent monitoring. This analysis then becomes the basis for ongoing monitoring. The baseline count limits may be slightly higher for low-risk operations than for high-risk operations. Subsequently, any significant change in the counts obtained, either as a single spike or a gradual rise in the cfu count, would require investigation into the cause.

When counts exceed the established baseline count by a determined amount (the action level), a written plan of action should be initiated. The plan would usually call for a repeat of the monitoring tests the next day and an investigation into the cause, and may include such actions as review of decontamination procedures, resanitization of the LAFW and the Buffer Room, a change to a different sanitizing agent, or retraining of operators. It should be remembered that microbial monitoring results are not available until after incubation, usually 48 hours, thus causing a delay in taking any corrective action. Therefore, trends should be detected as early as possible. Action levels would be slightly higher for low-risk operations than for high-risk operations.

The workspace in an LAFW is the only environment required to meet Class 100 (MCB-1) conditions, with the exception of specialized rooms (e.g., laminar flow rooms) specifically designed to achieve Class 100 conditions. To ensure that Class 100 conditions are met continuously, the LAFW (or room) should be certified after installation and recertified at least annually and after the unit is moved. This certification process includes testing for HEPA filter leaks and the laminar air-flow velocity. The microbial counts normally anticipated within the LAFW (or room) will average less than one per 10 cubic feet, even under dynamic testing conditions. However, culture media exposed to the airstream tends to dry and, therefore, should not be exposed for more than one hour. Table 3 provides examples of microbial environmental test limits, and is presented as a guide.[6]

TEST METHODS

A well-known test method is the exposure of settling plates, that is, petri dishes with solid nutrient agar medium congealed in the bottom section of the plate. These 100-mm diameter plates are simply opened and allowed to rest on a surface for a planned period of time. They do not sample a known volume of air; rather, viable particles collect on the agar surface as they fall from the environment or are impacted by the movement of air currents. Three-hour exposure of settling plates in a room is an appropriate, easy, and inexpensive way to obtain a representation of the con-

tamination that could be expected to settle from the air at the sampling site.

Well-known volume-of-air samplers include the slit-to-agar (STA) sampler and the Reuter centrifugal air sampler (RCS). The STA sampler utilizes a revolving nutrient agar plate under a slit orifice to impinge their sample particles on the surface of the nutrient agar in the plate. While the unit is portable, it requires a vacuum and an electrical source. The unit can be sanitized but not sterilized. The RCS draws air with an impeller into the head of the unit and centrifugally impacts any particles on a nutrient agar strip around the perimeter of the head. The unit samples in multiples of 40 liters per minute and is sanitizable and portable, with a self-contained battery power unit. Both of these units are relatively expensive but, unlike settling plates, have the advantage of quantitative sampling.

Surface sampling is most frequently done with contact plates[7] to detect accumulated microbial contamination on a flat surface. These plates are 60 mm in diameter and filled with nutrient agar medium to form a convex surface. The agar usually contains additives to help neutralize residues of disinfectants that may be on the test surface. The agar is pressed onto a flat surface lifting any microorganisms present onto the surface of the agar. This method can be considered to be relatively quantitative when contaminants are residing superficially on a flat, smooth surface. However, residual agar must be thoroughly removed from the test surface.

AN EXAMPLE OF AN ENVIRONMENTAL MONITORING PROGRAM

The following is a suggestion for one possible environmental monitoring program consisting of multiple tests to determine the baseline count and subsequent reduced testing for ongoing monitoring of the environmental control conditions.[8]

Settling plates should be uncovered at sites A–N (see Fig. 1) and exposed for 3 hours (except 1 hour at site "A"), both under static and dynamic conditions. This test should be repeated each day and each shift for at least one week, preferably two weeks. If STA or RCS air samplers are used, at least 10 cu. ft. (280 liters) air samples should be taken at sites B, D, E, J, K, and L. The nutrient agar plates or strips are then incubated at 30° to 35° for 48 hours and the colonies counted. These tests should be repeated about six months later. The average number of colonies at each site is computed to give baseline counts, being sure that housekeeping and other environmental control procedures are functioning at maximum efficiency.

Similarly, at the end of each shift and before any clean-up sanitization is done, perform surface sampling with contact plates at the same sites, being careful to remove any residual medium from the surfaces with an alcohol wipe. In addition, at least the index finger of each operator should be rolled on a contact plate.

The results of these evaluations are critically reviewed. Using the data given in Table 3 as an example, a reduced number of sites for monitoring, which give the best evidence of the level of microbial control maintained during facility operation, can be selected. Monitoring tests under dynamic conditions should then be performed at least weekly during the shift of highest activity at the selected sites (i.e., sites D, E, J, and L, or other sites that give evidence of being more representative of the true environmental control conditions). At least monthly another shift should be monitored in the same manner. Volume-of-air samples might be reduced to one site in each room weekly. However, the number of monitoring sites or the sampling frequency should be increased if there is any indication that the monitoring program is inadequate. Action levels are determined by making a reasoned judgment. A 50% increase above the baseline count is probably reasonable for high-risk operations. For low-risk operations an increase of 100% probably would be acceptable. However, whenever a rising trend appears to be in progress, the operations should be closely monitored

---

[6]These test limits were compiled from suggested values in Technical Monograph No. 2, the Parenteral Society (Great Britain), 1989, and other sources. They were also correlated with the USP proposed data in *Microbiological Evaluation and Classification of Clean Rooms and Clean Zones* ⟨1116⟩.

---

[7]Dishes meeting these specifications are obtainable from laboratory supply houses as Rodac brand, or use the equivalent.
[8]See also *Am. J. Hosp. Pharm.* 1980; 37:668.

Table 3. A Sample Dynamic Environmental Microbial
Monitoring Program.

Site	Baseline cfu	Low-risk Action Level	High-risk Action Level
Settling Plates*			
A	0,1	3	2
D	2,3	6	4
E	4,5	10	6
J	5	10	7
L	8	15	10
Contact Plates			
D	2,3	6	4
E	4,6	10	7
J	6	12	8
L	8	15	10
STA or Impaction Sampler**			
A	0,1	3	2
E	5	10	7
H	8	15	10

*Based on 3-hour exposure, except 1-hour for "A". See Fig. 1 for site locations.
**Based on 10 cu. ft. samples.

with more frequent sampling being performed to confirm whether or not a trend is occurring.

PROCESSING

Personnel Training and Evaluation

The pharmacy should follow a written program of training and performance evaluation designed to ensure that each person working in the aseptic area has the appropriate knowledge and skills necessary to perform the assigned tasks properly. Each person assigned to the aseptic area must successfully complete specialized training in aseptic technique and aseptic area practices.

Training should include didactic material and practical skills activities. Evaluation should include written testing and a written protocol of frequent routine performance checks involving random direct observation of critical operations and adherence to all aseptic area procedures and codes. Prompt appropriate action should occur to correct performance deviations, whether detected during a performance check or informally. At six-month intervals each person's continuing training needs should be reassessed, then documented, to ensure that skill levels are maintained.

Aseptic Technique

All critical operations are carried out by appropriately trained and qualified personnel in an LAFW using proper aseptic technique described in a written procedure (see the section *Suggested Standard Operating Procedures*). Aseptic technique is equally applicable to the preparation of sterile sensitizing and chemotoxic agents. However, it should be recognized that additional precautions must be used to protect the compounder and the compounding environment from the adverse effects of the agents being processed. A vertical laminar flow workbench (VLFW) with biohazard control capabilities, the protective capabilities of garb and gloves, sprayback and spill control techniques, the use of specialized compounding devices, and proper disposal are some of the additional measures to be considered.

Components

The pharmacy should follow written procedures to ensure that all items used to compound sterile drug products retain their purported or expected qualities at the time of use.

STERILE COMPONENTS

Commercially available sterile drug products, sterile ready-to-use containers and devices are examples of sterile components. A written procedure for unit-by-unit physical inspection preparatory to use should be followed to ensure that these components are sterile, free from defects, and otherwise suitable for their intended use.

NONSTERILE COMPONENTS

Drug components should meet compendial standards. Certificates of analysis from reputable manufacturers of bulk drug substances may be used to establish that each lot of bulk drug substance received by the pharmacy meets its specifications. Bulk drug substances stored properly in the pharmacy can be expected to retain their quality until the manufacturer's labeled expiration date. Bulk drug substances that are not labeled with a manufacturer's expiration date should be dated upon receipt, stored properly, dated when opening the container, used within a reasonable period of time, and visually inspected by the pharmacist upon use. The conditions under which containers of bulk drug substances are opened and the technique of the contents' withdrawal should be strictly controlled. Additionally, the devices used to withdraw the contents should be clean to preclude contamination of the remaining contents. The pharmacy may repackage bulk drug substances into smaller, suitable, and properly sealed containers (e.g., using a shrink seal) to minimize the risk of contamination. Upon receipt of each lot of bulk drug substance used to compound an HSD, the pharmacy should perform an inspection of the lot for any visual evidence of deterioration, other types of unacceptable quality, and wrong identity. Visual inspection of bulk drug substances should be performed routinely.

Because finished compounded HSDs are not usually tested for pyrogens, nonsterile bulk drug substances could impart pyrogenic properties to the finished product. Therefore, the pharmacy should have a procedure to ensure that the final product does not exceed specified endotoxin limits. See *Bacterial Endotoxins Test* ⟨85⟩ for procedural details concerning endotoxin testing.

Equipment

The pharmacy should ensure that equipment, apparatus, and devices used to compound an HSD are capable of consistently operating properly and within acceptable tolerance limits. Written procedures should be established and followed that include equipment calibration, annual maintenance, monitoring, and control. Routine maintenance checks should be documented. Personnel should be qualified through an appropriate combination of specific training and experience to operate or manipulate any item of equipment, apparatus, or device to which they will be assigned to use when preparing drug products for patients. Training should include the ability to determine whether any item of equipment is operating properly or is malfunctioning.

FINISHED PRODUCT RELEASE CHECKS AND TESTS

All HSDs should be subjected to appropriate checks or tests to ensure that only those HSDs free from defects and meeting all quality specifications will be distributed. An HSD should not be released until all quality specifications have been reviewed and it is determined that all release requirements are met.

Physical Inspection

All finished HSDs should be individually inspected in accordance with written procedures after compounding and, if not distributed promptly, prior to leaving the pharmacy. Immediately after compounding and as a condition of release, each product unit, where possible, should be inspected against lighted white and black backgrounds for evidence of visible particulates or other foreign matter. Pre-release inspection should also include container-closure integrity and any other apparent visual defect. Products with observed defects should be immediately discarded or marked and segregated from acceptable products in a manner that prevents their administration to patients. When products are not distributed promptly after preparation, a predistribution inspection should be conducted to ensure that an HSD with defects, such as precipitation, cloudiness, and leakage, which may develop between the time of release and the time of distribution, is not released.

Compounding Accuracy Checks

Written procedures for double checking compounding accuracy should be followed for every HSD prior to release. The double check system should meet state regulations and include label accuracy and accuracy of the addition of all drug products or ingredients used to prepare the finished product and their volumes or quantities. The used additive containers and, for those additives for which the entire container was not expended, the syringes used to measure the additive, should be quarantined with the final products until the final product check is completed. Syringe plungers should be drawn back to the volume mark used for each additive, if the additive volume was not checked prior to the addition. Automated pump settings should be verified just prior to or just after pumping and mixing. In addition, the volumes of each ingredient actually pumped should be checked to establish that the accuracy of the automated pump is within the limits set by the manufacturer. Written procedures for accountability of all drug product units used in the preparation of HSDs should be followed.

Additional finished product tests should be performed on *high-risk HSDs*, as follows.

Sterility Testing

Sterility testing should be performed on *Category II* high-risk HSDs promptly upon the completion of preparation. The sterility test, including the sampling scheme, should be conducted according to one of the USP methods (see *Sterility* ⟨71⟩). Membrane filtration is the method of choice where feasible. A method not described in the USP may be used if validation results demonstrate that the alternative is at least as effective and reliable as the USP membrane filtration method or the direct transfer method where the membrane filtration method is not feasible.

Normally, the HSD should not be released for patient use until test results show no evidence of microbial contamination of the product. However, when the HSD must be released on the same day of compounding prior to the completion of sterility testing, the HSD can be conditionally released. In such a case the pharmacy should have a procedure requiring daily observation of the media and requiring an immediate recall if there is any evidence of microbial growth. In addition, the physicians of those patients to whom a potentially contaminated HSD was administered should be notified as to the potential risk to the patient. Positive sterility test results should prompt an investigation of aseptic technique, environmental control, and other sterility assurance controls to identify and correct problems as much as possible.

Pyrogen Testing

Each HSD prepared from nonsterile drug components or from an intermediate compounded for a nonsterile component should be tested for pyrogen or endotoxin according to the recommended methods (see *Bacterial Endotoxins Test* ⟨85⟩). The product should not be released until it has been determined that the endotoxin limit specified for the product is not exceeded.

Potency Testing

The pharmacy should have a procedure for a pre-release check of the potency of the active ingredients in HSDs prepared from nonsterile bulk active ingredients. The procedure should include at least the following verifications by a pharmacist:

(1) The lot of the active ingredient used for compounding has the necessary identity, potency, purity, and other relevant qualities. For example, this can be established for official drug substances by comparing the information stated on the lot's certificate of analysis with the requirements specified in the USP monograph for the substance.

(2) All weighings, volumetric measurements, and additions of ingredients were carried out properly. This can be established by reviewing compounding records to ensure that these steps were confirmed and initialed by a second person during compounding.

(3) The compounding or control records include documentation that the fill volumes of all units available for release were checked and were correct.

(4) The final yield is confirmed to be consistent with the theoretical yield.

In addition, instrumental analysis of potency should be performed to support expiration dating periods greater than 30 days assigned to HSDs prepared from nonsterile drug substances.

STORAGE AND EXPIRATION DATING

Each finished drug product unit should bear labeling that specifies the product's storage requirements and expiration date, and where appropriate, the time of day beyond which the product is not to be used. Unless otherwise indicated, HSDs should be refrigerated until time of use, with allowance for adequate time to equilibrate to room temperature before administering to the patient. HSDs intended for administration promptly after compounding may be retained at room temperature from the time of compounding.

Even under the best of conditions, there is always the likelihood that unsuspected microorganisms might inadvertently gain entry into the HSD during aseptic processing. Thus, as an adjunct sterility assurance measure, HSDs not intended for prompt use should be stored at a temperature no greater than 4°, that is, at a temperature expected to inhibit microbial growth. The multi-day HSDs (injections prepared for administration by a portable infusion pump or reservoir) should be started promptly after preparation, and administration should be completed within 7 days. Those HSDs, such as 5-fluorouracil, that cannot be refrigerated after preparation should be used within 28 hours of preparation as further assurance of sterility.

Pharmacists should also consider the effect of "cumulative" room temperature storage on the physical–chemical stability and characteristics of the HSD. For example, an HSD may be removed from the refrigerator and allowed to equilibrate to room temperature, only to be replaced into the refrigerator. This could happen any number of times before the product is ultimately used by the patient. Thus, the original expiration date assigned by the pharmacist could easily be invalidated under these circumstances. A procedure should be in place that details what is to be done when this situation occurs. Should this situation arise, the pharmacist needs to determine what the actual stability of the product will be, keeping in mind the cumulative effects of room temperature storage upon the product. The drug product's manufacturer or other credible stability reference source should be consulted, particularly for expensive biotechnology or chemotherapeutic drugs.

Additionally, some HSDs may be subjected to elevated temperature conditions (e.g., body temperature) for continuous or novel drug delivery devices such as ambulatory infusion pumps, implantable infusion devices, and elastomeric infusion devices. Pharmacists should have adequate stability reference data to ensure that the product's potency characteristics are maintained when stored at these elevated temperatures during the labeled period of time chosen. HSDs may be frozen if adequate stability evidence to support freezing is available.

All light-sensitive products should be suitably protected from light from the time of preparation until the time of use or, where indicated, until the conclusion of administration.

Determining Expiration Dates

Where possible, the expiration date should be in accordance with allowances specified in the approved labeling. However, reliable, published stability information is sometimes lacking for many types of drugs. In these instances, pharmacists should consult with the drug's manufacturer to establish an expiration date. Because of compelling patient-care needs, a pharmacist may be unable to stay within the approved labeling and product guidelines stated in the package insert. For example, a higher concentration of drug may be prescribed; different diluent, container, etc., may be necessary; or the patient may require the HSD for longer periods of time. The pharmacist should communicate the deviations from the package insert to the manufacturer when requesting stability information. Otherwise, the pharmacist should ensure that the manufacturer's stability information is product specific, that is, the exact strength, diluent, fill volume, and container type (PVC bag, plastic syringe, elastomeric infusion device, etc.) will be used by the pharmacist when preparing the HSD. Pharmacists should obtain a letter from the manufacturer certifying the expiration dating period provided. Information provided by the manufacturer is usually for the HSD's chemical and physical stability only and would therefore not be relevant to sterility assurance imparted by the pharmacist each time the product is made. Therefore, it is the pharmacist's responsibility to ensure that compounding methods are validated to ensure final product sterility. Expiration dating not specifically referenced in the product's approved labeling should be limited to 30 days.

To ensure consistent practices in determining and assigning expiration dates, the pharmacy should have written policies and procedures governing the determination of the expiration dates for all of its compounded products. The following information may be helpful in providing a basis for these policies and procedures.

Product-specific, experimentally determined stability data based on sound stability evaluation protocols are preferable to published stability information for the prediction of expiration dates. Pharmacists should consult the general information chapter *Pharmaceutical Dosage Forms* ⟨1151⟩ for the appropriate stability parameters to be considered when initiating or evaluating a product-specific stability study. However, the use of professional judgment based on accumulated information may also be acceptable for determining expiration dates.

It should be recognized that the only truly valid evidence of stability for predicting expiration dating is from product-specific (appropriate bracketing is acceptable) experimental studies. Predictions based on other evidence, such as publications, charts, tables, etc., would result in theoretical expiration dates. Theoretically predicted expiration dating introduces varying degrees of assumptions and hence a likelihood of error, or at least inaccuracy. The degree of error or inaccuracy would be dependent upon the extent of differences between the HSD's characteristics (e.g., composition, concentration of ingredients, fill volume, container type and material, etc.) and the characteristics of the products from which stability data or information are to be extrapolated. Thus, the greater the doubt of the accuracy of theoretically predicted expiration dating, the greater the need to determine dating periods experimentally. Theoretically predicted expiration dating periods should be seriously considered for HSDs prepared from nonsterile bulk active ingredients having therapeutic activity, especially where these HSDs are expected to be compounded routinely. Semi-quantitative procedures, such as thin-layer chromatography (TLC), may be acceptable for many HSDs. However, quantitative stability-indicating assays, such as high-performance liquid chromatography (HPLC), would be more appropriate for certain critical HSDs. Examples include HSDs with a narrow therapeutic dosage range or a narrow therapeutic index where close monitoring or titering is required to ensure therapeutic effectiveness or to avoid toxicity; where a theoretically established expiration dating period is supported by only marginal evidence; or where a significant margin of safety cannot be verified for the proposed theoretical expiration dating period.

Additionally, conditions to which the finished product may be subjected during in-home use (e.g., in homes without air-conditioning in a hot climate) should be considered on a patient-by-patient basis. Thus, the possible need to shorten a general expiration date should be considered at the time of dispensing based on the particular circumstances of the patient.

In all instances where alternate informational resources are used to establish an expiration date for a drug product, the pharmacist should ensure that those resources have undergone critical evaluation in conjunction with the specific product for which an expiration date is established. Expiration dates predicted from alternate informational resources should be conservative and not extend beyond the realistic and practical patient care needs of the pharmacy. Pharmacists should subsequently maintain a record of the specific basis used to establish the expiration date for each compounded drug product. Pharmacists should utilize an exception log for products with expiration dates that fall outside of the pharmacy's established SOPs on stability and expiration dating. Alternatively, the exceptional reasons for changing the product's expiration date may also be documented in the patient's chart.

Monitoring Controlled Storage Areas

To ensure that product potency is retained through the expiration date, pharmacists must monitor the drug storage areas within the pharmacy. Controlled temperature storage areas in the pharmacy (refrigerators, 2° to 8°, freezers, -20° to -10°, and incubators, 30° to 35°, etc.) should be monitored at least once daily and the results documented on a temperature log. Additionally, pharmacy personnel should note the storage temperature when placing the product into or removing the product from the storage unit in order to monitor for any temperature aberrations. Suitable temperature recording devices may include a calibrated continuous recording device or an NBS calibrated thermometer that has adequate accuracy and sensitivity for the intended purpose and should be properly calibrated at suitable intervals. If the pharmacy uses a continuous temperature recording device, pharmacy personnel should verify at least once daily that the recording device itself is functioning properly.

The temperature sensing mechanism should be suitably placed in the controlled temperature storage space to reflect accurately its true temperature. In addition, the pharmacy should adhere to appropriate procedures of all controlled storage spaces to ensure that such spaces are not subject to significantly prolonged temperature fluctuations as may occur, for example, by leaving a refrigerator door open too long.

MAINTAINING PRODUCT QUALITY AND CONTROL AFTER IT LEAVES THE PHARMACY

Packing

The pharmacy is responsible for ensuring that the HSDs are suitably packed for transport. Packing should provide adequate control of the conditions under which HSDs are transported to the patient. Packing specifications, including configuration and materials, should be appropriate, as determined on a product-by-product basis, to maintain the storage conditions necessary to protect the product against adverse physical conditions such as temperatures beyond the range allowable for the HSD and, where indicated, exposure to light. Packing should retain adequate effectiveness for the duration of, and under the environmental conditions expected during, transit.

In-transit temperatures of HSDs should be maintained near the midpoint of the HSDs' specified upper and lower limits, recognizing that some temperature excursion, not to exceed the product's specified limits, is permissible during transit. Under no circumstances may excursions exceed the limits specified in the *General Notices* under *Storage Temperatures* for the defined temperature conditions.

The pharmacy should have and follow written procedures that specify packing techniques, configurations, and materials for groups of products with common storage characteristics and for specific products where unique storage conditions are required to retain adequate stability and product quality. It must be recognized that additional precautions should be used to protect the shipper, patient, and caregiver from adverse effects from any leakage of sensitizing or chemotoxic agents. Although written procedures should also ensure that biohazard controls are adequate for transit conditions and for meeting all OSHA and local requirements, this topic is beyond the scope of this chapter, and other references should be consulted.

The pharmacy should ensure that transit specifications and procedures are effective. For example, post-transit determinations of internal pack temperatures following several trial shipments of goods packed with new or modified materials, configurations, or techniques provide an indicator of packing suitability under actual transit conditions. Following the initial determination of packing suitability, occasional shipments should be subsequently checked, especially whenever transit conditions vary, such as from seasonal temperature changes or transit times. Because different packing configurations, pack size, internal packing matrices (e.g., insulated coolers or containers, styrofoam, bubble wrap, freezer packs, etc.) and pack thickness differ in their resistance to heat penetration or loss, packing should not vary from established procedures and specifications without evaluation.

Transit

Unlike the selection of the adherence to packing specifications, the pharmacy may lack complete control over transit time and conditions. However, the pharmacy can establish reasonable expectations of transit time and conditions and can carry out procedures to ensure that expectations are usually met. The determination of packing suitability is based on these expectations. Where possible, delivery personnel should be trained by the pharmacist on how to transport HSDs.

When common carriers are utilized, the pharmacy is responsible for choosing a reliable carrier capable of consistently fulfilling the pharmacy's requirements for delivery schedules, transit time duration, handling, care, external temperature controls, and special handling that may be required. The pharmacy should provide the carrier with a written statement of shipping requirements and should obtain from the carrier an assurance of capability and commitment for fulfilling these requirements before the pharmacy engages the carrier's services.

Delivery personnel, whether employees of the pharmacy, the parent organization, or the common carrier, should know the shipping requirements of each package consigned. Printed labels, prominently displayed on the exterior of each package, are usually sufficient. Supplementary printed instructions may be necessary in some instances.

The pharmacy should have an effective system for the routine evaluation of shipping performance. For example, the pharmacy might periodically review delivery receipts or conduct periodic shipment follow-ups by telephoning patients or caregivers. Delivery time, internal temperature (temperature indicators such as strips or probes inside packages provide objective evidence for determining the adequacy of temperature control), condition of goods upon receipt, and courteousness of personnel are some key determinants of acceptable shipping performance.

In The Home

The pharmacy's basic responsibilities for ensuring that HSDs in the home maintain their quality until administered include the following:
(1) The immediate labeling of the HSD container displays prominently and understandably the requirements for proper storage and expiration dating.
(2) Adequate information is obtained to assure the pharmacist that the storage conditions existing in the home are suitable for the HSD's specified storage requirements. (It is acceptable for the pharmacist to obtain this information through documentation by nursing or delivery personnel.)
(3) The patient has an acceptable temperature measurement device in the refrigerator and understands the importance of its use for maintaining proper storage temperature.
(4) A separate information sheet is issued and includes instructions for proper storage, interpretation of the expiration dating, and how to look for signs of unsuitability for use.

The patient or caregiver should be informed of the need to notify the pharmacy promptly of any actual or suspected malfunction of the refrigerator, freezer, or temperature measurement de-

vice. The pharmacy should assist patients or caregivers as necessary to ensure that proper storage conditions for HSDs are maintained with little or no interruption.

The pharmacy is responsible for ensuring that the home is visited at regular intervals to confirm compliance with appropriate drug storage conditions, cleanliness, separation of food and drug items, avoidance of improper re-use of multiple dose containers or supplies such as tubing or syringes, avoidance of the use of single-dose products as multiple-dose containers, and product inventory as indicative of product usage compliance. Inappropriately stored, exteriorly soiled, expired, or visibly defective drug products should be removed from the patient's possession, using the opportunity to instruct the patient or caregiver or to reinforce storage and handling responsibilities. Similarly, the home visit should also assess compliance with waste containment and disposal. The pharmacy may entrust the home visit to another health professional or paraprofessional.

PATIENT OR CAREGIVER TRAINING

A formal training program should be provided as a means to ensure understanding and compliance with the many special and complex responsibilities placed upon the patient or caregiver for the storage, handling, and administration of HSDs. The instructional objectives for the training program should include all home care responsibilities expected of the patient or caregiver and should be specified in terms of patient or caregiver competencies.

Upon the conclusion of the training program, the patient or caregiver should, correctly and consistently, be able to do the following:
(1) Describe the therapy involved, including the disease or condition for which the HSD is prescribed, goals of therapy, expected therapeutic outcome, and potential side effects of the HSD.
(2) Inspect all drug products, devices, equipment, and supplies on receipt to ensure that proper temperatures were maintained during transport and that goods received show no evidence of deterioration or defects.
(3) Handle, store, and monitor all drug products and related supplies and equipment in the home, including all special requirements related to same.
(4) Visually inspect all drug products, devices, and other items the patient or caregiver is required to use immediately prior to administration in a manner to ensure that all items are acceptable for use. For example, HSDs should be free from leakage, container cracks, particulates, precipitate, haziness, discoloration, or other deviations from the normal expected appearance, and the immediate packages of sterile devices should be completely sealed with no evidence of loss of package integrity.
(5) Check labels immediately prior to administration to ensure the right drug, dose, patient, and time of administration.
(6) Clean the in-home preparation area, scrub hands, use proper aseptic technique, and manipulate all containers, equipment, apparatus, devices, and supplies used in conjunction with administration.
(7) Employ all techniques and precautions association with HSD administration, for example, preparing supplies and equipment, handling of devices, priming the tubing, and discontinuing an infusion.
(8) Care for catheters, change dressings, and maintain site patency as indicated.
(9) Monitor for and detect occurrences of therapeutic complications such as infection, phlebitis, electrolyte imbalance, and catheter misplacement.
(10) Respond immediately to emergency or critical situations such as catheter breakage or displacement, tubing disconnection, clot formation, flow blockage, and equipment malfunction.
(11) Know when to seek and how to obtain professional emergency services or professional advice.
(12) Handle, contain, and dispose of wastes, such as needles,

syringes, devices, biohazardous spills or residuals, and infectious substances.

Training programs should include hands-on demonstration and practice with actual items that the patient or caregiver is expected to use, such as HSD containers, devices, and equipment. The patient or caregiver should practice aseptic and injection technique under the direct observation of a health professional.

The pharmacy is responsible for ensuring initially and on an ongoing basis that the patient or caregiver understands, has mastered, and is capable of and willing to comply with all of these home care responsibilities. This should be achieved through a formal, written assessment program. All specified competencies in the patient or caregiver's training program should be formally assessed. The patient or caregiver should be expected to demonstrate to appropriate health care personnel their mastery of their assigned activities before being allowed to administer HSDs unsupervised by a health professional.

Printed material such as checklists or instructions provided during training may serve as continuing post-training reinforcement of learning or as reminders of specific patient or caregiver responsibilities. Post-training verbal counseling should also be used periodically, as appropriate, to reinforce training and to ensure continuing correct and complete fulfillment of responsibilities.

PATIENT MONITORING AND COMPLAINT SYSTEM

The pharmacy must have written policies and procedures describing the monitoring of patients using HSDs and the handling of reports of adverse events.

Outcome Monitoring

The pharmacy is responsible for developing a patient monitoring plan, which includes written outcome measures and systems for routine patient assessment. The outcome monitoring system should provide information suitable for the evaluation of the quality of patient care and of pharmaceutical services. Examples of assessment parameters include infection rates, rehospitalization rates, incidence of adverse drug reactions, catheter complications, and other variables that may serve as meaningful indicators of the effectiveness and suitability of the home use of HSDs. In selecting suitable outcome measures, the focus should be on high-risk, high-volume, or problem-prone factors.

Reports

The pharmacy should have policies and procedures for the receipt, documentation, handling, and disposition of reports of patient problems, complaints, adverse drug reactions, drug product or device defects, and other adverse events reported by patients, caregivers, family members, pharmacists, or other health professionals. The pharmacy should have a procedure to ensure that the patient receives prompt and appropriate medical attention as necessary in response to all adverse incidents from HSDs or devices. When a complaint or problem prompts a suspicion that an HSD or a device may be defective, the pharmacy should also be able to identify and recall the potentially defective item to the patient level whenever appropriate.

Procedures should also include a mechanism for periodic review of reports received to determine any need for correction of underlying systems problems. All reports received should be maintained in a log, file, or binder dedicated for this purpose and readily retrievable as needed for subsequent analysis, legal or regulatory inquiry, or quality assurance audit. Standardized forms or formats for the reporting and recording of incidents, complaints, etc., should be used. Reports should be completed and signed by the individual receiving it or by the individual involved in the situation. Procedures should depict the classification, documentation, investigation, and resolution of all reports and should provide a mechanism for participation in various federal and state reporting programs such as USP or FDA programs for reporting reaction problems, or defects with drug products or medical devices.

THE QUALITY ASSURANCE PROGRAM

A provider of HSDs should have in place a formal Quality Assurance (QA) Program[9] intended to provide a mechanism for monitoring, evaluating, correcting, and improving the activities and processes described in this chapter. Emphasis in the QA Program should be placed on maintaining and improving the quality of systems and the provision of patient care. In addition, the QA program should ensure that any plan aimed at correcting identified problems also includes appropriate follow-up to make certain that effective corrective actions were performed.[10]

Characteristics of a QA plan include the following:

(1) Formalization in writing;
(2) Consideration of all aspects of the preparation and dispensing of products as described in this chapter, including environmental testing, validation results, etc.;
(3) Description of specific monitoring and evaluation activities;
(4) Specification of how results are to be reported and evaluated;
(5) Identification of appropriate follow-up mechanisms when action limits or thresholds are exceeded; and
(6) Delineation of the individuals responsible for each aspect of the QA program.

In developing a specific plan, focus should be on establishing objective, measurable indicators for monitoring activities and processes that are deemed high-risk, high-volume, or problem-prone. Appropriate evaluation of environmental monitoring might include, for example, the trending of an indicator such as settling plate counts. In general, the selection of indicators and the effectiveness of the overall QA plan should be reassessed on an annual basis.

---

[9]Other accepted terms that describe activities aimed at assessing and improving the quality of care rendered include Continuous Quality Improvement, Quality Assessment and Improvement, and Total Quality Management.

[10]The use of additional resources, such as the Accreditation Manual for Home Care from the Joint Commission on Accreditation of Healthcare Organizations, may prove helpful in the development of a QA plan.

Copied from the USP 23–NF 18
Copyright 1994
The USP Convention, Inc. Permission Granted

The USP 23–NF 18 is recognized as an official compendium under law. As such, its contents may have legal implications. The USP is revised continually. Readers are urged to consult the *USP 23–NF 18* and its *Supplements* directly.

Glossary

Aseptic preparation—The procedures designed to preclude contamination (of drugs, packaging, equipment, and supplies) by microorganisms during processing.

Batch preparation—The compounding of multiple sterile product units, in a single discrete process, by the same individuals during one limited period.[1]

Biological safety cabinet (BSC)—A containment unit suitable for the preparation of low- to moderate-risk agents when the product, personnel, and environment must be protected according to National Sanitation Foundation Standard 49.[2]

Calibration—The comparison of a measurement standard or instrument of unknown accuracy with one of known accuracy to detect, correlate, report, or eliminate (by adjustment) any variation in its accuracy.[3]

Cleanroom—An enclosed space, containing one or more clean zones, where the concentration of airborne particles is controlled.[3]

Clean zone—A defined space where the concentration of airborne particles is controlled to meet a specified airborne particulate cleanliness class.[3]

Closed-system transfer—The movement of sterile products from one container to another in which the container system and transfer devices remain intact throughout the transfer process except for the penetration of a sterile, pyrogen-free needle or cannula through a designated stopper or port to effect transfer, withdrawal, or delivery. Withdrawal of a sterile solution from an ampul in a Class 100 environment is generally acceptable; however, a rubber-stoppered vial (when available) is preferable.[1]

Component—Any ingredient intended for the compounding of a drug product, including ingredients that may not be part of the final product.[4]

Compounding—"The preparation, mixing, assembling, packaging, or labeling of a drug (including radiopharma-ceuticals) or device (i) as the result of a practitioner/patient/pharmacist relationship in the course of professional practice, or (ii) for the purpose of, or as an incident to, research, teaching, or chemical analysis and not for sale or dispensing. Compounding also includes the preparation of drugs or devices in anticipation of prescription drug orders based on routine, regularly observed prescribing patterns."[4]

Condensation nucleus counter (CNC)—An instrument for counting small airborne particles, approximately 0.01 μm and larger, by optically detecting droplets formed by condensation of a vapor on the particles.[3]

Controlled area—The space designated for preparing sterile products (e.g., cleanroom or buffer room).[1]

Critical area—Any space in the controlled area where products or containers are exposed to the environment.[5]

Critical surface—The surface that comes into contact with previously sterilized products or containers/closures.[5]

Discrete-particle counter (DPC)—An instrument, such as an optical particle or condensation nucleus counter, that can resolve responses from individual particles.[3]

Expiration date—The latest date (and time, when applicable) that a product is acceptable for use (i.e., the product should be discarded beyond this time). *Note:* An expiration date and time may arrive while an infusion is in progress. When this situation occurs, a pharmacist should determine whether to discontinue that infusion and replace the products. Organizational policies on this procedure should be clear.[6]

High-efficiency particulate air (HEPA) filter—A device composed of pleats of filter medium separated by rigid sheets of corrugated paper or aluminum foil that direct the air in a uniform parallel flow. HEPA filters remove 99.97% of all air particles 0.3 μm or larger. When these filters are used as a component of a horizontal or vertical laminar-airflow hood, an environment can be created consistent with standards for a Class 100 cleanroom.[7]

Home use sterile drug product (HSD)—A product requiring sterility (e.g., injectables and ophthalmics) that is prepared in and dispensed from a licensed pharmacy for administration by a patient, a family member, or other caregiver. This administration takes place in a setting other than an organized, professionally staffed health care facility.[6]

Manufacturing—The production, preparation, propagation, conversion, or processing of a drug or device, either directly or indirectly, by extraction from substances of natural origin or by chemical or biological synthesis. This process includes any packaging or repackaging of the substance or labeling or relabeling of its container and the promotion of such drugs or devices. Manufacturing also includes the preparation and promotion of commercially available products from bulk compounds for resale by pharmacies or practitioners and other persons.[4]

Quality assurance—The activities used to ensure that sterile drug products meet predetermined standards of quality.[1]

Quality control—The testing activities used to ensure that ingredients, components (e.g., containers), and final sterile products meet predetermined requirements for identity, purity, nonpyrogenicity, and sterility.[1]

Sterilizing filter—A device that produces a sterile effluent when challenged with a solution containing *Pseudomonas diminuta*, at a minimum concentration of 10^7 organisms/sq cm of filter surface.[5]

Temperatures (USP)—"Frozen" means temperatures between -20 and $-10°$ C (-4 and $14°$ F), "refrigerated" means between 2 and $8°$ C (36 and $46°$ F), and "room temperature" means between 15 and $30°$ C (59 and $86°$ F).[8]

Validation—Verification that a specific process consistently produces a product with predetermined specifications and quality attributes.[5]

REFERENCES

1. American Society of Hospital Pharmacists. ASHP technical assistance bulletin on quality assurance for pharmacy-prepared sterile products. *Am J Hosp Pharm.* 1993; 50:2386–98.

2. Model rules for sterile pharmaceuticals. Chicago, IL: National Association of Boards of Pharmacy; 1993:12.1–3.

3. Federal standard airborne particulate cleanliness classes in cleanrooms and clean zones. Washington, DC: U.S. General Services Administration; 1992 (Sept):1–48.

4. Good compounding practices applicable to state licensed pharmacies. Parts I and II. *Natl Pharm. Compliance News.* 1993; May:2–3 and Oct:2–3.

5. Center for Drugs and Biologics. Guideline on sterile drug products produced by aseptic processing. Rockville, MD: Food and Drug Administration; June 1987:10.

6. Sterile drug products for home use. In: United States pharmacopeia, 23rd rev./national formulary, 18th ed. Rockville, MD: United States Pharmacopeial Convention; 1994:1963–75.

7. Turco SJ. Extemporaneous preparation. In: Turco SJ, ed. Sterile dosage forms, their preparation and clinical application, 4th ed. Philadelphia, PA: Lea & Febiger; 1994:57–78.

8. General notices and requirements. In: United States pharmacopeia, 23rd rev./national formulary, 18th ed. Rockville, MD: United States Pharmacopeial Convention; 1994:11.